Minimally Invasive VITREOUS SURGERY

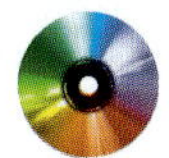

System requirement:

- Operating System – Windows XP or above
- Web Browser – Internet Explorer 8 or above, Mozilla Firefox and Safari
- Essential plugins – Java & Flash player
  - Facing problems in viewing content – it may be your system does not have java enabled.
  - If Videos don't show up – it may be the system requires flash player or need to manage flash setting
  - You can test java and flash by using the links from the troubleshoot section of the CD/DVD.
  - Learn more about flash setting from the link in the troubleshoot section.

Accompanying CD/DVD-ROM is playable only in Computer and not in DVD player.
CD/DVD has Autorun function – it may take few seconds to load on your computer. If it does not works for you then follow the steps below to access the contents manually:

- Click on my computer
- Select the CD/DVD drive and click open/explore – this will show list of files in the CD/DVD
- Find and double click file – "launch.html"

DVD Contents

1. **MIVS for ERM**
   Alay S Banker
2. **25 Gauge for IOL Drop***
   Saurabh Luthra
3. **Sutureless Silicon OIL Removal***
   Shalabh Sinha
4. **27 Gauge Vitrectomy**
   Yusuke Oshima
5. **Small Gauge Vitrectomy for Endophthalmitis**
   Lalit Verma, Gopal S Pillai
6. **MIVS in Diabetic Retinopathy***
   Cyrus Shroff
7. **20 Gauge MIVS in Drop Nucleus***
   Shalabh Sinha

---

* *No voice over*

Minimally Invasive VITREOUS SURGERY

20 Guage to 27 Gauge

Editor
Shalabh Sinha MBBS MS DNB
Vitreoretinal Surgeon
Krishna Vitreoretinal Surgery and Laser Center
Patna, Bihar, India

Foreword
PN Nagpal

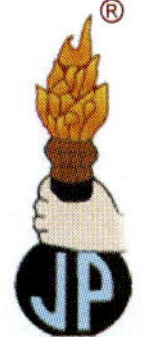

JAYPEE BROTHERS MEDICAL PUBLISHERS (P) LTD

New Delhi • London • Philadelphia • Panama

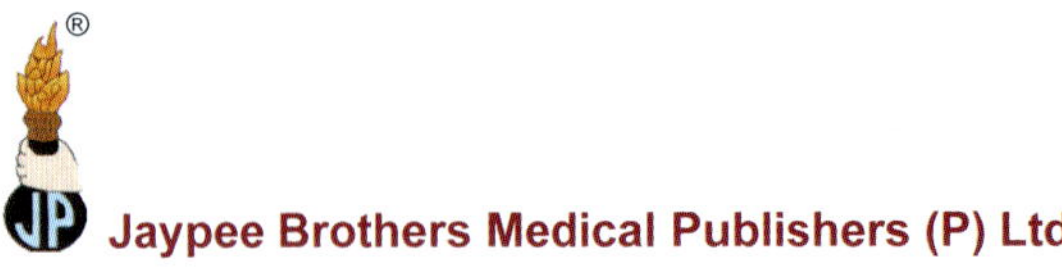

Jaypee Brothers Medical Publishers (P) Ltd

Headquarters

Jaypee Brothers Medical Publishers (P) Ltd
4838/24, Ansari Road, Daryaganj
New Delhi 110 002, India
Phone: +91-11-43574357
Fax: +91-11-43574314
Email: jaypee@jaypeebrothers.com

Overseas Offices

J.P. Medical Ltd
83, Victoria Street, London
SW1H 0HW (UK)
Phone: +44-2031708910
Fax: +02-03-0086180
Email: info@jpmedpub.com

Jaypee-Highlights Medical Publishers Inc.
City of Knowledge, Bld. 237, Clayton
Panama City, Panama
Phone: +507-301-0496
Fax: +507-301-0499
Email: cservice@jphmedical.com

Jaypee Brothers Medical Publishers Ltd
The Bourse
111 South Independence Mall East
Suite 835, Philadelphia, PA 19106, USA
Phone: + 267-519-9789
Email: joe.rusko@jaypeebrothers.com

Jaypee Brothers Medical Publishers (P) Ltd
17/1-B Babar Road, Block-B, Shaymali
Mohammadpur, Dhaka-1207
Bangladesh
Mobile: +08801912003485
Email: jaypeedhaka@gmail.com

Jaypee Brothers Medical Publishers (P) Ltd
Shorakhute, Kathmandu, Nepal
Phone: +00977-9841528578
Email: jaypee.nepal@gmail.com

Website: www.jaypeebrothers.com
Website: www.jaypeedigital.com

Inquiries for bulk sales may be solicited at: jaypee@jaypeebrothers.com

Minimally Invasive Vitreous Surgery: 20 Gauge to 27 Gauge

First Edition: **2013**

ISBN: 978-93-5090-379-7

Printed at: Ajanta Offset & Packagings Ltd., New Delhi

Dedicated to

My mother Late Dr Shiv Rani Sinha,
whose constant encouragement made me an eye surgeon.
She would have been extremely proud today.

My father, Dr Arun Kumar Sinha
an eye surgeon extraordinare
whose simple and ethical teaching made me a decent clinician.

My Guru Dr PN Nagpal
whose continuing support made me a better retinal surgeon.

All my teachers in school
Sherwood College, Nainital
Jawahar Lal Nehru Medical College, Belgaum
and CH Nagri Municipal Eye Hospital, Ahmedabad.

Dr Usha H Vyas
Dr Bakulesh Khamar and Dr Manish Nagpal.

My family, most of all my wife Dr Pallavi
and my wonderful kids, daughter Aishani and son Pranjal
for their love and affection
and without whose support this book would
never have seen the light of day.

Contributors

Abhishek Kothari MS FRCS
Vitreoretinal Services
Aravind Eye Hospital and
Postgraduate Institute of Ophthalmology
Coimbatore, Tamil Nadu, India

Ajit Babu Majji MD
Consultant Ophthalmologist
LV Prasad Eye Hospital
Hyderabad, Andhra Pradesh, India

Alay S Banker MS
Director
Banker's Retina Clinic and Laser Center
Ahmedabad, Gujarat, India

Amit Gupta MS
Vitreoretinal Services
Aravind Eye Hospital and Postgraduate Institute of Ophthalmology
Coimbatore, Tamil Nadu, India

Anshuman Sinha MD
Kamal Eye Clinic
Ranchi, Jharkhand, India

AP Lafetá MD
Vitreoretinal Department
Sint-Augustinus Hospital
Wilrijk, Belgium

Arindam Chakravarti MS
Aditya Jyot Eye Hospital Pvt Ltd
Mumbai, Maharashtra, India

Arup Chakrabarti MS
Chakrabarti Eye Care Center
Thiruvananthapuram, Kerala, India

Atul Kumar MD
Professor of Ophthalmology
Dr RP Center for Ophthalmic Sciences
All India Institute of Medical Sciences
New Delhi, India

Baruch D Kuppermann MD PhD
Chief of Retina Service
Gavin Herbert Eye Institute
University of California
Irvine, California, USA

Bhushan Khare DOMS
Khares Eye Institute
Pune, Maharashtra, India

C Claes MD
Vitreoretinal Department
Sint-Augustinus Hospital
Wilrijk, Belgium

Charu Gupta MS
Shroff Eye Center
New Delhi, India

Cyrus Shroff MD
Shroff Eye Center
New Delhi, India

Gopal S Pillai MD DNB FRCS
Professor of Ophthalmology and Chief
Vitreoretinal Surgery
Amrita Institute of Medical Sciences and
Research Center
Kochi, Kerala, India

Harsha Bhattacharya MS FRCS
Sankardeva Netralaya
Guwahati, Assam, India

Kapil Bhatia MD
Consultant and Ophthalmologists
LV Prasad Eye Institute
Hyderabad, Andhra Pradesh, India

Lalit Verma MD
Director
Vitreoretinal and Lasers
Center for Sight
New Delhi, India

Manish Nagpal MS DO FRCS
Retina Foundation
Shahibaug Underbridge
Ahmedabad, Gujarat, India

Meena Chakrabarti MS
Chakrabarti Eye Care Center
Thiruvananthapuram, Kerala, India

Narendran V DNB
Vitreoretinal Services
Aravind Eye Hospital and Postgraduate Institute of Ophthalmology
Coimbatore, Tamil Nadu, India

Pramod Bhende MS
Sankara Nethralaya
Chennai, Tamil Nadu, India

Priyank Garg MS
Assistant Professor and VR Surgeon
Department of Ophthalmology
LLRM Medical College
Meerut, Uttar Pradesh, India

Raja Narayanan MS
LV Prasad Eye Hospital
Hyderabad, Andhra Pradesh, India

Raju Sampangi MD DNB
Netraspandana Eye Hospital
Bengaluru, Karnataka, India

Ranjana DO
Drishti Eye Care and Research Center
Kankarbagh, Patrakar Nagar
Patna, Bihar, India

RK Akhaury MS DO
Drishti Eye Care and Research Center
Patna, Bihar, India

Rohan Chauhan MBBS DO
Rising Retina Clinic
Ahmedabad, Gujarat, India

Saurabh Luthra MS
Drishti Eye Center
Dehradun
Uttarakhand, India

Saurav Sinha MS FMRF
BB Eye Foundation
Kolkata, West Bengal, India

Shalabh Sinha MBBS MS DNB
Vitreoretinal Surgeon
Krishna Vitreoretinal Surgery and Laser Center
Patna, Bihar, India

Sharad Bhomaj MS DNB
Shanti Saroj Netralay
Miraj, Maharashtra, India

Shobhit Chawla MS
Medical Director and Chief
Vitreoretinal Services
Prakash Netra Kendra
Lucknow, Uttar Pradesh, India

SN Jha MD
Sir Ganga Ram Hospital
New Delhi, India

Sonia Rani John DNB
Chakrabarti Eye Care Center
Thiruvananthapuram, Kerala, India

Subhash Prasad MD
Divya Drishti Eye Center
Patna, Bihar, India

Subijay Sinha MD
Dr RP Center for Ophthalmic
All India Institute of Medical Sciences
New Delhi, India

Sudipta Das MS
Sankara Nethralaya
Chennai, Tamil Nadu, India

Sundaram Natarajan DO
Aditya Jyot Eye Hospital Pvt Ltd
Mumbai, Maharashtra, India

Suraj Pandya MBBS DO
Sarita Eye and Retina Center
Mumbai, Maharashtra, India

Varun Gogia MD
Dr RP Center for Ophthalmic
All India Institute of Medical Sciences
New Delhi, India

Yusuke Oshima MD PhD
Assistant Professor
Department of Ophthalmology
Osaka University Graduate School
of Medicine
Suita, Japan

Foreword

If we could enhance our sensitivity and listen to the cry of millions of innocent cells, the constituents of conjunctiva, sclera and uveal tissue, who were subjected to invasion by surgical penetration and destruction to create a sclerotomy at 3–4 places in order to get the instruments into the vitreous cavity to perform the vitrectomy and remove the pathology. Those innocent sclerotomy cells were asking (rather crying), "Why We" are being sacrificed. It is the "Basic Principles" of surgery in general that do the surgery to the extent the disease is and not make "Surgical Intervention" a disease. Surgery is trauma. We do attach a religious sanctity to it, but every cut kills cells and invites the same inflammation. Just as street accident trauma. Taking sutures is also traumatic, however, necessary at times.

So, it is the duty of every surgeon to reduce the surgical trauma as much as possible.

Simply putting, the Microincision Vitrectomy Surgery is an attempt to reduce the surgical trauma by reducing the guage of vitrectomy instruments and putting up a sutureless vitreous surgery.

How timely this multiauthor book is to help the vitrectomy surgeon to change from the conventional 20 guage to 23, to 25 and now 27 guage. I must congratulate Dr Shalabh Sinha and his many contributors which needs exercise to edit a book which is the need of the hour.

I am sure it will help convert the new and the other retinovitreous surgeons, who are sitting on the fence to change over to minimally invasive vitreous surgery (MIVS).

PN Nagpal MS FACS FDAAD
Director
Retina Foundation
Shahibaug Underbridge
Ahmedabad, Gujarat, India

Preface

Like the turning spokes of a wheel, change is permanent. Similarly, the field of ophthalmology has been constantly changing and adapting to the needs of the surgeons and their patients. Better engineering skills have driven machines to perform tasks unimaginable 20 years ago. We, as eye surgeons, and as retinal surgeons, have been gifted with a remarkable opportunity to live in a time, when surgical finesse is at its upward slope. Recent advances in microinvasive technology have provided us with the ability to do justice to our patients and aid in their early visual recovery. The coming years will be even more interesting with refinements in current technology.

This book was conceived three years ago, at the All India Ophthalmic Conference (AIOC), Kolkata, West Bengal, India, where I had felt the need for a book on *Minimally Invasive Vitreous Surgery: 20 Gauge to 27 Gauge.* I am extremely grateful to all the contributors of this book, who have tried their best at guiding the young retinal surgeons at the nuances of small gauge vitreous surgery. An enclosed interactive DVD would further aid the learning process for a young retinal surgeon.

Furthermore, I request all readers to help us in improving upon this maiden effort, by phone, email or in person. Any shortcomings in the book, I humbly beg pardon for.

Shalabh Sinha

Acknowledgments

I express my sincere gratitude to all the contributors for this book.

I thank Shri Jitendar P Vij (Group Chairman), Mr Ankit Vij (Managing Director) and Mr Tarun Duneja (Director-Publishing), and the entire team of M/s Jaypee Brothers Medical Publishers (P) Ltd, New Delhi, India, who have been extremely patient with me.

Contents

CHAPTER

1

Introduction and Anesthesia

Shalabh Sinha

INTRODUCTION

Minimally invasive surgery, whether it is in general surgery, or orthopedics or cardiac surgery, is the universal choice for patients as well as surgeons. There is little doubt that lesser the surgical trauma, the faster is the recovery for the patient. The proof for ophthalmology lies in phacoemulsification for cataract removal, a revolutionary surgical step that has proved itself over time. Vitreous surgery has only followed suite. Various gauges of instrumentations have now become available for the vitreous surgeon, apart from the conventional 20 gauge. The vitreous surgeon must choose and evaluate the MIVS procedure that would become his/her choice for the treatment of various vitreoretinal diseases. No one gauge may be suited for all patients and all diseases. There is of course a learning curve that the surgeon must go through. For a surgeon who is well-versed with conventional 20 gauge vitrectomy, a 23 gauge system would be most ideal. 25 or 27 gauge vitrectomy system could be adopted later depending upon the indication, the machine one is using and the comfort of the vitreous surgeon.

Reasons for Choosing MIVS

In primary surgery

1. Minimal conjunctival trauma—This is important in patients that already have a filtering bleb or who may need a glaucoma surgery at a later date.
2. Less patient discomfort or pain.
3. Faster visual rehabilitation—As there is less corneal astigmatism, and MIVS wounds heal quicker than conventional 20 gauge wounds.

In repeat surgery

1. Conjunctival peritomy in a previously operated eye can cause significant bleeding.
2. Scleral wounds remains healthy because no cautery is used. There are less chances of scleral necrosis or ectasia.

Advantages of Cannula

1. Protects the sclera and conjunctiva during intraoperative instrument exchanges.
2. Minimal traction at the vitreous base, and hence reduction in sclerotomy related iatrogenic retinal breaks.
3. Higher likelihood of a sealed/closed incision at completion of surgery.
4. Silicone oil removal is easier with nonvalved cannula system, even passively.
5. Ease of introducing instruments of appropriate gauge through the cannula, one does not have to search for the sclerotomy.

Advantages of Valves

1. Valved cannulas provide stable intraoperative intraocular pressure.
2. No fluid leak intraoperatively. This is valuable in eyes having undergone previous vitrectomy.
3. Less turbulence inside the vitreous cavity especially during instrument removal or exchange.
4. Least likelihood of vitreous or retinal incarceration into the cannula.
5. Least likelihood of intraoperative choroidal detachment.
6. Valved cannulas provide freedom from scleral plugs.

Misconceptions Regarding MIVS

It is faster than conventional 20 gauge surgery—False

While time was saved in not having to perform conjunctival peritomy, suturing the infusion cannula, or the sclerotomy and conjunctiva at completion of surgery, longer vitrectomy time balanced out time saved. This was with older generation cutters with reduced aspiration. Midlab cutter has a better aspiration rate than the older generation Alcon cutter. The new generation Alcon cutters have better aspiration rates and programmable duty cycle. It allows the surgeon to choose a particular mode such as "core vitrectomy" or "shave" depending upon where one is working.

Incisions need not be sutured—False

The threshold for placing a suture needs to be low. Any active leak must be addressed with placement of a suture. Sutures do not mean that the procedure has failed. It is what one does inside the eye that matters more with fine gauge instrumentation than the scleral suture.

Complicated cases cannot be done with MIVS—False

It is easier to perform surgery in tractional retinal detachment with narrow gauge instrumentation. The cutter becomes a multifunctional tool, making the use of scissors and forceps negligible. Bimanual membrane dissection can also be done using a suitable chandelier.

Patients requiring a buckle along with vitrectomy do not require the use of cannula—False

Valved cannulas provide all the benefits of using them as in a transconjunctival surgery. If silicone oil is used, there is minimal egress of silicone oil after removing the cannula. This ensures a complete fill.

Dropped nucleus or intraocular foreign body require a conventional 20 gauge vitrectomy—False

20 gauge valved cannula system is ideally suited for both the conditions for vitrectomy. A 23 gauge fragmatome needle is now available for dropped nuclei. One of the superior cannulas can be removed and the fragmatome needle can be passed through the same track to perform nucleus removal. The cannula can be placed back into the wound with a blunt insertor, and the procedure could be completed. For large foreign bodies in phakic or pseudophakic eyes one of the sclerotomies could be enlarged. If the patient is aphakic, a corneal tunnel incision could be fashioned for removal of the foreign body.

ANESTHESIA

The various modalities available for vitreoretinal surgery include local anesthesia and general anesthesia. Local anesthesia can be in the form of topical, sub-Tenon's, retrobulbar, peribulbar and parabulbar. The choice of the anesthesia must be based on the needs of the patient, the requirements of the surgeon and the skill of the anesthetic provider.[1]

Topical Anesthesia

Topical anesthesia is simple, quick and noninvasive.[2] Similar to phacoemulsification, retinal surgeons have been looking to provide this modality to their patients. The first report of topical anesthesia for posterior vitrectomy was by Yepez et al using 4% lidocaine drops in 20 gauge vitrectomy along with perioperative sedation. Mild pain was perceived during making of sclerotomy, cautery and conjunctival closure.[3] 23, 25 and 27 gauge MIVS are less invasive than conventional 20 gauge vitreous surgery and are ideally suited for topical anesthesia. Raju et al reported that 25 gauge vitrectomy could be safely performed using topical anesthesia in their patients with vitreous hemorrhage, endophthalmitis and retained cortex. Pain was felt during insertion of the cannula, in most patients.[4] Tang et al had a larger series of patients where they used topical anesthesia (Alcain) for their patients with macular disorders. 67.4% of patients tolerated the procedure well, but 28.3% required topical supplement during surgery and a further 4.3% required intravenous sedation.[5] The major difference from cataract surgery is that the cannula passes through the uveal tissue in the pars plana. Penetration of the uveal tissue and movement of the cannula during surgery causes pain. Short duration of surgery combined with minimal manipulations may be the ideal candidates for topical anesthesia. Satyen et al have suggested surgeons calculate the expected duration of surgery and only those with least time be subjected to topical anesthesia using 23 gauge vitreous surgery.[6] Theocharis et al have indicated that endolaser, scleral indentation and peribulbar anesthesia caused pain in their two year prospective study using topical 2% lidocaine drops and gel formulations. They have also found that 23 gauge MIVS was easier to perform than 25 gauge.[7] Lidocaine gel formulations can provide a longer lasting anesthetic effect. The anesthetic gel must be placed after 5% or 10% povidone iodine has been instilled in the conjunctival cul-de-sac. Ehab et al compared 2% lidocaine gel to retrobulbar anesthesia for 23 gauge vitrectomy for macular disorders. They found that local anesthesia with 2% lidocaine gel was as effective as retrobulbar injection without the risks of IOP elevation prior to surgery. Lack of akinesia did not pose a problem and did not prevent a successful outcome.[8]

Sub-Tenon's Anesthesia

Sub-Tenon's anesthesia is found to be safe and effective for retinal surgery. It was initially used as a technique to augment the effect of retrobulbar anesthesia.[9] Mark et al described it as an alternative technique to retrobulbar anesthesia. The authors used a 19 gauge blunt irrigating cannula to place anesthetic agent into the sub-Tenon's space, by opening the posterior Tenon's capsule. The technique was effective in 98% patients undergoing vitreoretinal surgery.[10] Li et al evaluated patients with sub-Tenon's anesthesia for retinal surgery. Patients involved in longer duration of surgery and those with painful procedures such as scleral buckle and cryopexy needed supplementation either in the form of local or intravenous medication.[11] The only problem with Sub-Tenon's anesthesia is increase in intraocular pressure and conjunctival chemosis. Chemosis may hamper placement of the microcannula. Hee et al studied the effect of volume used and found that 3–5 ml of anesthetic fluid was safe and effective. This was much less than the 11 ml of anesthetic solution used by Li et al. The authors also reported that posterior segment surgery lasting more than 3 hours or those requiring scleral buckling or cryopexy were more likely to require supplementation in the form of local anesthetic or intravenous sedation.[12] Vip et al used 5 ml anesthetic agent injections into the sub-Tenon's space in two quadrants to provide better anesthesia than single quadrant injection.[13] Sub-Tenon's anesthesia was found to be more effective than intravenous fentanyl in pediatric patients undergoing vitreo-retinal surgery. IV fentanyl group had more pain and required more ibuprofen postoperatively. The incidence of oculocardiac reflex was more in this group.[14]

Parabulbar anesthesia was described by Tarun Sharma et al. It comprised of a combination of orbicularis oculi injection, subconjunctival injection and sub-Tenon's irrigation. 69% patients did not require supplementation.[15]

Needle-based and nonneedle cannula-based sub-Tenon's anesthesia has been described by various authors in the literature.[16] A variety of rigid metallic cannulas and flexible cannulas have also been described. The choice is based on the surgeon and anesthetist preference.

Minor complications of sub-Tenons' anesthesia include chemosis, subconjunctival hemorrhage, retained visual sensations. Major complications are orbital hemorrhage, retinal and choroidal vascular occlusion, optic neuropathy and postoperative diplopia.[16] Globe perforation has been reported with sub-Tenon's anesthesia by Brett et al and they have pointed towards prior ophthalmic surgery, thinned sclera, excessive scarring as the various risk factors.[17]

Peribulbar Anesthesia

Peribulbar anesthesia is the more commonly employed procedure of local anesthesia for vitreoretinal surgery. The anesthetic agent is placed in the extraconal compartment in contrast to the retrobulbar technique where the drug is injected into the intraconal space. Peribulbar anesthesia is increasingly being adopted due to the major complications associated with retrobulbar anesthesia.

Peribulbar anesthesia for vitreoretinal surgery was described by Benedetti, et al.[18] The most commonly used anesthetic agents are 2% lignocaine and 0.5% bupivacaine. Ropivacaine and levobupivacaine are two newer anesthetic agents. Hyaluronidase is universally used regardless of the anesthetic agent. Sharma et al described the use of pH adjusted alkalinized 0.5% bupivacaine and found that it produced a better quality of anesthesia in comparison to a nonalkalinized mixture of 2% lignocaine and 0.5% bupivacaine.[19] Calenda et al used a mixture of bupivacaine 0.5%, lignocaine 2% and clonidine 1 mg/kg body weight and reported analgesia in 85% of patients. With sub-Tenon's supplemental infiltration the figure rose to 99% patients.[20]

Ropivacaine has also been used for peribulbar anesthesia in vitreoretinal surgery. Gioia et al evaluated 0.75% ropivacaine against a 1:1 combination of 2% lidocaine and 0.5% plain bupivacaine. 0.75% ropivacaine had similar onset of action and produced better postoperative analgesia.[21] Preemptive analgesia with 0.75% ropivacaine in 5 ml dosage given before pars plana vitrectomy via peribulbar injection was found to produce less postoperative pain and discomfort.[22] Another anesthetic agent 0.5% levobupivacaine, an S—enantiomer of racemic bupivacaine with limited cardio and neurotoxicity may be useful in elderly patients.[23] Ghali evaluated 0.75% levobupivacaine versus 0.75% ropivacaine in peribulbar anesthesia in vitreoretinal surgery. 0.75% levobupivacaine was found to provide more effective peribulbar anesthesia and better postoperative analgesia than 0.75% ropivacaine.[24]

Retrobulbar anesthesia has however, not been completely abandoned. Aksu et al compared the efficacy of 0.5% levobupivacaine, 0.5% bupivacaine and 2% lidocaine for retrobulbar anesthesia in three different groups of patients undergoing vitreoretinal surgery.[25] Combined retrobulbar and peribulbar anesthesia for vitreoretinal surgery has been reported using ropivacaine. The authors concluded excellent clinical efficacy as regards analgesia and muscle akinesia.[26] Lim et al have reported successful use of retrobulbar anesthesia only in pars plana vitrectomy and transconjunctival sutureless vitrectomy.[27]

The length of the needle used is also important. The standard practice is to use a 31 mm needle for retrobulbar and a 25 mm needle for peribulbar anesthesia. But using long needles puts the patient at risk for developing complications. Some complications can cause serious enough to be sight and life-threatening. Raid et al used a 15 mm needle for peribulbar anesthesia for posterior segment surgery. The modification adopted was the application of digital compression around the hub of the needle using the thumb and index finger during injection of the anesthetic agent. This allowed the anesthetic solution to spread deeper into the orbit and obtain desired akinesia. The authors found comparable degree of akinesia, rate of supplementation and surgeon satisfaction as with the 25 mm needle without the risks of complications associated with long needles.[28]

Local anesthesia is safer than general anesthesia where traction on the rectus muscle is required, as in scleral buckle. Grover et al reported increased incidence of oculocardiac reflex with general anesthesia, than with local anesthesia.[29]

Sedation

Sedation is often required to improve the patient comfort during placement of local anesthetic block. Monitored anesthetic care is a term used for patients who undergo surgery under local anesthesia and intravenous sedation along with monitoring of vital signs by anesthetist.

Benzodiazepines such as midazolam, lorezopam and diazepam are the most widely used for sedation. The main effects of benzodiazepines are sedation, hypnosis, decreased anxiety, anterograde amnesia, centrally mediated muscle relaxation and anticonvulsant activity. In addition to their action on the central nervous system, benzodiazepines have a dose-dependent ventilatory depressant effect and they also cause a modest reduction in arterial blood pressure and an increase in heart rate as a result of a decrease of systemic vascular resistance. However caution must be exercised when combining midazolam with fentanyl or other opioids.[30] It produces a potent drug interaction that places patients at a high risk for hypoxemia and apnea. Adequate precautions, including monitoring of patient oxygenation with pulse oximetry, the administration of supplemental oxygen, and the availability of persons skilled in airway management are recommended when benzodiazepines are administered in combination with opioids.[31]

Newer agents such as propofol and dexmedetomidine are considered safer than benzodiazepines. Propofol is an intravenous sedative hypnotic agent which rapidly and reliably causes loss of consciousness. It is also associated with a quick and 'smooth' recovery.[32] Abdul et al used combination of propofol and remifentanil as a continuous infusion in patients undergoing vitreoretinal surgery under local anesthesia. The authors concluded that the combination of the two drugs given as a continuous infusion before the local anesthesia was associated with lesser incidence of patient movement, breakthrough pain or discomfort, hemodynamic stability and higher surgeon satisfaction.[33] However propofol is both a cardiovascular and respiratory depressant. Dexmedetomidine is a potent α_2 adrenoceptor agonist with sedative, anxiolytic and analgesic action following intravenous administration.[34] Ashraf et al compared dexmedetomidine versus propofol for sedation in patients undergoing vitreoretinal surgery under sub-Tenon's anesthesia. The authors concluded that dexmedetomidine at similar sedation levels with propofol was associated with equivalent hemodynamic effects, maintaining an adequate respiratory function, similar time of discharge from PACU, better analgesic properties, similar surgeon's satisfaction, and higher patient's satisfaction.[35] Both propofol and dexmedetomidine have also been used in general anesthesia. While propofol is used to induce anesthesia, dexmedetomidine is used as a supplement to isoflorane during vitreoretinal surgery.[36]

Snoring during vitreoretinal surgery under local anesthesia with anesthetist monitored sedation may be associated with sudden head movement. This is seen more in sedation with continuous infusion of propofol. The sudden head movement may result in complications during surgery.[37]

GENERAL ANESTHESIA

General anesthesia is preferred in children and patients in whom retrobulbar/peribulbar block is contraindicated, such as a high myope, or those with compromised ocular blood flow. General anesthesia is also used in patients who are expected to have a prolonged surgical time, or who fail to achieve adequate analgesia and akinesia with regional anesthesia. Care must be taken to ensure that the patient is fit for general anesthesia, by an evaluation by the anesthesiologist or physician. Combining general anesthesia with local anesthesia can reduce the dosage of potent general anesthetic agent. Early recovery from general anesthesia and prolonged postoperative analgesia is evident with this technique.[38] This is advantageous in high risk patients especially the elderly. Another reason for combining peribulbar anesthesia with general anesthesia is in vitreoretinal surgery with scleral buckling. It is frequently associated with the oculocardiac reflex intraoperatively, as a result of traction on the rectus muscles. A high incidence of postoperative pain and postoperative nausea and vomiting are attributed to increased intraocular pressure due to expansion of the gas bubble or tight buckling or encirclage, when performed under general anesthesia. Insufficient akinesia resulting from partial blockade and patient discomfort during prolonged surgery involving scleral buckling are further limitations to the use of local anesthesia alone.

The combination of general anesthesia and peribulbar anesthesia may reduce these drawbacks.[39]

DRESSING AND DRAPING

Standard conventional draping protocol is followed. After appropriate anesthesia, operative field along with eyelids and lashes are meticulously cleaned with antiseptic solution. Cutting of eyelashes is optional and should be left to surgeons' discretion. Prior povidone-iodine (5%) instillation in the conjunctival sac (contact time of 5–10 minutes) and thorough scrubbing of the lid margins reduces the risks of bacterial contamination without adding to conjunctival or corneal toxicity. Use of 10% povidone-iodine was evaluated 5 minutes preoperatively and for painting the periocular skin. It was found to reduce the bacterial load in the conjunctiva.[40] Though the study was done for patient undergoing cataract surgery, this is of great importance in MIVS which theoretically has an increased likelihood of developing postoperative endophthalmitis.

Disposable drapes with adhesive center must be used. The eyelashes need not be trimmed. The adhesive drape keeps them away from the surgical field. The speculum must give a wide exposure of the eye, but must not press upon the eye.

Since most MIVS procedures are done under peribulbar anesthesia, special attention must be paid to the airway. Most elderly patients find the drape claustrophobic. Also those with chronic obstructive pulmonary disease need to be put on a combination of air and oxygen so as to not have them panting or gasping for breath.

REFERENCES

1. Charles S, Fanning GL. Anesthesia considerations for vitreoretinal surgery. Ophthalmol Clin North Am. 2006;19(2):239–43.
2. Gayer S, Kumar CM. Ophthalmic regional anesthesia techniques, Minerva Anestesiologica. 2008;74(1–2):23–33.
3. Yepez J, Cedeño de Yepez J, Arevalo JF. Topical anesthesia in posterior vitrectomy. Retina. 2000;20(1):41–5.
4. Raju B, Raju NS, Raju AS. 25 gauge vitrectomy under topical anesthesia: A pilot study. Indian J Ophthalmol. 2006;54(3):185–8.
5. Tang S, Lai P, Lai M, Zou Y, Li J, Li S. Topical anesthesia in transconjunctival sutureless 25 gauge vitrectomy for macular-based disorders. Ophthalmologica. 2007;221(1):65–8.
6. Deka S, Bhattacharjee H, Barman MJ, Kalita K, Singh SK. No patch 23 gauge vitrectomy under topical anesthesia: A pilot study. Indian J Ophthalmol. 2011;59(2): 143–45.
7. Theocharis IP, Alexandridou A, Tomic Z. A two year prospective study comparing lidocaine 2% jelly versus peribulbar anesthesia for 25G and 23G sutureless vitrectomy. Graefes Arch Clin Exp Ophthalmol. 2007;245(9):1253–8.
8. Zakzouk E El, Emerah S, Shouman A, Raafat M, Bahy H. A prospective study. Comparing Lidocaine 2% Jelly versus retrobulbar anesthesia in 23 G Suturless

Vitrectomy for Macular-Based Disorders: Efficacy and Intraocular Pressure. Life Science Journal. 2012;9(1):883–7.

9. Calvin E Mein, Harry W Flynn Jr. Augmentation of local anesthesia during retinal detachment surgery. Arch Ophthalmol. 1989;107(7):1084.
10. Mark A. Friedberg, Frank A. Spellman, A. Raymond Pilkerton, L. Edward Perraut, Jr, Robert F. Stephens. An alternative technique of local anesthesia for vitreoretinal surgery. Arch ophthalmol. 1991;109(11):1615–16.
11. Li HK, Abouleish A, Grady J, Groeschel W, Gill KS. Sub-Tenon's injection for local anesthesia in posterior segment surgery. Ophthalmology. 2000;107(1):41–6.
12. Hee Jin Sohn, Hyun Seung Moon, Dong Heun Nam, Hae Jung Paik. Effect of Volume Used in Sub-Tenon's anesthesia on efficacy and intraocular pressure in vitreoretinal surgery. Ophthalmologica. 2008;222:414–21.
13. Gill VS, Presland AH, Lord JA, Bunce C, Xing W, Charteris DG. Two-quadrant high-volume sub-Tenon's anesthesia for vitrectomy: A randomised controlled trial. Br J Ophthalmol. 2012;96:189–92.
14. Chhabra A, Sinha R, Subramaniam R, Chandra P, Narang D, Garg SP. Comparison of sub-Tenon's block with i.v. fentanyl for paediatric vitreoretinal surgery. Br J Anaesth. 2009;103(5):739–43.
15. Sharma T, Gopal L, Parikh S, Shanmugam MP, Badrinath SS, Mukesh BN. Parabulbar anesthesia for primary vitreoretinal surgery. Ophthalmol. 1997;104(3):425–8.
16. Kumar CM, Williamson S, Manickam B. A review of sub-Tenon's block: Current practice and recent development. Euro J Anaesthesiol. 2005;22(8):567–77.
17. Brett J Frieman, Mark A Friedberg. Globe perforation associated with sub-Tenon's anesthesia. American Journal of Ophthalmol. 2001;131(4):520–1.
18. Benedetti S, Agostini A. Peribulbar anesthesia in vitreoretinal surgery. Retina. 1994;14(3):277–80.
19. Sharma T, Lingam G, Shanmugam, Mahesh P, Bhende, Pramod, et al. Comparison of pH adjusted bupivacaine with a mixture of non-pH-adjusted bupivacaine and lignocaine in primary vitreoretinal surgery. 2002;22(2):202–7.
20. Calenda E, Quintyn JC, Brasseur G. Peribulbar anesthesia using a combination of lidocaine, bupivocaine and clonidine in vitreoretinal surgery. Indian J Ophthalmol. 2002;50(3):205–8.
21. Gioia L, Prandi E, Codenotti M, Casati A, Fanelli G, Torri TM, et al. Peribulbar anesthesia with either 0.75% ropivacaine or a 2% lidocaine and 0.5% bupivacaine mixture for vitreoretinal surgery: A double-blinded study. Anesth Analg. 1999;89(3):739–42.
22. Schönfeld CL, Hierneis S, Kampik A. Preemptive analgesia with ropivacaine for pars plana vitrectomy: Randomized controlled trial on efficacy and required dose. Retina. 2012;32(5):912–7.
23. Pacella E, Collini S, Pacella F, Piraino DC, Santamaria V, Blasi RA De. Levobupivacaine vs racemic bupivacaine in peribulbar anesthesia: A randomized double blind study in ophthalmic surgery. Eur Rev Med Pharmacol Sc. 2010;14(6):539–44.
24. Ghali AM. The efficacy of 0.75% levobupivacaine versus 0.75% ropivacaine for peribulbar anesthesia in vitreoretinal surgery. Saudi J Anesth. 2012;6:1:22–26.
25. Aksu R, Bicer C, Ozkiris A, Akin A, Bayram A, Boyaci A. Comparison of 0.5% levobupivacaine, 0.5% bupivacaine, and 2% lidocaine for retrobulbar anesthesia in vitreoretinal surgery. Eur J Ophthalmol. 2009;19(2):280–4.
26. Seidenari P, Santin G, Milani P, David A. Peribulbar and retrobulbar combined anesthesia for vitreoretinal surgery using ropivacaine. Eur J Ophthalmol. 2006;16(2):295–9.

27. Lim TH, Humayun MS, Yoon YH, Kwon YH, Kim JG. The efficacy of retrobulbar block anesthesia only in pars plana vitrectomy and transconjunctival sutureless vitrectomy. Ophthalmic Surg Lasers Imaging. 2008;39(3):191–5.
28. W Riad, E Abboud1, E Al-Harthi, E Kahtani, N Ahmed. Superficial extraconal blockade for vitreoretinal surgery. Saudi J Anaesth. 2010;4(3):174–77.
29. Grover VK, Bhardwaj N, Shobana N, Grewal SPS. Oculocardiac reflex during retinal surgery using peribulbar block and nitrous narcotic anesthesia. Ophthalmic Surgery and Lasers. 1998;29:207–12.
30. Olkkola KT, Ahonen J, Midazolam and Other Benzodiazepines. Modern Anesthetics, Handbook of Experimental Pharmacology. 2008;182,III:335–60.
31. Bailey PL, Pace NL, Ashburn MA, Moll JW, East KA, Stanley TH. Frequent hypoxemia and apnea after sedation with midazolam and fentanyl. Anesthesiology. 1990;73(5):826–30.
32. Fulton BR, Faulds D. Propofol. An update of its use in anaesthesia and conscious sedation. Drugs. 1995;50(3):513–19.
33. Abdul Kader MM, Ghali AM. Combined use of remifentanil and propofol to limit patient movement during retinal detachment surgery under local anesthesia. Saudi J Anaesth. 2010;4(3):147–51.
34. Bhana N, Goa KL, McClellan KJ. Dexmedetomidine. Drugs. 2000;59(2):263–8.
35. Ghali A, Abdul Kader Mahfouz, Tapio Ihanamäki, Ashraf M. El Btarny. Dexmedetomidine versus propofol for sedation in patients undergoing vitreoretinal surgery under sub-Tenon's anaesthesia. Saudi J Anaesth. 2011;l5(1):36–41.
36. Lee YY, Wong SM, Hung CT. Dexmedetomidine infusion as a supplement to isoflurane anaesthesia for vitreoretinal surgery. Br J Anaesth. 2007;98(4):477–83.
37. McCannel, Colin A, Olson, Eric J, Donaldson, Mark J, et al. Snoring is associated with unexpected patient head movement during monitored anaesthesia care vitreoretinal surgery. Retina.
38. Koenig A, Weber H, Spitznas M. Combination of local anesthesia and intubation anesthesia in ophthalmic surgery—a gentle anesthetic technic for high risk patients. Anasth Intensivther Notfallmed. 1983;18(3):121–4.
39. Ghali AM, Btarny AM El. The effect on outcome of peribulbar anaesthesia in conjunction with general anaesthesia for vitreoretinal surgery. Anaesthesia. 2010;65(3):249–53.
40. Martin M, Nentwich, Mohammed Rajab, Christopher N, Ta, Lisa He, Martin Grueterich, et al. Application of 10% povidone iodine reduces conjunctival bacterial contamination rate in patients undergoing cataract surgery. Eur J Ophthalmol. .2012;22(4):541–6.

CHAPTER

2

Technological Support for MIVS

Kapil Bhatia, Ajit Babu Majji, Meena Chakrabarti

INTRODUCTION

As with cataract surgery, pars plana vitrectomy has also come a long way. With the advances in technology, the incisions have become smaller and smaller. From large limbal wound of intracapsular cataract extraction, we have come to microincision cataract (1.5 mm) surgery. Similarly from 20 gauge (0.89 mm) vitrectomy, microincision vitrectomy surgery (MIVS) involving 23 gauge, 25 gauge, and 27 gauge vitrectomy has become available to vitreoretinal surgeons, allowing them to reduce the size of scleral incisions to a fraction of what was possible with standard vitrectomy and in this way provide more rapid postoperative rehabilitation and a reduced risk of complications. Eugene De Juan Jr, with his 25 gauge system and then Claus Eckardt, with his 23 gauge system in 2005 made this transconjunctival sutureless technique popular.[1-3] Advantages of microincision vitrectomy include greater postoperative comfort and reduced ocular hyperemia. In addition, most procedures do not require sutures, so there is faster postoperative recovery.[3-5] The revolution in microincision vitrectomy is mainly due to refinements in the technology and advent of modern instrumentation, e.g. high speed 23 and 25 gauge cutters, disposable scissors, forceps and improved light source (Xenon), which has increased the safety and efficacy of the microincision vitrectomy.

25, 23 Gauge Vitrectomy Instruments

Various instruments for 25, 23 gauge vitrectomy have been developed recently. The trocars and the vitreous cutter are the instruments which require special mention apart from the various other instruments available.

Trocar-Cannula System

Trocar-Cannula system are the mainstay of sutureless stable wound in both 23 and 25 gauge vitrectomy. It plays a key role in minimizing damage to the wound. This is essential to prevent leakage of fluid. They are available in different colors, or colored markings by which we can differentiate 23 and 25 gauge trocars (Alcon system—Orange color cannula collar indicates 23 gauge and blue collar indicates 25 gauge cannula). They help in making

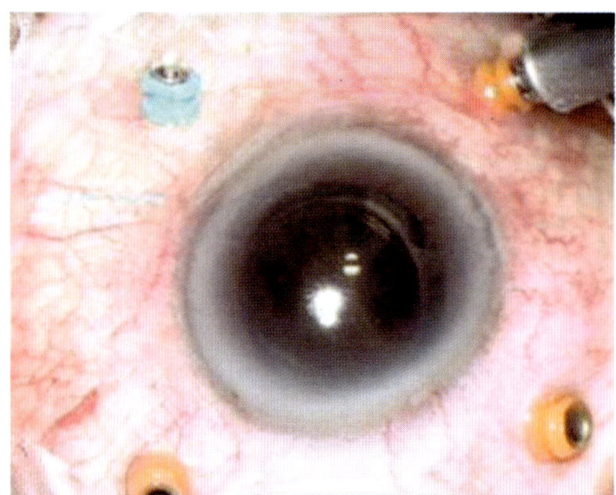

Fig. 2.1A: Alcon 25 gauge system—collar blue, Alcon 23 gauge system—collar orange (*Courtesy*: Dr Manish Nagpal)

simultaneous entry through conjunctiva and sclera, hence ensure correct configuration and placement of the sclerotomy so as to achieve a self-sealing wound at the completion of surgery. This is achieved by creating an oblique wound so as to ensure a valve like effect and misaligning the conjunctival and scleral entry sites by displacing the conjunctiva over the scleral surface before creating the wound. The cannula has a length of four millimeters. Longer cannulas of 6 mm are also available for select indications, wherein the choroid may be thicker, such as postoperative endophthalmitis. The outer diameter of the cannula is 0.55 mm to 0.60 mm for 25 gauge and 0.75 mm for 23 gauge vitrectomy system. These cannulas have an inbuilt collar to manipulate during surgery. The funnel, shaped external opening on the collar helps in plugging the system and ease for entry of surgical instruments. Cannulas have either a thin polyamide or titanium or stainless steel core. While the polyamide cannulas are primarily disposable and should not be reused, the titanium or stainless steel cannulas can be reused.

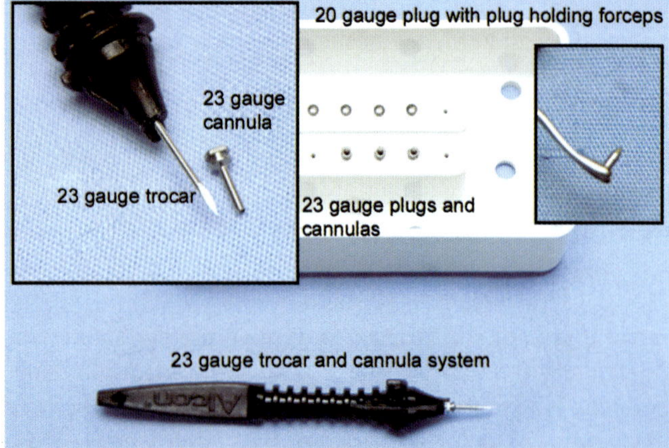

Fig. 2.1B: 23 gauge older generation trocar and titanium cannula system to create self sealing sclerotomy ports. Figure shows 20 (inset right) and 23 gauge scleral plugs to close the ports

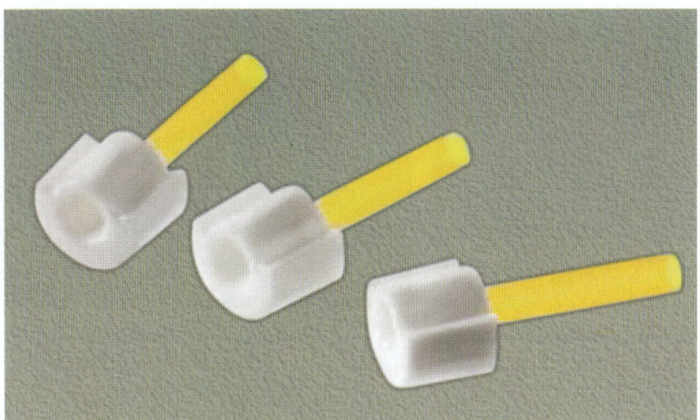

Fig. 2.1C: Baush and Lomb TVS polyamide cannula

Entry of sharp trocar with overlying cannula can be directly perpendicular (as in 25 gauge vitrectomy incisions), or it can be two step, first oblique and then perpendicular (23 gauge vitrectomy incisions). The straight conduits of the scleral wound and the conjunctival wound may increase the risk of postoperative infection. Therefore, it is extremely important to displace the conjunctiva when trocars are inserted into the sclera through the conjunctiva to prevent straight conduits.[3] This can be done either with the forceps holding and fixing the conjunctiva or by using the pressure plate. The Reichel-Chun forceps (Epsilon, USA) is specially designed to aid in placement of the cannula while giving a good grip on the conjunctiva. Various pressure plates are now available for the surgeon to choose from, beginning with the one introduced by DORC along with the 23 gauge cannula system. The Josephberg-Hilton Trocar Fixation Plate (ASICO, Westmont, IL) is used in a multifunctional manner while making the incision. The pressure plate forceps have incorporated calipers to measure distance from the limbus and have serrations on the undersurfaces, allowing a good hold on the conjunctiva for misalignment over the proposed scleral entry. The pressure plate forceps allow a stable fixed globe while making the biplanar incision. The pressure plate forceps' inner margins slide into the groove of the cannula, allowing easy trocar withdrawal without disturbing the integrity of the cannula.[7] The Dugel entry plate (Peregrine Surgicals, USA), has a groove for guiding the trocar at a fixed angle thus allowing a consistent wound construction. The pressure plate is most useful for a 25 gauge or 23 gauge disposable MVR blade creation of a sclerotomy for two step introduction of the cannula. The two entries through the conjunctiva and sclera are kept in the same plane by the use of the pressure plate.

The force required to insert the trocar cannula system was greater with the older generation system. The MVR blade design or the razor blade design of Synergetics system requires a far lesser amount of force to create the same incision.[8] The newer Edge Plus system of Alcon and the ESA system from Bausch & Lomb have addressed the issue, and need least amount of force

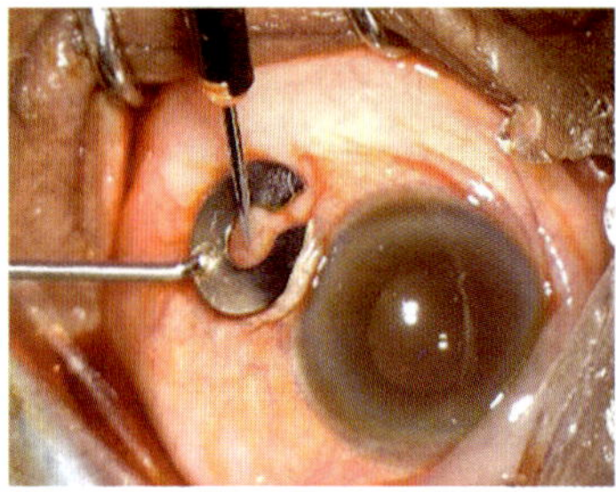

Fig. 2.1D: ASICO pressure plate (*Courtesy*: Dr Manish Nagpal)

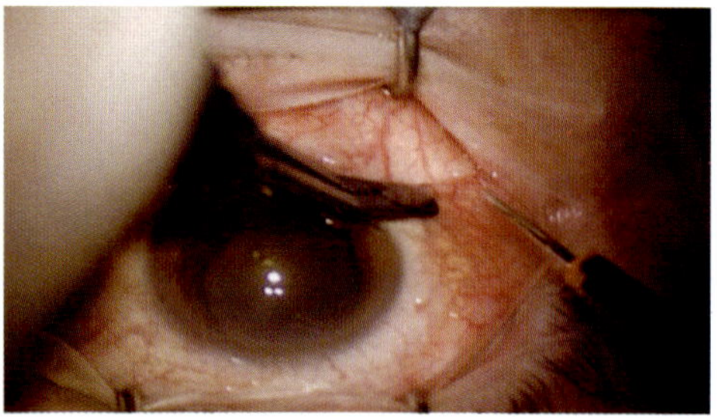

Fig. 2.1E: Reichel-Chun forceps (*Courtesy*: Epsilon)

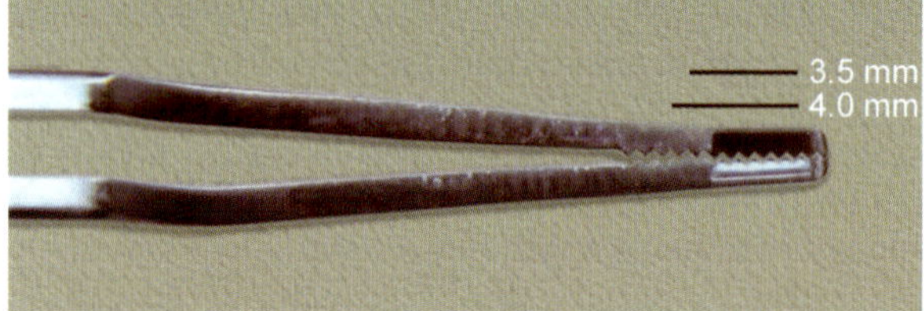

Fig. 2.1F: Reichel-Chun forceps (*Courtesy*: Epsilon)

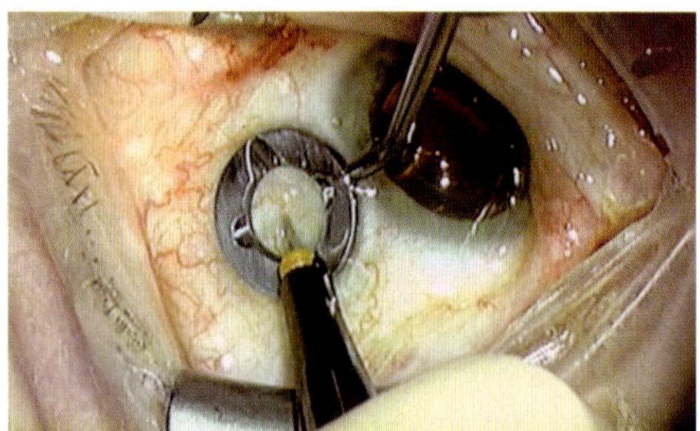

Fig. 2.1G: Dugel entry plate

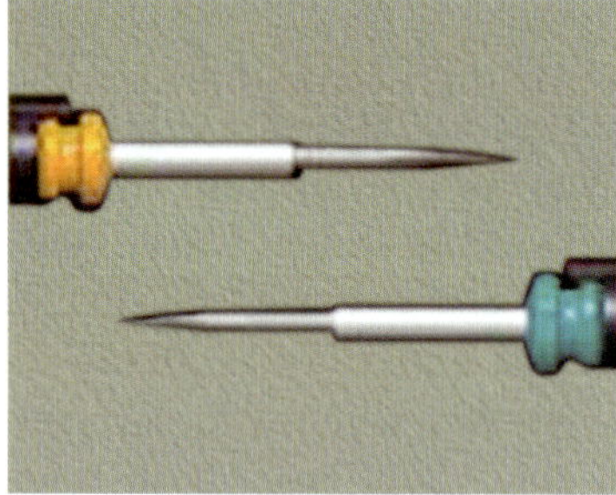

Fig. 2.1H: Alcon trocar edge plus 23 and 25 gauge

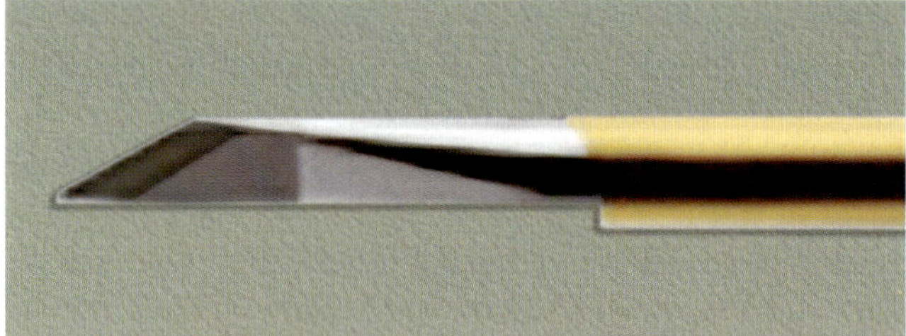

Fig. 2.1I: Synergetics razor blade design trocar

to insert the cannula. Rise in the intraocular pressure can occur during the insertion of the trocar cannula system through the sclera.[9] The lesser the force used to insert the trocar cannula, the least would be the rise in intraocular pressure. This is important when operating in eyes that have a compromised blood flow such as in diabetics or in open globe injury or in combined cataract and vitreous surgery. Twisting maneuver has been found to reduce the chances of rise in IOP.[10] This should be done once the scleral tunnel has been made and the cannula needs to pass into the track. Concerns however are of twisting the vitreous fibrils and causing peripheral vitreous traction and the possibility of formation of retinal breaks.

VALVED CANNULA

Like phacoemulsification, working in a closed environment that maintains intraocular pressure (IOP) at a consistent level during vitreous surgery is highly desirable. Complications due to fluid egress are noted with the non-valved variety. Peroperative IOP control is superior with the use of valved cannulas over one without, as it creates a closed globe that avoids risk of leakage. Routine use of valved cannulas eliminates the need for closing the cannula with sclerotomy plugs. Unvalved cannulas, in the absence of an instrument or plug, create a great deal of intraoperative leakage that may attract intraocular tissue toward the internal port of the cannula. Variations in preoperative IOP can cause serious complications such as choroidal/retinal hemorrhage or tissue incarceration into the cannulas.[11]

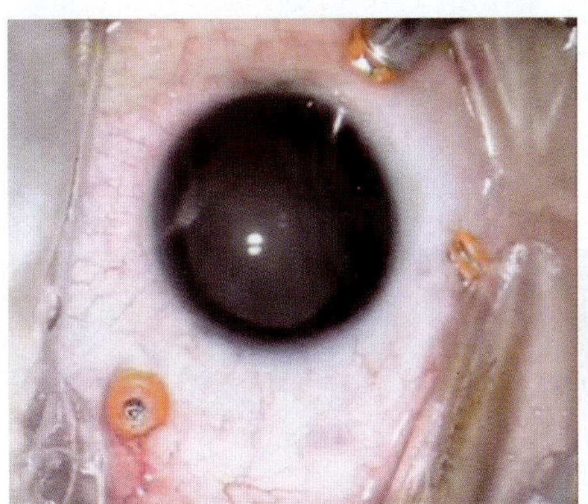

Fig. 2.1J: Alcon valved cannula (*Courtesy*: Dr Manish Nagpal)

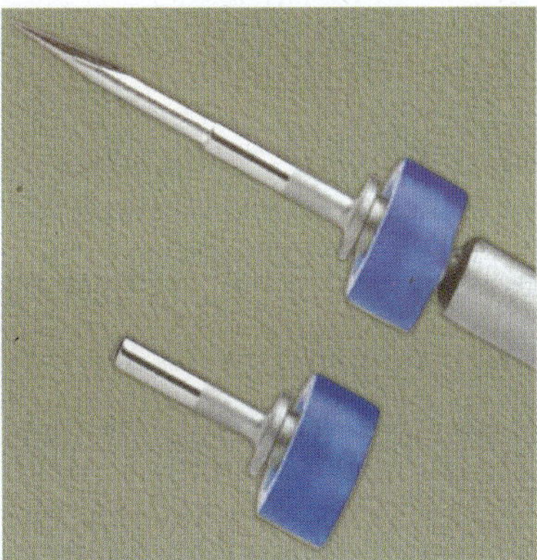

Fig. 2.1K: DORC valved cannula

For air—silicone oil exchange, either the valve is removed (as in the DORC system), or a vent is used (as in the Alcon system) to avoid IOP spike during this procedure. In the event of PFCL—Silicone oil exchange, passive aspiration of the perfluorocarbon liquid with a silicone tipped flute is possible without the need for valve removal or the use of vent.

INSERTION TROCAR

The insertion trocar can be blunt or sharp. The two step incision uses a blunt trocar whereas the one step incision uses a sharp trocar. The two step incision requires the use of a disposable MVR blade. MVR blades are either straight

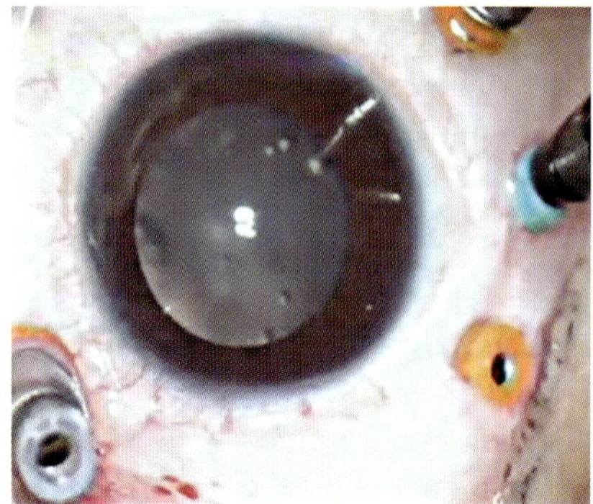

Fig. 2.1L: Vent for valved cannula (*Courtesy*: Dr Manish Nagpal)

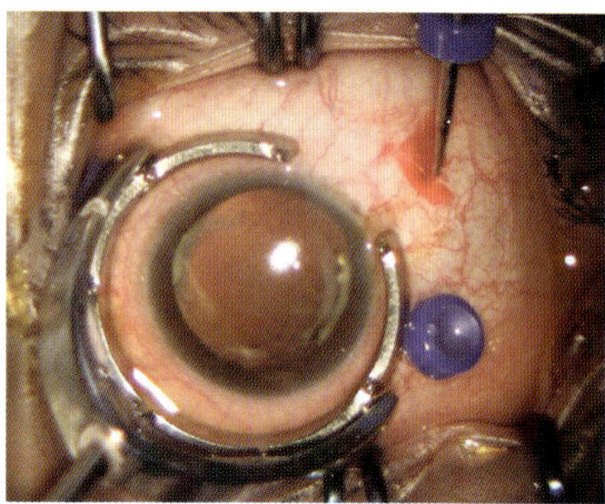

Fig. 2.1M: DORC blunt 2 step trocar and Fine Thorton ring

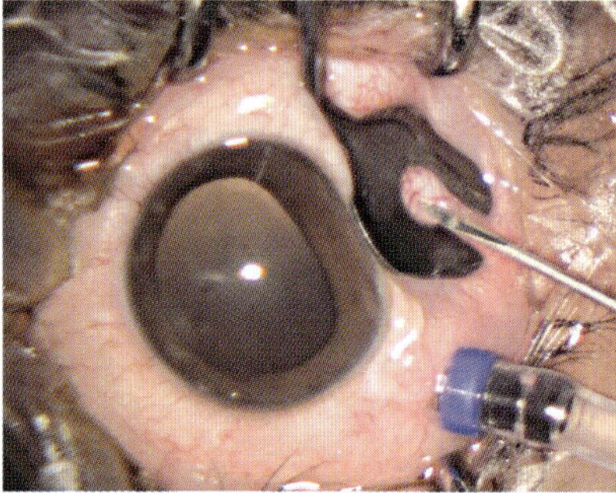

Fig. 2.1N: Straight MVR and Epsilon pressure plate

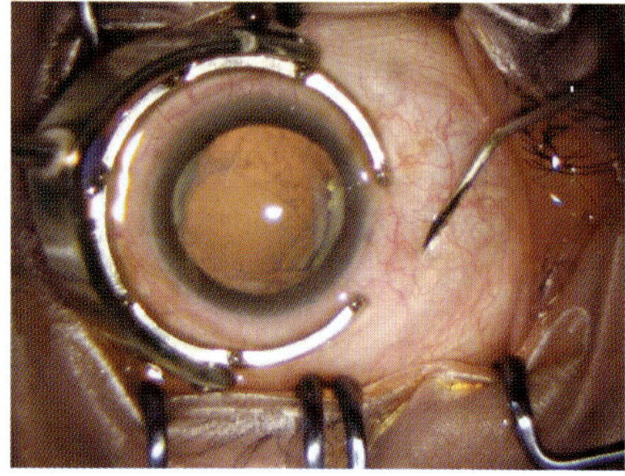

Fig. 2.1O: Bent MVR and Fine Thorton ring

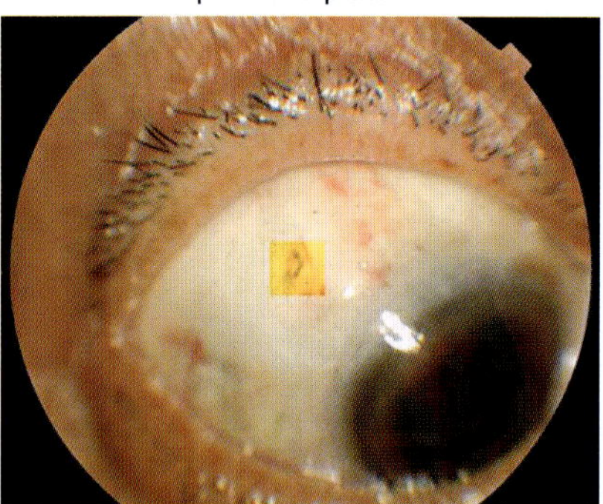

Fig. 2.1P: Chevron incision

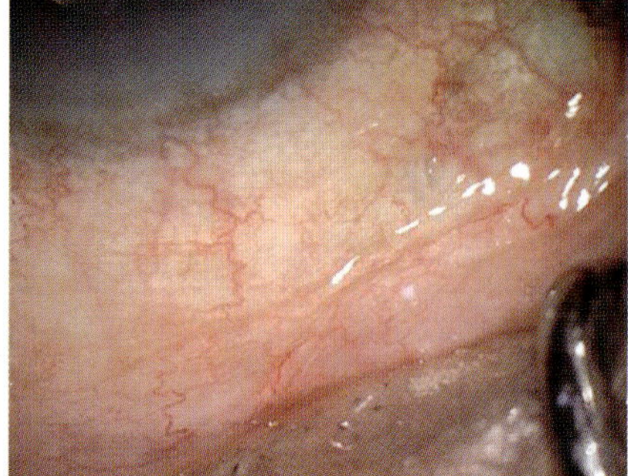

Fig. 2.1Q: Linear incision (*Courtesy*: Dr Manish Nagpal)

or angled, depending upon the choice of the operating surgeon. The sharp (9.6–10 mm) tipped solid (Alcon) or hollow bore (Bausch & Lomb) inserter had a continuous bevel attached with the microcannula. These trocars gave a biplaner but chevron-shaped incision. The MVR blade or the razor blade design of the synergetics system create a linear incision, which is superior to the chevron incision. The new Edge Plus trocars—cannula system (Alcon Laboratories, Inc.) and solid ESA system from Bausch & Lomb delivers a smooth, one-step entry for 23 and 25 gauge systems with excellent wound architecture using a linear incision. Rizzo et al had presented a new device, for trocar insertion. It provides the ability to have a fixed angle of entry, globe fixation and conjunctival retraction. Superior incisions can be created by the use of this injector system.[12]

INFUSION CANNULA

As regards the two system's respective infusion cannulas, that of the 25 gauge system is a metallic tube with an inner diameter 0.42 mm, whereas that of the 23 gauge is a steel tube with an inner diameter 0.56 mm, which contributes to the 23 gauge system's superior flow dynamics. The infusion cannula is composed of a 5 mm metallic tube, which fits through the microcannula array.

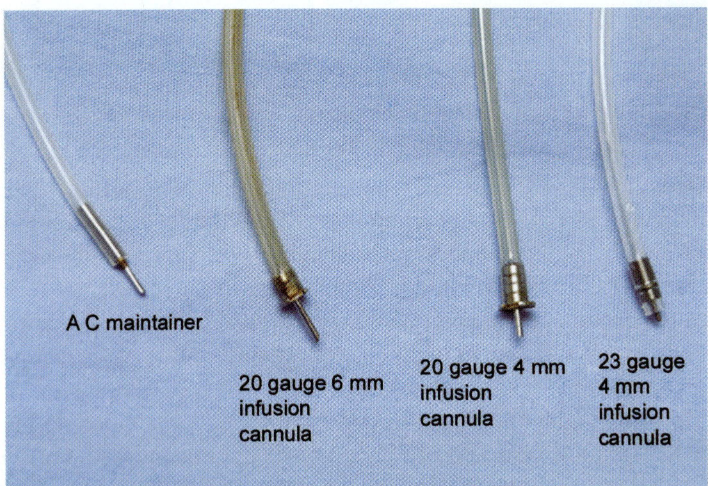

Fig. 2.2: Infusion cannulas used in 20 and 23 gauge system and anterior chamber maintainer. Note the sleeve around in 23 gauge cannula

VITREOUS CUTTERS

There are two different kinds of vitreous cutters, the pneumatic cutter driven by air pressure and the motor-driven cutter. The vitreous cutters of both systems have pneumatic driven diaphragm which provide radial reciprocal guillotine cutting. Both the 23 gauge and 25 gauge systems have the same lightweight probe, weighing four grams without tubing and 39 grams with tubing. Newly designed high speed cutters do not have spring (to drive the guillotine). It reduces vibrations giving better stability and precision cutting. These cutters have a maximum cutting speed limit of as fast as 2,500 rpm as in the 20 gauge system. The Oertli system provides a cut rate of 6000 cpm, the Alcon constellation 7500 cpm and midlab vit enhancer ultimate 8000 cpm. High speed cutting reduces the traction transmitted to the retina allowing surgeons to work closer to the mobile retina and vitreous base safely.[13] With ever increasing cutting rates it is necessary to increase the suction to maintain adequate flow rate. There are two setting options, proportional and 3D setting

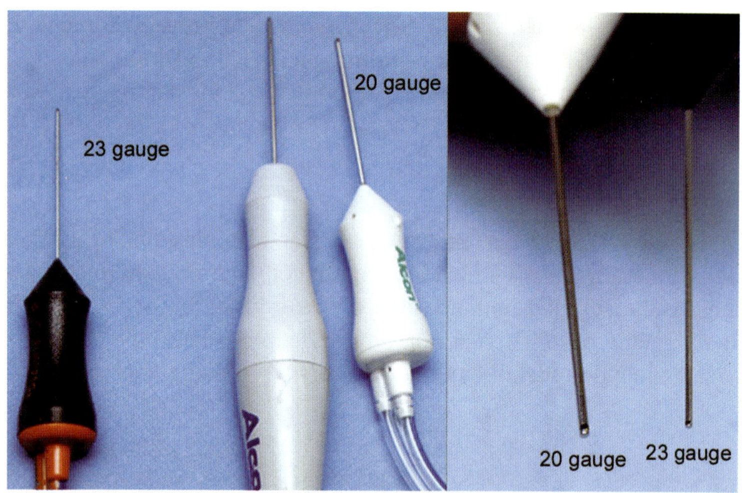

Fig. 2.3: 23 and 20 gauge vitrectomy cutters. Note the port of the cutter in 23 gauge located nearer to the tip

(Dual Dynamic Drive). In proportional setting, suction is variable depending on position of foot switch but cutting rate is fixed. In 3D setting, both cutting and suction can be independently controlled with foot switch. 3D setting further enhances the safety while working closer to the retina.

Because of the narrow aperture of the vitreous cutter, the aspiration rate is smaller than that of the 20 gauge cutter. Therefore, the aspiration vacuum is usually set to 500–600 mm Hg instead of 200 mm Hg to achieve enough aspiration flow.[3,6] The aperture of the vitrectomy cutter is closer to the tip of the vitreous cutter in the 25 and 23 gauge system compared with the 20 gauge system, allowing the surgeon to remove most of the membrane with a 25 and 23 gauge vitreous cutter without performing delamination using scissors. But these cutters have some inherent disadvantages also. The shafts of the instruments used during 25 gauge vitrectomy are much softer than those of the 20 gauge instruments.[14] A 23 gauge probe is only a fourth as stiff as a 20 gauge probe, it is over twice as stiff as a 25 gauge probe. The increasing use of smaller gauge systems has led to the finding that there is decreased flow performance during vitreous removal in 25 gauge vitrectomy relative to standard 20 gauge vitrectomy. This may be a rate-limiting step influencing the total surgical time.

The flow rate is affected by a number of factors, one of which is the duty cycle of the cutter. The duty cycle is the percentage of time the cutter port is open relative to each cutting cycle. When the port is open, the aspiration pressure draws some vitreous into the cutter. During cutting, a chunk of vitreous is removed from the main 'block' of vitreous. As the cut rate increases, at any given flow rate, the amount of vitreous in each bite is reduced. Reducing the aspiration pressure will decrease the traction on the remaining vitreous or retina. Availability of variable '*duty cycle*' (percent time that the port is open during one complete cutting cycle) in newer machines, allows to have variable but adequate flow rate and still can maintain very high cut rate. With increased port size and port closer to the tip in these cutters, the flow rate could be increased further. '*Aspiration flow limit*' is another feature complimentary to variable duty cycle and high cut rate. Once set, it maintains continuous state of fluidic stability in the eye, preventing sudden decrease in intraocular pressure and pulsatile traction on the retina. Other factors affecting flow rate are the nature of the removed substance, variable parameters such as vacuum applied and cutting rate, drive mechanism (pneumatic or electric), blade movement (axial or rotational), and the internal diameter of the vitrector.[14]

Flow analysis was undertaken in 20, 23, and 25 gauge systems using porcine vitreous.[14] Analysis of the percentage of vitreous flow rate/balanced salt solution (BSS) flow rate at different aspiration and cut rates showed an ascending curve providing evidence of flow obstruction at all cut rates, in all three systems. In the 20 gauge electric system, at faster cut rates, vitreous was removed faster and had less resistance, due to smaller pieces being removed. The 25 gauge electric system also had higher vitreous flow rates at high cut rates. Assessment of the 23 gauge pneumatic system revealed decreased duty cycle and incomplete aperture opening at 1500 cpm with resultant low flow. This trend also occurred in 20 and 25 gauge pneumatic cutters, with higher absolute flow when utilizing the larger gauge systems. Magalhaes et al compared infusion and extrusion volumes of three different 25 gauge systems.[15] Average infusion rates were 167.23 μL/s with the Bausch and Lomb (Millennium™), 190.53 μL/s with Alcon (Accurus™), and 250.09 μL/s with DORC (Associate™), respectively. These values increased with raised bottle height. With the cutter off, the Bausch and Lomb and Alcon systems had lower aspiration flow rates than the DORC system. They also had a variation in aspiration flow rate of < 10% between a cut rate of 0 cuts/min and 1100 cuts/min compared to > 50% in the DORC system, demonstrating lower power but greater flow stability. These findings may be of benefit when considering which system is best suited to a particular surgical procedure. Increased infusion rate and aspiration power may be of benefit in order to remove posterior hyaloid or clots in young patients. The wider safe vitrectomy zone (when infusion rate is higher than aspiration rate) may be required when dissecting membranes such as in diabetic eye disease. However, a close watch on the intraocular pressure is desirable since the blood flow to the optic nerve head is compromised in diabetic eye disease.

OTHER DISPOSABLE INSTRUMENTS

Many other instruments, including the diathermy probe, laser probes, extendable curved Pick forceps, aspirating pick, various kinds of forceps, vertical scissors, curved scissors, and silicone tipped blushed back-flush needles are now available in market.[16] The tensile strength of the disposable forceps in 23 gauge has been improved to where these instruments mimic their 20 gauge counterparts. The instrumentation for MIVS is more fragile and delicate, and may be easily damaged with reuse. That is why disposable instruments are gaining popularity recently. The GRIESHABER DSP line for small-gauge vitreoretinal surgical instruments with revolutionary style has led to relative ease of maneuvering them during microincision vitrectomy surgeries. Better instruments have revolutionized the smaller gauge surgeries. 23 gauge fragmatome needle has been introduced by DORC. However, we do not have phacofragmatome available for 25 gauge vitrectomy. Continuous development and better instruments in future might replace 20 gauge vitrectomy with 23, and 25 gauge vitrectomy.

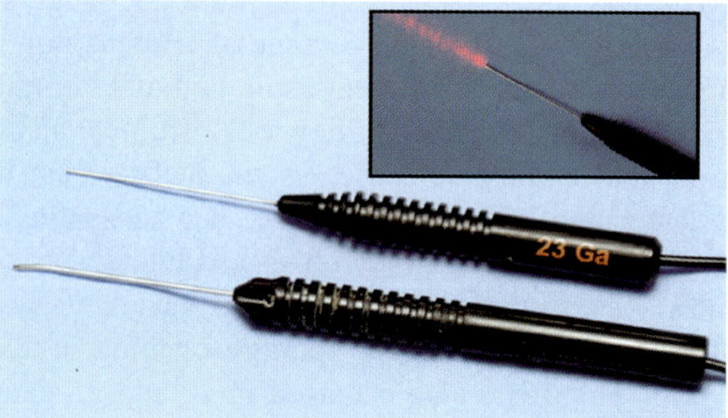

Fig. 2.4: Endophotocoagulation probes of 20 and 23 gauge systems. Both straight and bent probes available in both systems

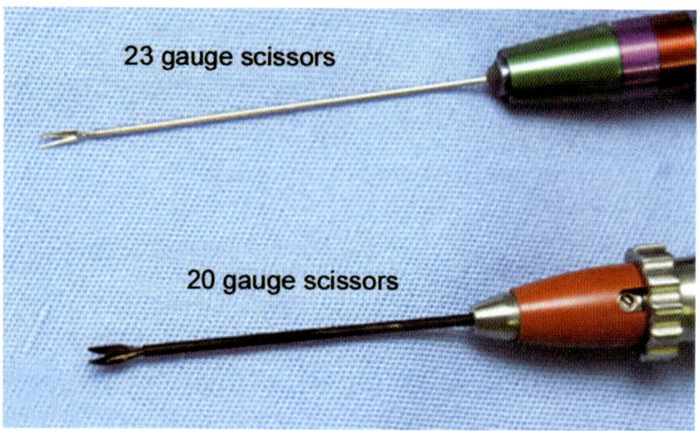

Fig. 2.5A: 230 and 23 gauge, Intravitreal scissors for membrane cutting

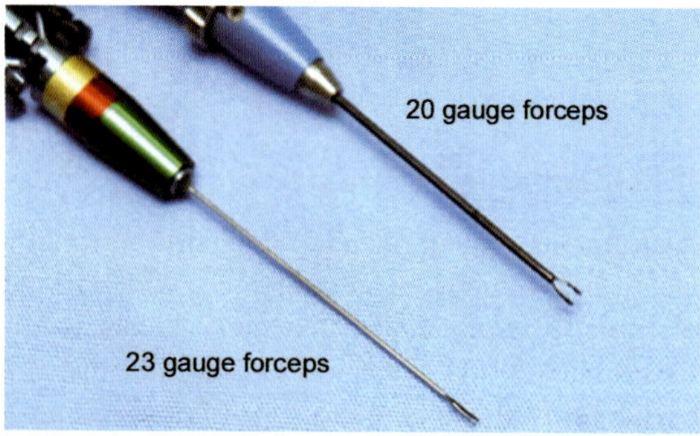

Fig. 2.5B: 230 and 23 gauge, Intravitreal forceps for membrane peeling

ENDOILLUMINATION

For the past decade, most retina surgeons have relied on the light sources integrated into the vitrectomy systems for their endoillumination requirements: dual-output halogen illumination or the dual-output metal halide illumination. Clinically, these sources of illumination provided a safe viewing environment with adequate illumination for most tasks using a standard 20 gauge light probe. Unfortunately, these illumination sources lacked the power to provide adequate viewing for lighted instrumentation, wide-angle probes, and chandelier systems, which is why they failed to gain mainstream popularity.

The introduction of wide-angle viewing systems was coupled with the development of more powerful light sources. While increased power allows for improved illumination, it is also associated with a higher risk of retinal phototoxicity. Retinal toxicity is thought to be secondary to photochemical exposure to shorter wavelength light, particularly ultraviolet and visible blue light.[17] This can disrupt the blood-retinal barrier function and hence blue-light–blocking filters are used.[18-20]

CONE OF ILLUMINATION

The cone angle of illumination on the original endoilluminator for the 25 gauge system was narrow. The power on the halogen systems was weak, making it seem like we were operating in the dark. Since then, we have seen three improvements:

1. **Chandelier systems** became easier and more prevalent.
2. **Endoilluminators** became more rigid in the 25 gauge systems; the cone angles nearly doubled for better illumination. The increased rigidity of the new second-generation 25 gauge endoilluminators gives the surgeon a better feel for moving the eye, particularly for the surgeon who is transitioning from 20 gauge to 25 gauge procedures. This light probe provides a cone angle of 79º, compared with its original 40º angle. The transmission capacity was also increased by nearly 50%, and a shaft stiffness increase of nearly 70%.
3. **The horsepower of the new illuminating boxes**—The Accurus High Brightness Xenon Illuminator (Alcon, Fort Worth, Texas) and the Synergetics Photon Illuminator (MISS Ophthalmics, Corby, Northamptonshire, UK) introduce much more light into the eye.

The first Xenon light source to come to market was the Synergetics Photon, which features a Xenon dual-output illumination source with an integrated laser pathway capability referred to as "bull's eye technology". Its increase in power capabilities is significant with 25 gauge probes and lighted instruments that are capable of higher illumination levels than those previously achievable with 20 gauge probes on maximum illumination. In addition, because of its tremendous power capabilities, very high levels of illumination can be driven

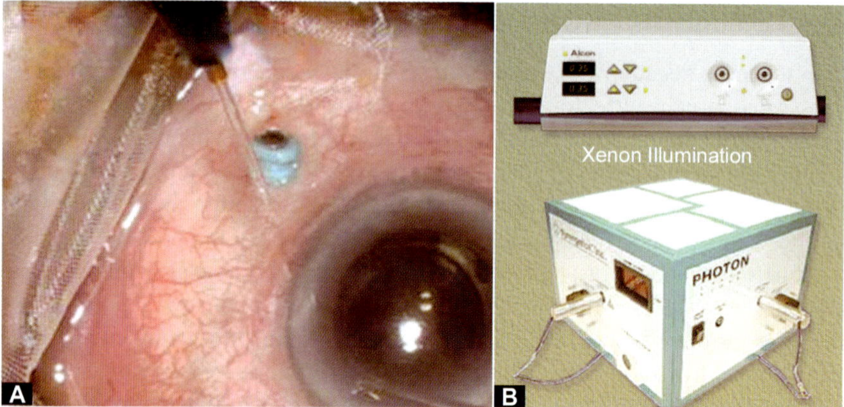

Figs 2.6A and B: (A) 25 gauge chandelier (*Courtesy*: Dr Manish Nagpal); (B) Alcon and Photon Xenon System

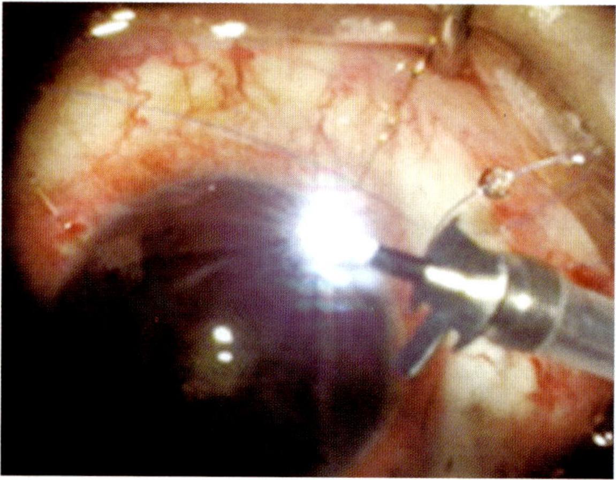

Fig. 2.6C: Synergetics lighted infusion cannula

through smaller gauge fibers, making 20 gauge and 25 gauge illuminated infusion cannulas and 25 gauge chandeliers clinically useful.

With the xenon illumination system, one gets exceptionally bright white light that is filtered for both ultraviolet and infrared energy with the xenon system. It has been shown that we can drive more light into the posterior segment using the xenon box with a 25 gauge endoilluminator than with a 20 gauge endoilluminator with halogen illumination.

Alcon conducted a rabbit study comparing halogen, xenon and metal halide light sources with a fixed exposure of light near the surface of the rabbit retina. The study found halogen and xenon to be equivalent, which is reassuring because most of our experiences are with halogen, and now, xenon. They showed that at 90 minutes versus 120 minutes, and then again at the 1 hour to 1.5 hour light exposure, there were no significant differences between the halogen and xenon sources. At exposure durations longer than

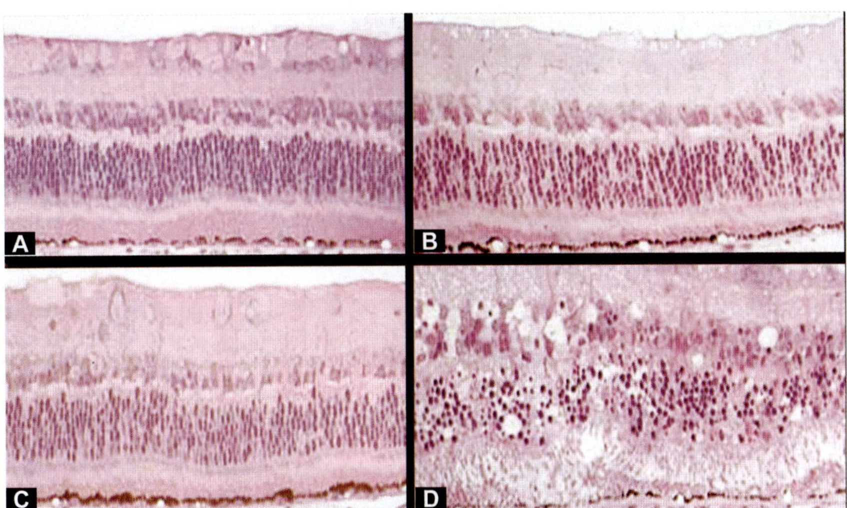

Figs 2.7A to D: Normal and 1.5 hour light exposed retina with a fixed position endoilluminator. Images show a normal rabbit retina (A), a Tungsten-halogen exposed retina (B), a xenon-bypass exposed retina (C) and a metal-halide exposed retina (D) (Adapted from Data on file, Alcon Research Ltd)

120 minutes, however, all types of light, whether halogen, xenon or metal halide, will cause more damage.

Chandelier lighting systems introduce more light into the eye, allowing for excellent illumination and better outcomes. The diffuse illumination of the chandelier provides an important overview of the pathology during the vitrectomy. Diffuse illumination allows the surgeon to more thoroughly identify areas of remote traction during this maneuver, thereby reducing the chance of creating an iatrogenic retinal break.

One of the major advantages of chandelier illumination is that it provides the ability to perform bimanual dissection. Regardless of the type of chandelier used, it is important that the fiber be aimed posteriorly. Autoclavable metal vascular clips are an excellent way to secure the fiber in the desired direction.

Chandelier illumination also allows the surgeon to perform scleral depression. The surgeon can simply plug one cannula and use his free hand to manipulate and depress the globe. This is quicker and safer for removing peripheral vitreous and blood than scleral depression performed by a surgical assistant. In phakic eyes, the surgeon has the option of temporarily moving the infusion line to one of the superior cannulas to allow access to the inferior periphery with less risk to the crystalline lens.

One disadvantage of chandelier illumination, compared with a conventional light pipe, is a diminished ability to see clear vitreous or to distinguish transparent epiretinal membranes. These are not relevant challenges in most diabetic vitrectomies, but occasionally a conventional light pipe has to be used to better identify the internal limiting membrane, which is typically peeled from the macula if there is obvious macular distortion or edema.

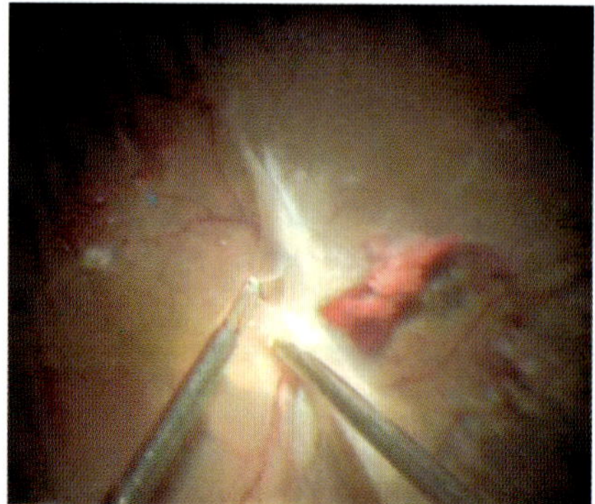

Fig. 2.8A: Bimanual surgery (*Courtesy*: Dr Manish Nagpal)

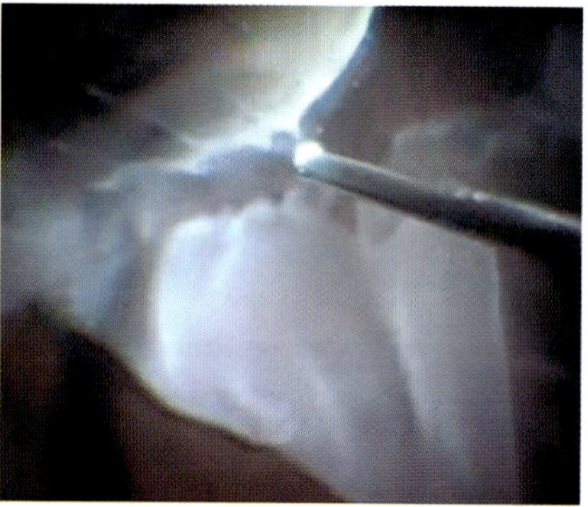

Fig. 2.8B: Scleral depression with chandelier illumination (*Courtesy*: Dr Manish Nagpal)

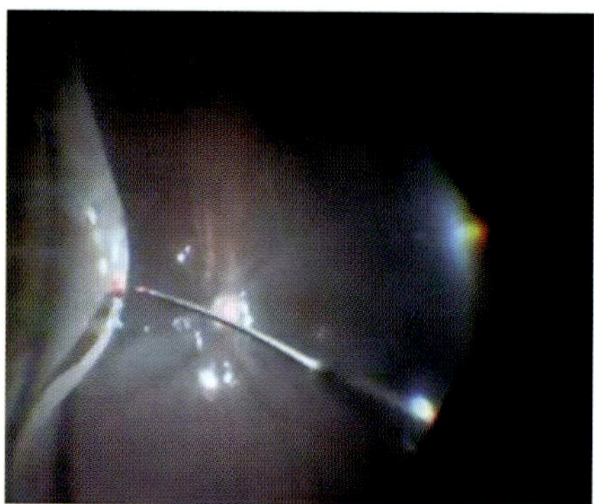

Fig. 2.8C: Scleral depression and laser (*Courtesy*: Dr Manish Nagpal)

LED ENDOILLUMINATORS

An ophthalmic endoilluminator utilizing five LEDs is a new innovation. LEDs are designated R, G, B, A, and W and represent red, green, blue, amber and white LEDs, respectively. The endoilluminator also includes controller collimating lenses dichroic beam splitters condensing lens and endoilluminator assembly.

The light from the five LEDs R, G, B, A, and W is collimated by collimating lenses. The collimated light is combined into a single beam by the dichroic beam splitters. The beam is focused by condensing lens. The focused beam is carried by an optical fiber in the endoilluminator assembly.

The five LEDs R, G, B, A, and W can be of any type. Typically, LEDs R, G, B, A, and W are chosen for the wavelength of light they produce. The eye's natural lens filters the light that enters the eye. In particular, the natural lens absorbs blue and ultraviolet light which can damage the retina. Providing light of the proper wavelength can greatly reduce the risk of damage to the retina through aphakic hazard, blue light photochemical retinal hazard, and similar light toxicity hazards.

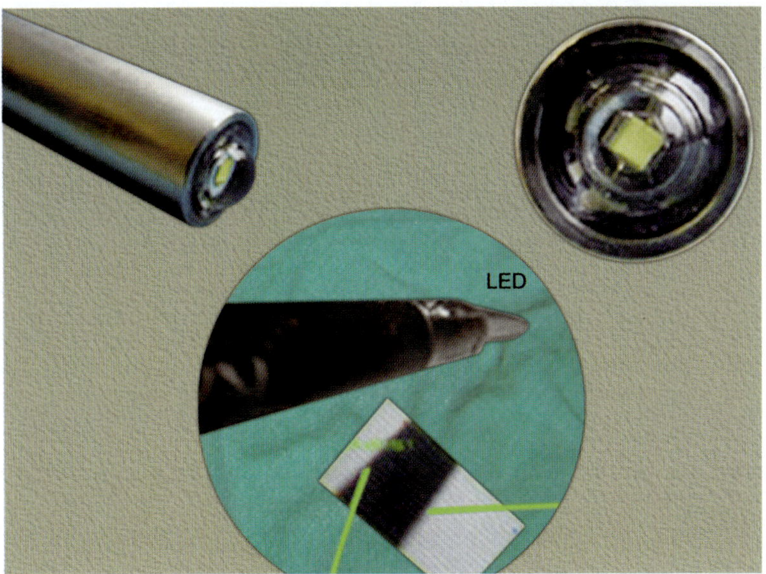

Fig. 2.9: Light emitting diode endoilluminator

LEDs provide greater flexibility in operation and light output. Pulse width modulation or amplitude modulation can be used to allow the appearance of continuous light while reducing heat generation. In addition, LEDs are highly efficient light sources—approximately 10–12% of current driven through an LED is converted into light.

More power is great but the question, of course, is can it be given to us safely? The safety of an endoilluminator light source is usually determined by measuring its aphakic retinal hazard function. Phototoxicity created by exposure to an endoilluminator can be either thermal or photochemical in nature. Thermal phototoxicity is usually not a concern with endoilluminators, but more of a concern with endoscopes. Essentially when we worry about phototoxicity we are worrying about ultraviolet (UV) or blue light toxicity. Through the work of Ham and colleagues on rhesus monkeys, we know the action spectrum or relative risk of UV or blue light toxicity when the retina is exposed to various wavelengths of UV or blue light.[17] The action spectrum that Ham and colleagues defined was then used to create an aphakic hazard curve, which is a relative risk of phototoxicity associated with a given wavelength of light. To determine the aphakic retinal hazard function of a light source, its chromatic curve (or output at each wavelength) is measured and then the amount of light it generates under the aphakic retinal hazard curve is multiplied and summed together.

Phototoxicity threshold has been studied extensively to maximize exposure time and minimize risk when developing light sources for vitrectomy. Standard light sources available on a 20 gauge fiber optic light probe include

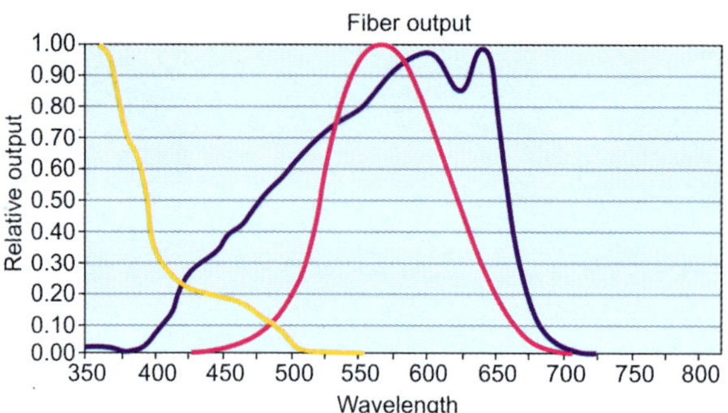

Fig. 2.10: Aphakic retinal hazard curve and chromatic curve for the Alcon Accurus halogen at high 3. (Ham WT Am J Ophthalmol. 1982; 93: 299–306.)

tungsten-halogen and metal halide available in the Alcon Accurus (Fort Worth, Texas) and Bausch & Lomb Millennium (Rochester, NY). These light sources typically have a maximum illumination of 10 lumens, which is roughly halved when used with lighted instruments, wide-angle probes, and chandelier systems through a standard 20-g light probe, leading to a significant drop in illumination.[21] The recent development of xenon light sources provides increased power output, with increased illumination in smaller gauge probes and chandelier systems. To reduce the risk of retinal phototoxicity, safety measures have been advocated. These include the recommended use of a 475 μm long pass filter to block blue light, the lowering of the power output, and perhaps most importantly, increasing the distance between the light probe and the retina. Xenon light has been shown to have similar safety profiles in comparison to tungsten-halogen and improved safety relative to metal halide light sources[21-23]as demonstrated by Yasuo Yanagi et al.[24] The purpose of the study was to investigate the brightness of the xenon/bandpass light in vitrectomy and assess its phototoxic effects using A2E-laden retinal pigment epithelial (RPE) cells. The total luminous flux and spectral irradiance of 20 and 25 gauge endoilluminators connected to xenon lamps were measured and compared to those of 20 and 25 gauge endoilluminators connected to a halogen lamp. *In vitro*, A2E-laden cells were evenly exposed to xenon/bandpass light for 5 to 30 min positioned at 1 cm and 2 cm for a standard light probe and an implantable "chandelier" light probe, respectively, above the cells, and the cell viability was assessed using WST-1 assay.

The cell viability was compared with cells exposed to 30 min of halogen light projected through a 20 gauge endoilluminator. The maximal total luminous flux of xenon/bandpass light emitted through the 20 gauge endoilluminator was 2.8 times higher than that of the halogen light. The total luminous flux of the 25 gauge endoilluminator was 0.6–1.1 times greater than the 20 gauge endoilluminators connected to the halogen light. The viability of the A2E-laden cells after exposure to the xenon/bandpass light was no different than that of the cells exposed to the halogen light when the total luminous flux of these lights was at the same level. Xenon/band pass light from an implantable "chandelier" light probe induced A2E-mediated RPE damage to a similar extent as that of the halogen light through a 20 gauge endoilluminator. Thus, A2E-mediated phototoxicity of xenon/bandpass light is comparable to that of halogen light.

One of the advantages of a xenon light source is the option to use it as an ancillary light in combination with wide-angle illuminators and instruments such as forceps or tissue manipulators. Another major advantage is that it can be used as the sole light source in a chandelier system, allowing bimanual surgery helpful in proliferative vitreoretinopathy (PVR) membrane dissection or peripheral and anterior vitreous base dissection. These also offer a wider angle of illumination, which is useful in 360° scleral depression. Given the increased working distance from the retina, this can significantly decrease retinal phototoxicity. Some currently available options include the Tornambe Torpedo (Insight Instruments, Buffalo, NY), the 25 gauge Awh Chandelier (Synergetics, O'Fallon, Mo), and fourth-port 25 gauge plug-in chandeliers such as the DORC Neptune Dual Chandelier (Kingston, NH). Regarding the xenon sources one word of caution: The brightness of the bulbs diminishes over-time, putting your patient at risk for phototoxicity when you replace a spent bulb with a new one but don't change the setting.

Xenon sources, plus the second generation endoilluminator, at 78°, provide an effective divergence angle for facilitating a view of the vitreous. Anything wider than that would be like driving with your high beams turned on in a fog. It makes it more difficult to see transparent vitreous, and more difficult to see the internal limiting membrane (ILM).

Vitreoretinal Endoscopes

Wide-angle viewing systems and powerful light sources allow access to the far peripheral retina and ciliary body, but they often require scleral depression. Ophthalmic endoscopes can provide complete assessment of the pars plana in its natural state without scleral depression, and they can extend surgical control where standard microscopic views are limited. In complicated cases of proliferative vitreoretinopathy and iris neovascularization, where a small pupil, hyphema, or opaque posterior capsule can prevent complete visualization—even with standard and panoramic contact lenses—ophthalmic endoscopy can augment control in the retroirideal area.[25-29] When used in conjunction with intraoperative fluorescein angiography, vitreoretinal endoscopy can identify pathologic areas in the pars plana and aid in intraoperative evaluation and further surgical treatment of complicated diabetic retinopathy. Endoscopy can also facilitate the management of complications of cataract surgery. It is used to visualize retained lens fragments that can be embedded in the vitreous base and to provide precise haptic placement in posteriorly dislocated intraocular lens implants. The learning curve can be steep as the surgeon's view is via television screen and therefore lacks stereopsis. However, new technology with high-definition televisions and 3 D software can now provide high-resolution stereoscopic views.[30]

REFERENCES

1. de Juan E Jr, Hickingbotham D. Refinements in microinstrumentation for vitreous surgery. Am J Ophthalmol. 1990;109:218–20.
2. Eckardt C. Transconjunctival sutureless 23 gauge vitrectomy. Retina. 2005;25:208–11.
3. Fujii GY, de Juan E Jr, Humayun MS, et al. Initial experience using the transconjunctival sutureless vitrectomy system for vitreoretinal surgery. Ophthalmol. 2002;109:1814–20.
4. Lakhanpal RR, Humayun MS, de Juan E Jr, et al. Outcomes of 140 consecutive cases of 25 gauge transconjunctival surgery for posterior segment disease. Ophthalmol. 2005;112:817–24.
5. Tewari A, Shah GK, Fang A. Visual outcomes with 23 gauge transconjunctival sutureless vitrectomy. Retina. 2008;28:258–62.
6. Fujii GY, de Juan E Jr, Humayun MS, et al. A new 25 gauge instrument system for transconjunctival sutureless vitrectomy surgery. Ophthalmol. 2002;109:1807–13.
7. Manish Nagpal, Rituraj Videkar. Wound Construction in MIVS. Surgical pearls for the ideal small-gauge incision for vitrectomy. Retina Today February 2010.
8. Makoto Inoue, Kei Shinoda, Akito Hirakata, Twenty-three gauge cannula system with microvitreoretinal blade trocar. Br J Ophthalmol. 2010;94:498–502.
9. José Dalma-Weiszhausz, Maximiliano Gordon-Angelozzi, Orlando Ustariz-Gonzalez, Ana Maria Suarez-Licona. Intraocular pressure rise during 25 gauge vitrectomy trocar placement. Graefes archive for clinical and experimental ophthalmol. 2008;246(2):187–9.
10. Pei-Chang Wu, Ing Soo Tiong, Yao-Chi Chuang, Hsi-Kung Kuo. Twisting maneuver for sutureless vitrectomy trocar insertion to reduce intraoperative intraocular pressure rise. Retina. 2011:31(5):887–92.
11. Carl Claes. Expanding the Scope of MIVS—Substantial improvements in technology have increased the capabilities of surgeons and the indications for small-incision surgery. Retinal Physician 2011, Alcon Novartis.
12. Rizzo S, Genvesi-Ebert F. Micro Incisional Vitrectomy (MIVS): A new device for trocar insertion. Acta Ophthalmologica. 2008;86:0. Issue supplement s243.
13. Fang SY, Deboer CM, Humayun MS. Performance analysis of new generation vitreous cutters. Graefes Arch Clin Exp Ophthalmol. 2008;246:61–7.
14. Magalhaes O Jr, Chong L, DeBoer C, et al. Vitreous dynamics: Vitreous flow analysis in 20, 23, and 25 gauge cutters. Retina. 2008;28:236–41.
15. Magalhaes O Jr, Maia M, Maia A, et al. Fluid dynamics in three 25 gauge vitrectomy systems: Principles for use in vitreoretinal surgery. Acta Ophthalmol. 2008;86:156–9.
16. Masahito Ohji, Yasuo Tano. New instruments in vitrectomy. Vitreoretinal surgery: Essentials in ophthalmol. 2007;7:85–98.
17. Ham WT, Mueller HA, Ruffolo JJ, et al. Action spectrum for retinal injury near ultraviolet radiation in the aphakic monkey. Am J Ophthalmol. 1982;93:299–306.
18. Van Best JA, Putting BJ, Oosterhuis JA, et al. Function and morphology of the retinal pigment epithelium after light-induced damage. Microsc Res Tech. 1997;36:77–88.
19. Putting BJ, Van Best JA, Vrensen GF, et al. Blue-light-induced dysfunction of the blood-retinal barrier at the pigment epithelium in albino versus pigmented rabbits. Exp Eye Res. 1994;58:31–40.

20. Putting BJ, Zweypfenning RC, Vrensen GF, et al. Blood-retinal barrier dysfunction at the pigment epithelium induced by blue light. Invest Ophthalmol Vis Sci. 1992; 33:3385–93.
21. Chow DR. Shedding some light on current endoillumination. Retinal Physician. 2005;2:37–9.
22. Van den Biesen PR, Berenschot T, Verdaasdonk RM, et al. Endoillumination during vitrectomy and phototoxicity thresholds. Br J Ophthalmol. 2000; 84:1372–75.
23. Data on file, Alcon Research Ltd.
24. Yasuo Yanagi, Aya Iriyama,Woo-Dong Jang, Kazuaki Kadonosono. Evaluation of the safety of xenon/bandpass light in vitrectomy using the A2E-laden RPE model Graefe's Arch Clin Exp Ophthalmol. 2007;245:677–81.
25. Ciardella AP, Fisher YL, Carvalho C, et al. Endoscopic vitreoretinal surgery for complicated proliferative diabetic retinopathy. Retina. 2001;21:20–7.
26. Terasaki H, Miyake Y, Awaya S. Fluorescein angiography of peripheral retina and pars plana during vitrectomy for proliferative diabetic retinopathy. Am J Ophthalmol. 1997;123:370–76.
27. Uram M. Endoscopic fluorescein angiography. Ophthalmic Surg Lasers. 1996; 27:849–55.
28. Chan CK, Agarwal A, Agarwal S. Management of dislocated intraocular implants. Ophthalmol Clin North Am. 2001;14:681–93.
29. Boscher C, Lebuisson DA, Lean JS, et al. Vitrectomy with endoscopy for management of retained lens fragments and/or posteriorly dislocated intraocular lens. Graefes Arch Clin Exp Ophthalmol. 1998;236:115–21.
30. Miyake K, Ota I, Miyake S, et al. Application of a newly developed, highly sensitive camera and a 3-dimensional high-definition television system in experimental ophthalmic surgeries. Arch Ophthalmol. 1999;117:1623–29.

CHAPTER

3

Faster Visual Recovery in MIVS

Raja Narayanan, Anshuman Sinha, Baruch D Kuppermann

In 2003, Eckardt promoted the use of 23 gauge vitrectomy which combines the benefits of both 20 gauge and 25 gauge vitrectomy. The advantages of a transconjunctival sutureless approach such as increased patient comfort, decreased operative times,[1,2] and decreased corneal astigmatism[3] have been well known and reported in the literature. It has also been hypothesized that the visual recovery is faster after sutureless small gauge vitrectomy. The disadvantages of small gauge vitrectomy include higher risk of hypotony, endophthalmitis, and lack of complete instrumentation such as fragmatome. Hypotony[4] and endophthalmitis[5] are some of the major complications reported are sutureless vitrectomy. In conventional 20 gauge vitrectomy, suturing the sclera and overlying conjunctiva may result in added patient discomfort and increased corneal astigmatism. In sutureless vitrectomy systems, the flow rate is also reduced, owing to the smaller diameter available for flow.

The 23 gauge group had a much faster visual recovery compared to the 20 gauge group with majority of the 23 gauge patients recovering almost their entire potential vision by the first postoperative week. The final visual acuity was also better in the 23 gauge group but was not statistically significant compared to the 20 gauge group. One reason why the visual recovery may be faster in the 23 gauge group could be the reduced postoperative corneal astigmatism reported in small gauge vitrectomy.[3,6,7] In all the previous studies, the induced astigmatism in the 20 gauge group was higher in the early postoperative period but significantly reduced by 1 month. Shinoda et al[8] reported faster visual recovery in cases of macular hole at 1 week after 25 gauge vitrectomy. Another reason for the early visual recovery in the 23 gauge system in our series could be the lesser flow of intraocular irrigating solution. Shinoda et al[8] had demonstrated that the amount of intraocular irrigating solution was much less in the 25 gauge system (244 ml) compared to the 20 gauge system (416 ml). The low flow system is likely to produce less inflammation and edema of ocular tissues compared to a higher flow system. Increased intraocular inflammation in 20 gauge system due to sutures may also be a factor in the delayed visual recovery in the 20 gauge system.

We performed a retrospective study of comparing the rate of visual recovery after 23 gauge and 20 gauge vitrectomies for various indications.[9] The most common indications for surgery in the 20 gauge and 23 gauge groups, respectively, were: Nonresolving vitreous hemorrhage due to diabetic retinopathy (16,14), retinal vein occlusion (7,8), epiretinal membrane (4,3). One patient in each group had silicone oil injection at the time of surgery, and 1 patient in the 20 gauge group had simultaneous cataract surgery with intraocular lens implantation.

The mean BCVA on postoperative day 1 and week 1 was significantly higher in the 23 gauge group compared to the 20 gauge group. The mean BCVA on postoperative day 1 was 0.05±0.09 (Snellen equivalent 20/400) versus 0.16±0.18 (Snellen equivalent 20/125) in the 20 gauge and 23 gauge groups respectively (p=0.004). The mean BCVA on week 1 was 0.12±0.20 (Snellen equivalent 20/160) versus 0.30±0.27 (Snellen equivalent 20/63) in the 20 gauge and 23 gauge groups respectively (p=0.002). The mean BCVA at 6 weeks was minimally better in the 23 gauge group (Snellen equivalent 20/60) than the 20 gauge group (Snellen equivalent 20/70), though it was not statistically significant.

Gain in BCVA

The BCVA at baseline, 1 day and 1 week were calculated as a proportion of the final BCVA at 6 weeks. There was no difference in the baseline BCVA between the 2 groups. The mean BCVA at 1 week was 43% of the final BCVA in the 20 gauge group compared to 83% (p=0.0001) of the final BCVA in the 23 gauge group. At 1 week, most of the patients in the 23 gauge group had a visual acuity close to their final BCVA. The mean surgical time in the 23 gauge group (33±13 minutes) was also significantly less compared to the 20 gauge group (44±22 minutes; p=0.03).

In conclusion, faster visual recovery can be obtained after 23 gauge vitrectomy compared to 20 gauge vitrectomy.

REFERENCES

1. Misra A, Ho-Yen G, Burton RL. 23 gauge sutureless vitrectomy and 20 gauge vitrectomy: A case series comparison. Eye. 2009;23:1187–91.
2. Yanyali A, Celik E, Horozoglu F, et al. 25 gauge transconjunctival sutureless pars plana vitrectomy. Eur J Ophthal. 2006;16:141–7.
3. Okamoto F, Okamoto C, Sakata N, et al. Changes in corneal topography after 25 gauge transconjunctival sutureless vitrectomy versus after 20 gauge standard vitrectomy. Ophthalmol. 2007;114:2138–41.
4. Gupta OP, Ho AC, Kaiser PK, et al. Short-term outcomes of 23 gauge pars plana vitrectomy. Am J Ophthalmol. 2008;146:193–7.
5. Kunimoto DY, Kaiser RS. Incidence of endophthalmitis after 20 and 25 gauge vitrectomy. Ophthalmol. 2007;114:2133–7.
6. Hikichi T, Matsumoto N, Ohtsuka H, et al. Comparison of one year outcomes between 23 and 20 gauge vitrectomy for preretinal membrane. Am J Ophthalmol. 2009;147:639–43 e1.
7. Kadonosono K, Yamakawa T; Uchio E, et al. Comparison of visual function after epiretinal membrane removal by 20 gauge and 25 gauge vitrectomy. Am J Ophthalmol. 2006;142:513–5.
8. Shinoda H, Shinoda K, Satofuka S, et al. Visual recovery after vitrectomy for macular hole using 25 gauge instruments. Acta Ophthalmol. 2008;86:151–5.
9. Narayanan R, Sinha A, Reddy R, Krishnaiah S, Kuppermann BD. Faster visual recovery after 23 gauge vitrectomy compared to 20 gauge vitrectomy. Retina. 2010;30 (9)1511–4.

CHAPTER

4

Microincision Vitrectomy—Incisions

Abhishek Kothari, Narendran V, Amit Gupta

INTRODUCTION

Surgeons across specialities in medicine have embraced minimally invasive techniques for their procedures in the last twenty years. In ophthalmology, a transition in cataract surgery to ever smaller incisions has been closely followed by a similar trend in the vitreoretinal field. Better understanding of vitreoretinal diseases, superior instrumentation and a desire to reduce surgery times and hasten postoperative recovery have all spurred the increasing adoption of microincision vitrectomy for ever expanding indications.

MICROINCISION WOUNDS

Self-sealing wounds that cause minimal disturbance of the ocular coats are the essence of minimally invasive vitreous surgery. Hence, proper wound construction is vital to the success of microincision vitrectomy. An ideal incision should be simple to construct, facilitate maneuvers during surgery, and maintain integrity in the postoperative period prevent egress of intraocular contents (fluid, gas) and ingress of extraocular material (contaminants).

ATTRIBUTES OF MIVS INCISIONS

An important principle in wound construction for microincision vitrectomy is misalignment of the conjunctival and scleral wounds. This ensures coverage of the sclerotomy by intact conjunctiva and provides additional safety.

For the purpose of description, a microincision wound can be said to have two parts the entry incision and the intrascleral tunnel. MIVS wounds are commonly of two types (Figure 4.1). They may have scleral entry incision parallel to the limbus (circumferential) with the intrascleral tunnel running anteroposterior (radial). The other type has the scleral entry perpendicular to limbus (radial) and the intrascleral tunnel parallel to it (circumferential). Circumferential scleral entry incisions are in line with the scleral fibers, and would cause less damage than radial incisions, which will cut across the same. With the same logic, anteroposterior (radial) tunnels would result in separation of scleral fibers whereas circumferential tunnels would cut across

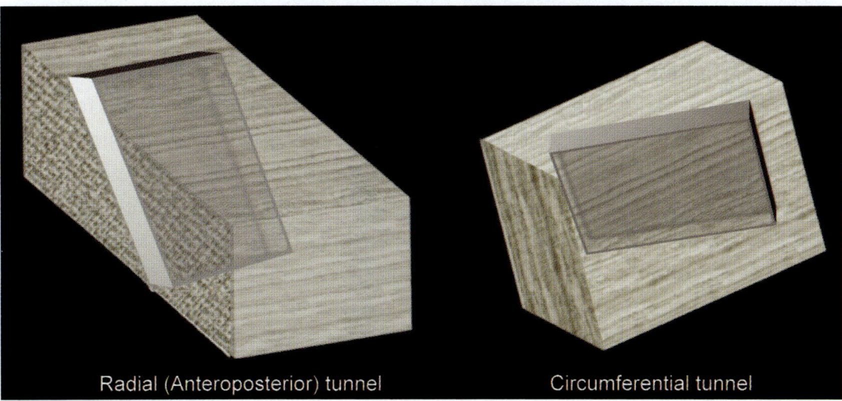

Fig. 4.1: Two MIVS wounds with respect to scleral fiber arrangement. Scleral incision (dark line) is parallel to the scleral fibers and tunnel (gray) runs between circumferential collagen lamellae in radial tunnel wounds. Scleral incision cuts across scleral fibers and tunnel divides collagen lamellae in circumferential tunnel wounds

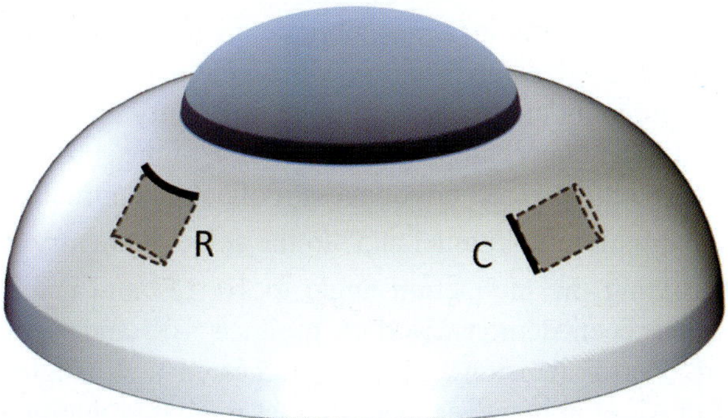

Fig. 4.2: Commonly employed MIVS wounds. Bold line—Scleral entry incision; shaded area- intrascleral tunnel; dotted ellipse – internal entry; R—Radial or anteroposterior tunnel; C—Circumferential tunnel

scleral fibers throughout the extent of the tunnel. The consequence would be better apposition and safety with a combination of circumferential entry and radial tunnels. However, there is a risk of inadvertent damage to the ora if the interior opening of such a wound emerges close to it. The risk is especially higher in the one-step technique of incision with the trocar-cannula assembly. Here, the trocar blade extends well beyond the microcannula and has to be inserted to its full length to place the microcannula in the wound. Additionally, this type of wound carries a risk of injury to the lens in phakic patients. This type of wound is less commonly employed.

Another attribute to be considered is the obliqueness of the tunnel through the sclera, i.e. the angle that the tunnel makes with the external or internal scleral surface. Simple trigonometry shows us that increasingly oblique tunnels are longer (Figure 4.2) and hence, more securely air/water tight. The tunnel can be uniplanar or multiplanar.

MIVS WOUND VARIANTS

Several variations of microincision vitrectomy wounds have been proffered. Initial reports of 25 gauge surgery described straight incisions. Here, the trocar was introduced straight into the vitreous cavity. These incisions were more likely to have leakage related problems. Singh A et al have shown India ink particles within the wound in straight incisions even with conjunctival displacement.[1] Hagemann and Lopez-Guajardo et al proposed inserting trocars with a 30° inclination to the sclera, leading to a radial scleral entry and tunnel parallel to limbus with 30° oblique path.[2] Rizzo et al subsequently reported their technique of making scleral incisions with circumferential entry wound and anteroposterior tunnel.[3] The external entry wound was made at 3 mm from the limbus, with the tunnel 30° oblique to the sclera and vitreous entry at 4 mm. Ultrasound biomicroscopy studies have confirmed the superiority of both the oblique techniques compared to the straight incision. Both the oblique techniques were found satisfactory, with better safety profile with Rizzo's approach.

For 23 gauge vitrectomy incisions, oblique incisions with an angle of 45° to the sclera have been given up for those with an inclination of 30°. The earlier practice of straightening the trocar during the final entry into the vitreous has also been found to be unnecessary. This is because of the substantially longer length of tunnel with increased obliqueness. Pollack had initially suggested a biplanar incision with initial tunnel at 5° to the sclera and entry into vitreous at 30°.[4] Decreasing the inclination angle to 10–15° and entering without straightening has been demonstrated to produce safe and airtight wounds (the so-called 'Zorro' incision). Pollack suggested a 9° angle of cannula insertions.[5] Lin AL et al however reported that increased duration of surgery > 45 minutes and nonmacular diagnosis were likely to cause wound leaks in spite of the extremely oblique incisions.[6] Similar to that described for 25 gauge wounds, Taban M et al studied 25 and 23 gauge incisions using spectral domain OCT and histopathology with variable IOP to simulate real life situations. Angled entries with 25 and 23 gauge incisions provided better wound apposition with higher IOP.[7] Rizzo et al had also developed an injector system for giving a consistent angle of 5–10° for cannula placement and had found it to be very effective.[8]

MIVS WOUND CONSTRUCTION

Two techniques have been described for wound construction in small gauge vitrectomy. The one-step technique utilizes a trocar-cannula set. This is an assembly of a sharp trocar over which the microcannula is mounted. The trocar is introduced obliquely through the sclera to create the incision and the microcannula is left behind in place as the trocar is withdrawn. The Alcon™ system has a caliper at the end opposite to the trocar, which helps in measuring the distance from limbus for the sclerotomy without the need to change instruments. The first generation trocars were beveled. Introduction of these required some force and sclerotomies produced could be irregular. The newer trocar design is similar to conventional MVR blades. These blades encounter less resistance during incision and result in easier insertion and better wounds. Makato et al have reported a better wound construction and lesser incidence of hypotony using the MVR trocar—cannula system over the conventional trocar cannula system in 23 gauge MIVS.[9]

The two-step technique was originally described by Eckardt for 23 gauge surgery.[10] The first step involves using a stiletto blade to create the initial sclerotomy. This is followed by the placement of a microcannula into the sclerotomy over a blunt inserter. This method produces stable self-sealing wounds. However, it has certain disadvantages-need for two instruments, difficulty in finding the conjunctival opening during microcannula insertion and double conjunctival punctures. A pressure plate is mandatory to allow the conjunctiva to remain retracted and the scleral opening to be easily seen. There is an advantage of using a blunt inserter, if the cannula dislodges at any point during surgery. The cannula can be inserted over the blunt inserter and replaced in its previous tract. A sharp trocar is more likely create a second scleral incision near the previous one. UBM analysis in 23 gauge MIVS was undertaken at 8–10 days postoperatively by Teixeria et al comparing a single step incision to a 2 step incision. No difference in the site diameter of the two wounds could be seen.[11] Gutffeisch compared 20, 23 one step, 23 two step and 25 gauge incisions on UBM. Subconjunctival blebs were seen most often with 25 gauge followed by single step 23 gauge incisions. Vitreous incarceration in the wound was found in more eyes with 25 gauge followed by 20 gauge and single step 23 gauge incisions. Wound were open at day 30 in all 20 gauge incisions, 30% in the single step 23 gauge and 10% of 2 step 23 gauge and 25 gauge incisions.[12]

Shape of Incision

The first generation single step Alcon trocars produced a chevron shaped incision. Kyung See Choi et al compared the incisions of 23 gauge using the conventional trocar with the MVR blade.[13] A chevron incision was created with the conventional blade. A V shaped incision was seen with the bevel up and a reverse V with the bevel down. A slit shaped incision was seen with the MVR blade. V shaped incisions were more prone to leaks than the others. The razor blade design of the Synergetics system and the 2 step incisions with the DORC system produced the slit or linear shaped incisions. This led to refinement in the Alcon system which too produced the linear incisions with their Edge Plus design.

Technique of Incision Making

The conjunctiva is held by a forceps and displaced laterally for about 2–3 mm. It is best to hold the conjunctiva (preferably with Tenon's tissue) just posterior to the proposed incision site and bring it upto the limbus just ahead of this site. Holding anterior to the site of incision helps in exerting counter-pressure while introducing the trocar and prevents torsion of the globe. Holding the conjunctiva at the opposite limbus or behind the incision site leads to excessive torsion and conjunctival tearing while incisions are made. Alternatively, a pressure plate can be used. Care is needed in elderly patients and those with thin conjunctiva as there is propensity for the conjunctiva to tear while performing the incision. Cotton tipped applicators may be used to stabilize the globe in these cases. A sharp trocar prevents undue pressure and rotation of the globe while making the incision.

A description of the standard oblique incision follows. The incision is made with the blade of the trocar perpendicular to the limbus. The trocar is held at an angle of 30° (or even less) tangential to the sclera in a direction parallel to the limbus and introduced in that direction to create an oblique tunnel in the sclera. After introducing the trocar fully, the plastic hub of the microcannula is held in place as the trocar is withdrawn, leaving it in place in the sclerotomy. Creation of a biplanar tunnel requires tilting up the trocar midway during insertion to the desired angle, prior to entry into the vitreous cavity. The practice of oblique initial entry followed by tilting up of the trocar handle 90° to enter the vitreous cavity perpendicular to the sclera serves no additional purpose and may result in leaky sclerotomies. Hence, a fully oblique pass is recommended.

For anteroposterior tunnels (Rizzo et al), the blade is positioned parallel to the corneal limbus to create circumferential scleral wound 3 mm from the limbus. It is then introduced posteriorly towards the posterior pole to create radial tunnel in the sclera.

During incision making, the trocars are directed towards either the inferior pole of the eye (6 o'clock) or the superior pole (12 o'clock) (Figure 4.3). We prefer to direct the trocars towards the 6 o'clock position for the superior sclerotomies. Most of the vitreous surgery would happen with instruments (cutter, endoilluminator, etc.) entering the superior ports directed towards the inferior pole. Tunnels with a similar orientation would, therefore, tend to get distorted less intraoperatively. Tunnels pointing towards 12 o'clock would be subject to more twisting and distortion during surgery, and be more likely to leak without sutures.

The infusion cannula is secured first through a sclerotomy made preferably in the inferotemporal quadrant. A tactile click of the infusion tip in the 23 gauge microcannula indicates firm connection. This is essential to prevent the infusion cannula coming loose during globe manipulation during surgery. The tip of the infusion cannula is visualized in the vitreous cavity with a fibreoptic light source held inside the limbus with one hand and the microcannula

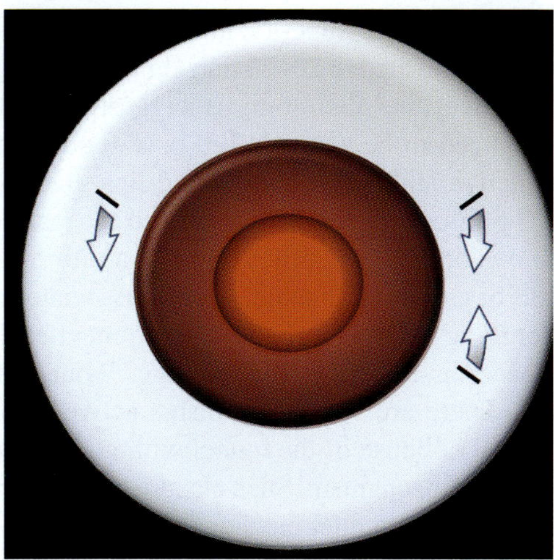

Fig. 4.3: Direction of Insertion of the trocar for creating MIVS wounds

depressed with the other. Once correct placement is confirmed, the infusion can be turned on. Doing this prior to the other sclerotomies is especially helpful in eyes with hypotony, low scleral rigidity or those that are previously vitrectomised. Eyes with total retinal detachment, with or without choroidal detachment, and myopic eyes pose difficulty in inserting the first cannula due to hypotony. A small amount of balanced salt solution may be injected into the vitreous cavity using a 30 gauge needle to make the eye normotensive before inserting the first cannula.

Active sclerotomies are made in the superotemporal and the superonasal quadrants. These sclerotomies are preferably placed one clock hour above the horizontal. In some cases, the superonasal sclerotomy site has to be chosen depending on the available approach for instruments. For patients that have a prominent brow or nasal bridge or sunken orbits, the usual site may have to be moved more superiorly. Distance from the limbus depends on the phakic status of the patient (phakic eyes: 3.5 mm to 4 mm; aphakic or pseudophakic eyes: 3 mm).

INCISION CLOSURE

Vitreous from the inner end of the microcannula is removed well during surgery. The infusion is clamped transiently or infusion pressure is lowered sufficiently during microcannula removal to minimize chances of vitreous prolapse through the wound. The light probe is introduced through the microcannula into the vitreous cavity and the microcannula pulled out slowly over the same. The light probe is then slowly withdrawn and gentle pressure and massage is done over the sclera. Investigators have recently shown that the scleral tunnel needs to be compressed using a solid instrument to allow apposition of the scleral walls and closure of the wounds. This should be done for 30–60 seconds. After both superior microcannulae are removed in this fashion, the pressure is elevated to 20–25 mm Hg to check the wound integrity. A conjunctival bleb over the sclerotomy is suggestive of its leaking nature. These sclerotomies need to be sutured. 7–0 or 8–0 absorbable single suture through the conjunctiva and the scleral wound lips gives good closure with patient comfort. The infusion cannula is removed the last. If there is leakage from this sclerotomy and subsequently hypotony, a suture is placed and globe reformed with BSS or gas, as applicable. Factors associated with wound leaks include eyes undergoing resurgery, multiple instrument exchanges, extensive vitrectomy with base dissection and young age. Wounds in these eyes are preferably sutured. There are two mechanisms active in preventing wound leaks. The mechanical collapse of the tunnel with good apposition of its roof and floor is an important mechanism. Such closure occurs more frequently with the anteroposterior or radial tunnel incisions. Though complete apposition is desirable in every case, this does not always occur. The other mechanism preventing leaks is the surface tension of the intraocular vitreous replacement. If the surface tension of the vitreous substitute exceeds the intraocular pressure acting across the sclerotomy, it will remain as a single bubble and withstand leaking. In BSS filled eyes, this factor is negligible and tunnel collapse is the only factor preventing leaks. These eyes are, therefore, more prone to have wound leaks with microincision wounds than gas filled eyes as gas has a substantially high surface tension. Silicone oil has a low surface tension compared to gas, and eyes with this substitute are also more likely to have wound leaks causing ineffective tamponade and subconjunctival silicone oil (especially with 1000–1300 centistokes). These eyes are probably better off with sutured wounds, more so with 23 gauge surgery. No significant difference in pre and postoperative intraocular pressure was found using a releasable 8.0 nylon suture technique in both 20 gauge and 23 gauge transconjunctival surgery.[14] EH Ryan has shown the use of 6.0 plain gut "tape" suture for closure of 23 gauge incisions instead of the vicryl suture.[15] Polyethylene glycol hydrogel polymer sealant and tissue glue for closure of the sclerotomy was found to be very effective in preventing wound leakage.[16,17]

Confirmation of wound stability using the Terry Barraquer applanation tonometer to check the intraocular pressure is more reliable than digital palpation with the finger. A desired IOP of 15–21 mm Hg can be achieved with a sealed incision, and confirmed with this applanation tonometer at completion of the MIVS procedure. These incisions are least likely to leak.[5]

CONCLUSION

The development of microincision vitrectomy has enabled vitreoretinal procedures with minimal morbidity and an early rehabilitation for patients. The keystone of this type of surgery is the 'minimally invasive' wound. Understanding wound architecture and proper wound construction goes a long way to ensure the success and safety of microincision surgery.

REFERENCES

1. Singh Ajay, Chen, Julie A, Steward, Jay M. Ocular Surface Fluid Contamination of Sutureless 25 gauge vitrectomy incisions; Retina: April 2008;28(4):553–7.
2. Lorenzo Lopez-Guajardo, Jesus Pareja-Esteban, Miguel Angel Teus-Guezala. Oblique sclerotomy technique for prevention of incompetent wound closure in transconjunctival 25 gauge vitrectomy. American Journal of Ophthalmology. 2006;14(6):1154–6.
3. Stanislao Rizzo, Federica Genovesi-Ebert, Andrea Vento, Sofia Miniaci, Federica Cresti, Michele Palla. Modified incision in 25-gauge vitrectomy in the creation of a tunneled airtight sclerotomy: an ultrabiomicroscopic study. Graefe's Archive for Clinical and Experimental Ophthalmol. 2007;245(9):1281–8.
4. Rizzo S, Genovesi-Ebert F, Augustin AJ. Small-Gauge Incision Techniques: The Art of Wound Construction. Retina Today, January/February 2008.
5. Pollack JS. Preventing 23 gauge Vitrectomy Wound Leaks. September 2010 Insert RetinaToday.com
6. Lin Albert L, Ghate Deepta A, Robertson Zachary M, O'sullivan Patrick Sean, May Warren L, Chen Ching-Jygh. Factors affecting wound leakage in 23 gauge sutureless pars plana vitrectomy. Retina. 2011;31(6):1101–8.
7. Taban M, Ventura AA, Sharma S, Kaiser PK. Dynamic evaluation of sutureless vitrectomy wounds: An optical coherence tomography and histopathology study. Ophthalmol. 2008;115(12):2221–8.
8. Rizzo S, Genovesi-Ebert F. Micro Incisional Vitrectomy (MIVS): a new device for trocar insertion. Acta Ophthalmologica. 2008;86(243).
9. Makoto Inoue, Kei Shinoda, Akito Hirakata; Twenty-three gauge cannula system with microvitreoretinal blade trocar. Br J Ophthalmol. 2010;94:498–502.
10. Eckardt C. Transconjunctival sutureless 23 gauge vitrectomy. Retina. 2005;25:208–11.
11. Teixeira A, Allemann N, Yamada AC, Uno F, Maia A, Bonomo PP. Ultrasound biomicroscopy in recently postoperative 23 gauge transconjunctival vitrectomy sutureless self-sealing sclerotomy. Retina. 2009;29(9):1305–9.
12. Gutfleisch M, Dietzel M, Heimes B, Spital G, Pauleikhoff D, Lommatzsch A. Ultrasound biomicroscopic findings of conventional and sutureless sclerotomy sites after 20, 23, and 25 gauge pars plana vitrectomy. Eye (Lond). 2010;24(7):1268–72.
13. Choi KS, Kim HD, Lee SJ. Sclerotomy site leakage according to wound shape in 23 gauge microincisional vitrectomy surgery. Current Eye Research. 2010;35(6):499–504.
14. Song Yumi, Shin Yong Woon, Lee Byung Ro. Adjunctive use of a novel releasable suture technique in transconjunctival vitrectomy. Retina. 2011;31(2):243–9.
15. Edwin H, Ryan Jr. Transconjunctival Plain Gut "Tape" for 23 Gauge Sclerotomy Closure. Arch Ophthalmol. 2011;129(8):1070–2.
16. Singh A, Hosseini M, Hariprasad SM. Polyethylene glycol hydrogel polymer sealant for closure of sutureless sclerotomies: A histologic study. Am J Ophthalmol. 2010;150(3):346–51.e2.
17. Batman C, Ozdamar Y, Aslan O, Sonmez K, Mutevelli S, Zilelioglu G. Tissue glue in sutureless vitreoretinal surgery for the treatment of wound leakage. Ophthalmic Surg Lasers Imaging. 2008;39(2):100–6.

CHAPTER

5

25 Gauge Vitrectomy Overview

Saurabh Luthra

Sutureless vitrectomy has now become an essential part of the armamentarium of a vitreoretinal surgical setup.

25 gauge (25 gauge) Vitrectomy (transconjunctival sutureless vitrectomy system or TSV) was first described by De Juan and colleagues in 2002.[1] They found it practical and safe for a variety of vitreoretinal procedures and concluded that it hastened postoperative recovery and decreased operating time and postoperative inflammatory response.[2] But it was not until the same group reported a larger case series with good results that this technique became popular.[3] Though 25 gauge vitrectomy was found to be better suited for procedures requiring minimal intraocular manipulation, expanded indications were described by combining with 20 gauge (20 gauge) devices,[4] and the concept of "hybrid vitrectomy" came about. With the development of 23 gauge (23 gauge) vitrectomy (first described by Eckardt[5] in 2005) and very recently the 27 gauge (27 gauge) vitrectomy described by Tano and colleagues,[6] a wide variety of options are now available for sutureless vitrectomy.

Using ultrasound biomicroscopy (UBM), the sclerotomy wounds of 25 gauge vitrectomy have been found to be completely healed by 4 weeks postoperatively compared with 8 weeks for 20 gauge vitrectomy.[7,8] Concurrently, the surgically induced keratometric astigmatism was significantly lesser and reduced faster in the 25 gauge vitrectomy compared with 20 gauge vitrectomy (recovering to preoperative baseline within 1 month in 25 gauge and 2 months in 20 gauge).[8] Wound construction is critical in the postoperative wound stability. Oblique sclerotomy incisions with tunneling to create a valve have been reported to be superior and safer to straight incisions in several studies.[9,10] Also conjunctival displacement to misalign conjunctival and scleral wounds helps to reduce wound leakage and hypotony with its resulting complications.

Though initially the indications for 25 gauge vitrectomy were mostly limited to macular surgery such as macular holes and epimacular membranes,[11] subsequently the procedure has been used in a wide variety of conditions like submacular hemorrhage in wet AMD,[12] Terson's syndrome,[13] "floaterectomy" for vitreous floaters,[14] choroidal tumor biopsy,[15] angle closure glaucoma,[16] phacoemulsification associated vitreous loss,[17,18] and posterior capsulectomy following congenital cataract surgery.[19]

Over the years, the indications for 25 gauge vitrectomy have expanded to include rhegmatogenous retinal detachment,[20,21] silicone oil removal,[22] and even complex vitreoretinal cases.[23]

Though complications of retinal break post 25 gauge vitrectomy have been reported,[24] however, 25 gauge vitrectomy was found to be safer than 20 gauge vitrectomy[25] probably due to protection of the vitreous base by the cannulas.

Postoperative endophthalmitis has been reported after 25 gauge vitrectomy.[26-28] There were initial concerns with 25 gauge vitrectomy about increase in incidence of postoperative endophthalmitis compared with 20 gauge vitrectomy. However, a recently published meta-analysis found that the various studies that reported this were not homogenous and hence the evidence is inconclusive.[29] All cases of endophthalmitis reported after 25 gauge vitrectomy were seen in those eyes in which partial fluid-air exchange was not done at the completion of surgery. The higher surface tension of air compared with that of fluid reduces or eliminates wound leaks which may lead to hypotony and vitreous wicks thereby protecting against endophthalmitis. Also air prevents subconjunctival antibiotics from entering the eye which protects against retinal toxicity. For partial fluid-air exchange, more than two-thirds fill and not one-third fill as previously reported is advocated, as the inferotemporal sclerotomy will also be covered when patient is seated or standing. Other measures to reduce the chances of postoperative endophthalmitis include (1) preoperative use of 10% betadine in the cul-de-sac and lid scrubbing reduces the conjunctival bacterial load, (2) angled or beveled incisions as in 23 gauge, (3) near complete vitrectomy, (4) light pipe assisted cannula removal to reduce the chances of vitreous wick, (5) extrainsufflation of air or gas to maintain a stable intraocular pressure.[30]

Another issue with 25 gauge vitrectomy was tool flex. This has been overcome by improvements in design. The second generation Alcon endoilluminator and laser probes are 57% stiffer than the first generation ones. Also, the new Alcon DSP Forceps and Scissors are 2 mm shorter and significantly stiffer than their first generation predecessors (Figure 5.1).

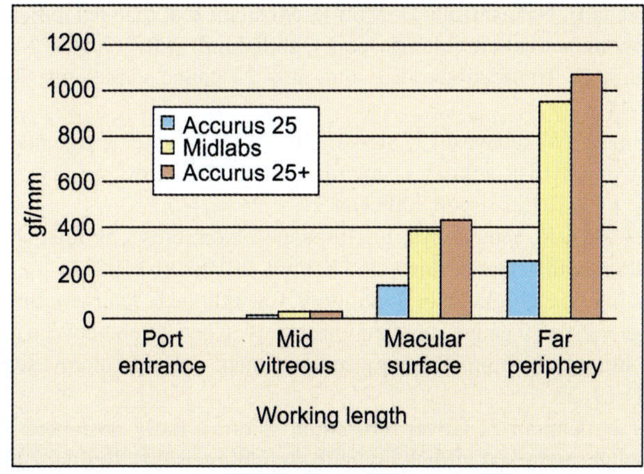

Fig. 5.1: Stiffness comparison. *Source*: Alcon laboratories, inc

Advantages of 25 gauge tools: Portbased flow limiting reduces iatrogenic retinal breaks due to sudden elastic deformation of epiretinal membrane and smaller port closer to the cutter tip facilitates easier and safer access to the membrane. A lot of times, this obviates the need for additional instruments like the forceps and scissors.

New System for 25 Gauge Transconjunctival Pars Plana Vitrectomy

In the June issue of the *American Journal of Ophthalmology*, surgeons using a new nontrocar system for 25 gauge transconjunctival pars plana vitrectomy reported no intraoperative or postoperative complications in a series of 14 patients. The system (NIDEK Corp.) consists of a contact lens ring with four projections containing 1 mm holes (located 3 mm from the ring's edge), a wedge-shaped 25 gauge. infusion cannula, and two plugs. The ring is fixed with 7–0 silk sutures at the 3 and 9 o'clock positions on the limbus. Using the 25 gauge needle, the surgeon creates three conjunctival and scleral incisions at the projection holes located inferotemporally, superonasally and superotemporally. Suturing of the sclerotomies is not required.

Source: Tei M, Shimamoto T, Yasuhara T, Komori H, Oda H, Kinoshita S. A new nontrocar system for 25 gauge transconjunctival pars plana vitrectomy. Am J Ophthalmol 2005;139:1130-3.

REFERENCES

1. Fujii GY, De Juan E Jr, Humayun MS, Pieramici DJ, et al. A new 25 gauge instrument system for transconjunctival sutureless vitrectomy surgery. Ophthalmology. 2002; 109(10):1807–12; discussion 1813.
2. Fujii GY, De Juan E Jr, Humayun MS, Chang TS, et al. Initial experience using the transconjunctival sutureless vitrectomy system for vitreoretinal surgery. Ophthalmology. 2002;109(10):1814–20.
3. Lakhanpal RR, Humayun MS, de Juan E Jr, Lim JI, et al. Outcomes of 140 consecutive cases of 25 gauge transconjunctival surgery for posterior segment disease. Ophthalmol. 2005;112(5):817–24.
4. Shimada H, Nakashizuka H, Mori R, Mizutani Y. Expanded indications for 25 gauge transconjunctival vitrectomy. Jpn J Ophthalmol. 2005;49(5):397–401.
5. Eckardt C. Transconjunctival sutureless 23 gauge vitrectomy. Retina. 2005;25(2): 208–11.
6. Oshima Y, Wakabayashi T, Sato T, Ohji M, et al. A 27 gauge instrument system for transconjunctival sutureless microincision vitrectomy surgery. Ophthalmol. 2010; 117(1):93–102.e2. Epub 2009 Oct 31.
7. You C, Wu X, Ying L, Xie L. Ultrasound biomicroscopy imaging of sclerotomy in children with cataract. Eur J Ophthalmol. 2010;20(6):1053–8.
8. Avitabile T, Castiglione F, Bonfiglio V, Castiglione F. Transconjunctival sutureless 25 gauge versus 20 gauge standard vitrectomy: Correlation between corneal topography and ultrasound biomicroscopy measurements of sclerotomy sites. Cornea. 2010; 29(1):19–25.
9. Acar N, Kapran Z, Unver YB, Altan T, et al. Early postoperative hypotony after 25 gauge sutureless vitrectomy with straight incisions. Retina. 2008;28(4):545–52.

10. Inoue M, Shinoda K, Shinoda H, Kawamura R, et al. Two-step oblique incision during 25 gauge vitrectomy reduces incidence of postoperative hypotony. Clin Experiment Ophthalmol. 2007;35(8):693–6.
11. Guyomarch J, Delyfer MN, Korobelnik JF. Outcomes of 110 consecutive 25 gauge transconjunctival sutureless pars plana vitrectomies. J Fr Ophtalmol. 2008;31(5): 473–80.
12. Arias L, Monés J. Transconjunctival sutureless vitrectomy with tissue plasminogen activator, gas and intravitreal bevacizumab in the management of predominantly hemorrhagic age-related macular degeneration. Clin Ophthalmol. 2010;18(4):67–72.
13. Errera MH, Barale PO, Ounnoughene Y, Puech M, et al. 25 gauge transconjunctival vitrectomy in a case of bilateral epiretinal membrane associated with a Terson syndrome. J Fr Ophtalmol. 2009;32(4):268–72. Epub 2009 Mar 27.
14. Weber-Varszegi V, Senn P, Becht CN, Schmid MK. "Floaterectomy" pars-plana-vitrectomy for vitreous opacities. Klin Monbl Augenheilkd. 2008;225(5):366–9.
15. Sen J, Groenewald C, Hiscott PS, Smith PA, et al. Transretinal choroidal tumor biopsy with a 25 gauge vitrector. Ophthalmol. 2006;113(6):1028–31.
16. Miura S, Ieki Y, Ogino K, Tanaka Y. Primary phacoemulsification and aspiration combined with 25 gauge single-port vitrectomy for management of acute angle closure. Eur J Ophthalmol. 2008;18(3):450–2.
17. Shimada H, Nakashizuka H, Hattori T, Mori R, et al. Bimanual anterior vitrectomy using a 25 gauge high-speed cutter to manage vitreous loss during phacoemulsification. Int Ophthalmol. 2009;29(4):253–5. Epub 2008 Mar 13.
18. Chalam KV, Shah VA. Successful management of cataract surgery associated vitreous loss with sutureless small-gauge pars plana vitrectomy. Am J Ophthalmol. 2004;138(1):79–84.
19. Hong S, Seong GJ, Kim SS. Posterior capsulectomy using a 25 gauge microincision vitrectomy system for preventing secondary opacification after congenital cataract surgery: Outcome upto 4 years. Can J Ophthalmol. 2009;44(4):441–3.
20. Kunikata H, Nishida K. Visual outcome and complications of 25 gauge vitrectomy for rhegmatogenous retinal detachment; 84 consecutive cases. Eye (Lond). 2010; 24(6):1071–7. Epub 2010 Apr 16.
21. Kapran Z, Acar N, Altan T, Unver YB, et al. 25 gauge sutureless vitrectomy with oblique sclerotomies for the management of retinal detachment in pseudophakic and phakic eyes. Eur J Ophthalmol. 2009;19(5):853–60.
22. Kapran Z, Acar N. Removal of silicone oil with 25 gauge transconjunctival sutureless vitrectomy system. Retina. 2007;27(8):1059–64.
23. Riemann CD, Miller DM, Foster RE, Petersen MR, et al. Outcomes of transconjunctival sutureless 25 gauge vitrectomy with silicone oil infusion. Retina. 2007;27(3):296–303.
24. Okuda T, Nishimura A, Kobayashi A, Sugiyama K. Postoperative retinal break after 25 gauge transconjunctival sutureless vitrectomy: Report of four cases. Graefes Arch Clin Exp Ophthalmol. 2007;245(1):155–7. Epub 2006 May 19.
25. Scartozzi R, Bessa AS, Gupta OP, Regillo CD. Intraoperative sclerotomy-related retinal breaks for macular surgery, 20 vs 25 gauge vitrectomy systems. Am J Ophthalmol. 2007;143(1):155–6. Epub 2006 Sep 1.
26. Sommerville DN, Hainsworth DP. Bacterial endophthalmitis following 25 gauge transconjunctival sutureless vitrectomy. Clin Ophthalmol. 2008;2(4):935–6.
27. Mason JO 3rd, Yunker JJ, Vail RS, White MF Jr, et al. Incidence of endophthalmitis following 20 gauge and 25 gauge vitrectomy. Retina. 2008;28(9):1352–4.

28. Taylor SR, Aylward GW. Endophthalmitis following 25 gauge vitrectomy. Eye (Lond). 2005;19(11):1228–9.
29. Bahrani HM, Fazelat AA, Thomas M, Hirose T, et al. Endophthalmitis in the era of small gauge transconjunctival sutureless vitrectomy–Meta-analysis and review of literature. Semin Ophthalmol. 2010;25(5-6):275–82.
30. Lakhanpal RR. Improving the Safety of small gauge vitrectomy air tamponade may reduce complication risk. RetinaToday. January 2011.

CHAPTER

6

23 and 25 Gauge Vitrectomy: An Overview

Pramod Bhende, Sudipta Das

INTRODUCTION

In the history of surgery in all medical and surgical superspecialities there has been a guiding force to lessen invasive procedures to have a better intraoperative and postoperative patient care. The early 21st century showed a marked proliferation in the development of endoscopic instrumentation and procedures in the field of general surgery. The advantages of smaller surgical incision have resulted in faster postoperative recovery.[1-4]

In ophthalmology, the trend started with wide spread acceptance of phacoemulsification surgery popularizing over extracapsular techniques. These along with reducing the surgery time, had faster postoperative recovery and better patient compliance.[5]

Vitreoretinal surgery has experienced an astounding evolution since 1960s, when vitrectomy was performed with a cellulose sponge and manual scissors. Then in the field of vitreoretinal surgery, 20 gauge instruments had been used classically for years. Though 19–20 gauge instruments have been used to have self-sealing pars plana sclerotomies by scleral tunnel incisions,[6-12] yet the recent developments in the transconjunctival sutureless vitrectomy (TSV) systems subsequently renamed and popularly known as microincision vitrectomy system (MIVS), claimed to produce multiple beneficial effects starting from reduced conjunctival and scleral trauma to improved operative efficiency and smoother postoperative recovery.[7-9,11,13,14]

IDEOLOGY

Vitreoretinal instruments are traditionally 19 gauge (1.0 mm) or 20 gauge (0.9 mm) which requires conjunctival and scleral opening with subsequent suturing. The ideology behind 25 gauge vitrectomy was that 25 gauge needles being used transconjunctivaly to give intraocular injections via pars plana in self-sealing manner.[14] In 25 gauge vitrectomy three polyamide microcannulas are inserted through the conjunctiva and sclera in the region of pars plana.[14,15] First an infusion line and subsequently the other vitreoretinal instruments are then introduced into the vitreous cavity through these microcannulas. These narrow instrumentation do not require any conjunctival or scleral incision to be sutured, thus providing minimal surgical trauma and brief recovery times.[9,16-19] The sclerotomies in 25 gauge are only 0.5 mm in diameter, whereas the sclerotomies in 20 gauge vitrectomy are about 0.9 mm wide. However, some negative aspects of 25 gauge vitrectomy as higher incidence of hypotony, vitreous hemorrhage, endophthalmitis, flexibility of the instrumentation and lower cutter efficiency have appeared over time.[9,16-20] To overcome these problems with 25 gauge instruments, 23 gauge system with the aim of combining the advantages of using cannulas without sutures and the benefits of a large caliber, stiffer instruments with more efficient cutters and illumination probes came into the perspective of vitreoretinal surgeries.[13,21]

HISTORY

The selection of optimal instrumentation for advanced vitreoretinal procedures have become increasingly challenging over years. Robert Machemer[22] pioneered the modern technique for vitreoretinal surgery. He performed vitrectomy using 17 gauge (1.5 mm diameter) multifunctional instrument capable of cutting and aspirating the vitreous gel at the same time. In 1974, O'Malley[23] invented a smaller cutter with diameter of 0.9 mm (20 gauge) and subsequently the classic three port, 20 gauge vitrectomy system which is being utilized for over past 35 years in different vitreoretinal surgeries in around the world. These current 19 or 20 gauge vitrectomy systems do not allow self-sealing incisions but requires suturing of both sclera and conjunctiva after the surgery.

In the 1980s, Visitec introduced the first 23 gauge cutter for vitreous biopsy. In the year 1990, Eugene DeJuan & Hickingbotham[24] developed 25 gauge vitreoretinal instruments like vitreous cutter, vitreous membrane dissector and microforceps. It was followed by Stanley Chang and group who introduced 23 gauge system in 1995. However, these 25 and 23 gauge systems were not adopted by industry at that time for various reasons.

In 2002, the 25 gauge sutureless entry-site alignment system was modified and reintroduced by Fujii and coworkers[14] followed by modified 23 gauge system in 2005 by Stanley Chang and Claus Eckhardt. With this, microincision surgery (MIVS) began to establish in the V-R subspecialty. Though initial instruments had few structural and functional problems, subsequent modification made instrument more rigid thereby increasing their utility with expanding indications.

Recent advances and successful clinical experience have ushered in a new era of sutureless vitrectomy. As 25+ gauge vitrectomy and very recently 27 gauge (0.40 mm)[25] system (DORC) has evolved, there are further improvements in instrument design and function.

VITRECTOMY MACHINE PARAMETERS

The 25 gauge infusion cannula has a smaller size and diameter. The infusion rate is low in this system compared to a 20 gauge system by a mean factor of 6.9.[15] In the similar way, the aspiration rate in a 25 gauge cutter is proportionally decreased due to its smaller port and diameter by a mean factor of 6.6.[15] As the port area and the inner diameter are smaller in the 25 gauge cutter compared to the 20 gauge, the aspiration rate in a 25 gauge system must be increased in order to achieve sufficient aspiration. In the same way, maximum cut rate is required to achieve optimal fragmentation of intraocular tissue and to reduce aspiration port line obstruction. Thus, the infusion bottle height set at 40 cm appears to be adequate with an aspiration setting (500 mm Hg) in the Bosch and Lomb *Millennium* System. This setting produces an infusion rate of 0.09 ml/sec with an aspiration rate of around 0.087 mL/sec when measured in in vitro system.[15] As vitreous humor is significantly more viscous than normally used infusion fluid like Balanced Salt Solution (BSS) or Ringer Lactate (RL), the aspiration rates are reduced in vivo in MIVS system. This difference actually allows a greater safety margin against hypotony during aspiration. Following are the machine parameters in Alcon system (Table 6.1).

TABLE 6.1: Alcon probe comparisons

	20 gauge	23 gauge	25 gauge
Maximum cut rate	2500 CPM	2500 CPM	1500–2500
Stiffness (grams/sq mm)	130 gm	35 gm	14 gm
Tip to port distance	0.017 mm	0.009 mm	0.013 mm
Flow at 0 CPM	19 cc/min @ 150 mm of Hg	19 cc/min @ 450 mm of Hg	10 cc/min @ 600 mm of Hg
Flow at maximum cut rate (with BSS)	4 cc/min @ 150 mm of Hg	7 cc/min @ 450 mm of Hg	4 cc/min @ 600 mm of Hg

In 23 gauge system, in contrast to the 20 gauge system, the wounds are less traumatic. Sutures are not necessary to close the conjunctiva or sclera. This reduces the operating time, speeds recovery and eliminates suture induced astigmatism and postoperative discomfort. In comparison to 25 gauge instrument, the larger 23 gauge caliber offers two conveniences, a higher flow rate which results in faster vitrectomy and a higher tensile strength which reduces the likelihood of instrument bending or breakage enabling greater rotation of the eye.[26] To maximize the flow rate, the ideal vitreous cutter would have the highest duty cycle, larger internal diameter, a sharp guillotine and a high cut rate of at least 1500 cycles per minute (CPM).[27]

With the *Constellation* (Alcon) and Stellaris PC (B & L), the vitrectomy probe can even go faster at 5000 CPM. Among the recent advancements, the Accurus 25+ probe offers a high-performance, lightweight probe at 2500 CPM, the same as with the 23 and 20 gauge probes. The 25+ probe, because of its design changes, has higher inflow at high cutting rates, reaching a flow of 7 cc/min at 600 mm Hg at 2500 CPM compared with the previous 25 gauge vitrectomy probe that had a flow rate of around 4 cc/ min at 600 mm Hg at 1500 CPM. With the *Constellation*, the flow rate is even higher, reaching up to 8 cc/min at 650 mm of Hg at 5000 CPM. A stiffening sleeve has also been added to the new probe to closely mimic the feel and handling of larger gauge instruments and the port has been moved closer to the probe's tip to deliver greater control for vitreous base shaving and membrane dissection while working close to the retina. Furthermore, the duty cycle of the 25+ system has been enhanced to attain levels of 50%, compared with approximately 30% with the standard probe. This makes a dramatic difference and more efficient inflow characteristics of the new system. As already emphasized, the flow rate inside the vitrectomy probe is dependent on the viscosity of the aspirated liquid, the vacuum pressure, the internal lumen diameter of the vitrectomy probe and the duty cycle.

ADVANTAGES OF MIVS

Procedure does not involve conjunctival or scleral suturing, so it has no associated suture related inflammatory reactions and, in most cases, leaves the eye free of pain and irritation.[28] It cuts down the operation time and there is almost complete lack of postoperative complaints during rehabilitation time. There is no induced astigmatism.[29] However, Kellnerl et al when compared 25 gauge system with 20 gauge system, found that duration of surgery was comparable between the two systems—the shorter time needed for wound opening and closure in the 25 gauge group being equalized by the longer vitrectomy duration.[28]

Use of microcannula offers several advantages. It protects the sclerotomy and sclera around the sclerotomy; during repeated insertion and withdrawal of the instruments. It would not be torn, or shredded, nor would it be enlarged as it would be during a traditional vitrectomy. The cannula has smaller lumen and greater length hence less vitreous can escape through it thereby minimizing the risk of vitreous incarceration at the sclerotomy sites. The cannulas also permit interchangeability of instruments between entry sites. Ultrasound biomicroscopy (UBM) and histopathological studies have shown that there is minimal wound gape on postoperative day one and the site is undetectable within 2 weeks, compared with a 6–8 weeks of healing time for 20 gauge sclerotomies. UBM further demonstrated that sclerotomy sites with oblique cannula insertion heal much more rapidly than the standard direct cannula insertion. Introduction of *'Valved microcannula'* (Alcon, DORC) further improved the fluidics during surgery. It maintains intraocular pressure during instrument exchange, reduces the wastage of irrigation fluid and further reduces the risk of vitreous incarceration and prolapse.

DECISION MAKING

Case Selection

Choosing the correct gauge for vitrectomy is generally case dependent and MIVS system is excellent where the requirement of extensive tissue manipulation is less. Combining different gauge systems for different steps of surgery in a same eye is also an option.

In case of anticipated scleral buckle or encirclage, 20 gauge system is preferred as 360° conjunctival opening is needed in these eyes. In eyes with severe proliferative vitreoretinopathy (PVR), bad proliferative diabetic retinopathy (PDR) and severe posterior segment trauma, 20 gauge system is preferred. In eyes with nuclear fragments inside the vitreous and there is need to use fragmatome, 20 gauge instruments are preferred. In retained intraocular foreign body, 20 gauge system is preferred to facilitate easy removal of the foreign body.

PREFERRED INDICATION OF MIVS

With increasing experience, the indications for MIVS are ever increasing. Cases normally recommended for MIVS are epiretinal membrane peeling, macular hole, persistent diabetic macular edema, vitreous hemorrhage with or without minimum tractional retinal detachment, uncomplicated rhegmatogenous retinal detachment, endophthalmitis and cases with coexistent filtering bleb.[14] The 25 gauge system is very useful in minimal manipulative macular hole or macular pucker surgery with posterior vitreous detachment.[30]

The 23 gauge system has shown statistical significant visual improvement in eyes with epiretinal membrane, macular hole, diabetic macular edema and nonclearing vitreous hemorrhage not associated with extensive tractional retinal detachment.[31,32] Primary vitrectomy for retinal detachment with 23 gauge had comparable outcome with 20 gauge vitrectomy with shorter surgical time.[33] 23 gauge vitrectomy system alone or in combination with 20 gauge fragmatome was found to be safe and efficacious in the management of posteriorly dislocated lens or lens fragments.[34] Bimanual 23 gauge transconjunctival sutureless vitrectomy was found to be safe and effective in patients with complicated vitreoretinopathies including diabetic tractional detachment, complicated rhegmatogenous retinal detachment and massive subretinal hemorrhage.[35]

In newborn and premature infants with narrow palpebral fissures and smaller eyes with persistent hyaloidal system, lens sparing vitrectomy for stage 4 and selected stage 5 retinopathy of prematurity and uncomplicated tractional detachments MIVS is a better option. All three cannulas can be adequately located in the limited surgical space without damaging the lens or any other intraocular structure.

Is it safe?

Incidence of iatrogenic peripheral retinal breaks was found to be less in macular diseases with 23 gauge MIVS than 20 gauge vitrectomy.[36] Le Rouic et al have found 23 gauge MIVS to be safer than 20 gauge vitrectomy for macular diseases, in terms of lower rates of postoperative retinal detachment.[37] Misra et al reported considerably less risk of raised IOP in the 23 gauge group in comparison to 20 gauge for a variety of retinal pathologies.[38] 23 gauge transconjunctival vitrectomy can be performed safely in patients with postoperative endophthalmitis.[39]

LIMITATIONS OF MIVS

With reduced length of cutter and other instruments, it is difficult to reach posterior pole in eyes with larger axial length. It is more important now with newer generation of stiff 25+ instruments which further reduces effective length of instrument. Eyes with dense fibrous proliferation in severe proliferative diabetic retinopathy, proliferative vitreoretinopathy, and stage V retinopathy of prematurity are difficult to handling with small gauge vitrectomy system.[30]

With long trocar blade, there is increased risk of retinal injury in eyes with anteriorly displaced retina, e.g. stage V retinopathy of prematurity and severe anterior PVR. The other limitations include, decreased illumination with the older machines, still relatively more flexibility of the instruments, difficult and time consuming silicone oil injection and removal and unavailability of fragmotome.

SUMMARY

Since the inception of 20 gauge vitrectomy in 1970, for the last 30–35 years, this system has been well-tolerated and highly effective in the field of vitreo-retinal surgeries. The development of transconjunctival, sutureless 25 and 23 gauge vitrectomy systems have provided surgeons with new options in the surgical treatment of vitreoretinal diseases. Proper case selection is imperative, as the smaller scale of the instruments and decreased fluidics work most efficiently when extensive manipulation of intraocular tissue or significant membrane dissection is not required.

Although, continuing innovations in microincision instrumentation and techniques are raising the possibility of applying microincision approach to virtually all indications where standard 20 gauge vitrectomy system is presently being used, our experience to date with sutureless 25 and 23 gauge vitrectomy is limited. The benefits of shorter operating time and improved postoperative patient comfort are important, but represent short-term clinical outcomes. But these advantages must be weighed against the potential drawbacks in view of the most rational and evidence based practice in the field of vitreoretinal surgery. There still is no data demonstrating long-term visual benefit compared to 20 gauge surgery.

It is beyond doubt that there will be always indications for 20, 23, and 25 gauge vitrectomy surgery. For complicated cases like complex membrane peeling with or without tractional retinal detachment, retinal detachment with extensive PVR changes, nucleus removal, silicone oil removal, where extensive intraocular manipulation is needed, versatility of conventional 20 gauge instruments still makes them the first choice for most posterior segment surgeons. The 25 gauge system requires appropriate case selection. However, all-round utility and better stability of 23 gauge instruments seems to combine the best features of both 20 and 25 gauge systems and may be the preferred system for majority of the indications for VR surgery.

REFERENCES

1. Breedveld P, Stassen Hg, Meijer DW. Observations in laparoscopic surgery: Overview of impeding effects and supporting aids. J Laparoendosc Adv Surg Tech A. 2000;10:231–41.
2. Dunn MD, Clayman RV. Laparoscopic management of renal cystic disease. World J Urol. 2000;18272–77.
3. Koh CH, Janik GM. Laparoscopic microsurgery; current and future status. Curr Opin Obstet Gynecol. 1999;11:401–07.
4. Lundell L. Antireflux surgery in the laparoscopic era. Baillieres Best Pract Res Clin Gastroenterol. 2000;14:793–810.
5. Kraff MC, Sanders Dr Planned extracapsular extraction versus phacoemulsification IOL implantation: A comparison of concurrent series. J Am Intraocul Implant Soc. 1982;8:38–41.
6. Chen JC. Sutureless pars plana vitrectomy through self-sealing sclerotomies. Arch Ophthalmol. 1996;114:1273–75.
7. Jackson T. Modified sutureless sclerotomies in pars plana vitrectomy [letter]. Am J Ophthalmol. 2000;129:116–17.
8. Kwok AK, Tham CC, Lam DS. Modified sutureless sclerotomies in pars plana vitrectomy. Am J Ophthalmol. 1999;127:731–33.
9. Lam DS, Chua JK, Leung AT. Sutureless pars plana anterior vitrectomy through self-sealing sclerotomies in children. Arch Ophthalmol. 2000;118:850–51.
10. Milibak T, Suveges I. Complications of sutureless pars plana vitrectomy through self-sealing sclerotomies. Arch Ophthalmol. 1998;116:119.
11. Rahman R, Rosen PH, Riddell C, Towler H. Self-sealing sclerotomies for sutureless pars plana vitrectomy. Ophthalmic Surg Lasers. 2000;31:462–66.
12. Schmidt J, Nietgen GW, Brieden S. Selbstverschliessende, nahtlose Sklerotomie zur Pars planaVitrektomie. Klin Monatsbl Augenheilkd. 1999;215:247–51.
13. Eckardt C. Transconjunctival sutureless 23 gauge vitrectomy. Retina. 2005;25: 208–11.
14. Fujii GY, De Juan E Jr, Humayun. Initial experience using the transconjunctival sutureless vitrectomy system for vitreoretinal surgery. Ophthalmol. 2002;109:1814–20.
15. Fujii GY, De Juan E Jr, Humayun. New 25 gauge instrument system for trans conjunctival sutureless vitrectomy surgery. Ophthalmol. 2002;109:1807–12.
16. Chen E. 25 gauge transconjunctival sutureless vitrectomy. Curr Opin Ophthalmol. 2007;18:188 –93.

17. Ibarra MS, Hermel M, Prenner JL, Hassan TS. Longer-term outcomes of transconjunctival sutureless 25 gauge vitrectomy. Am J Ophthalmol. 2005;139:831–36.
18. Lakhanpal RR, Humayun MS, de Juan E Jr. Outcomes of 140 consecutive cases of 25 gauge transconjunctival surgery for posterior segment disease. Ophthalmol. 2005;112:817–24.
19. Meyer CH, Rodrigues EB, Schmidt JC, Horle S, Kroll P. Sutureless vitrectomy surgery. Ophthalmol. 2003;110:2427–8.
20. Gupta OP, Weichel ED, Regillo CD. Postoperative complications associated with 25-gauge pars plana vitrectomy. Ophthalmic Surg Lasers Imaging. 2007;38:270–75.
21. Barbara P, Guido P, Federicka R. Postoperative complications and intraocular pressure in 943 consecutive cases of 23 gauge transconjunctival pars plana vitrectomy with one year follow-up. Retina. 2010;30:107–11.
22. Machemer R, Buettner H, Norton E.W. Vitrectomy: a pars planar approach. Trans Am Acad Ophthalmol Otolaryngol. 1971;75:813–20.
23. O'Malley C, Heintz RM Sr. Vitrectomy with an alternative instrument system. Ann Ophthalmol. 1975;7:585–88,591–4.
24. De Juan E Jr, Hickingbotham D. Refinements in microinstrumentation for vitreous surgery. Am J Ophthalmol. 1990;109:218–20.
25. Oshima Y, Wakabayashi T, Sato T. A 27 gauge instrument system for transconjunctival sutureless microincision vitrectomy surgery. Ophthalmol. 2010;117:93–102.
26. McGregor N, Michael H, Singh J, et al. 23 gauge vitrectomy in 100 eyes; Short-term visual outcomes and complications. Retina. 2008;28:1193–1200.
27. Hubschman JP. Comparison of different vitrectomy systems. J Fr Ophthalmol. 2005; 28:606–09.
28. Kellner L, Wimpissinger B, Stolba U. 25 gauge vs 20 gauge system for pars plana vitrectomy: A prospective randomised clinical trial. Br J Ophthalmol. 2007;91:945–48.
29. Okamoto F, Okamoto C, Sakata N. 25 gauge transconjunctival sutureless vitrectomy does not induce significant changes in corneal topography and exerts little influence on the optical quality of the cornea. Ophthalmol. 2007;114:2138–41.
30. Gaudric A, Haouchine B, Massin P. Macular hole formation: New data provided by optical coherence tomography. Arch Ophthalmol. 1999;117:744–51.
31. Fine HF, Iranmanesh R, Iturralde D, Spaide RF. Outcome of 77 consecutive cases of 23 gauge transconjunctival vitrectomy surgery for posterior segment disease. Ophthalmol. 2007;144:1197–1200.
32. Lott MN, Manning MH, Singh J. 23 guage vitrectomy in 100 eyes: Short-term visual outcomes and complications. Retina. 2008;28:1193–1200.
33. Min Kyu Shin, Ji Eun Lee, Boo Sup Oum. Comparison Between 20 gauge and 23 gauge Vitrectomy System in Primary Vitrectomy for Rhegmatogenous Retinal Detachment, J Korean Ophthalmol Soc. 2009;50(3):405–11.
34. Minhee Cho, RV Paul Chan. 23 gauge pars plana vitrectomy for management of posteriorly dislocated crystalline lens. Clin Ophthalmol. 2011;5:1737–43.
35. Park KH, Woo SJ, Hwang JM, Kim JH, Yu YS, Chung H. Short-term outcome of bimanual 23 gauge transconjunctival sutureless vitrectomy for patients with complicated vitreoretinopathies. Ophthalmic Surg Lasers Imaging. 2010; 41(2):207–14.
36. Nakano, Tetsuro, Uemura, Akinori, Sakamoto, Taiji. Incidence of iatrogenic peripheral retinal breaks in 23 gauge vitrectomy for macular diseases. Retina. 2011;31(10):1997–2001.

37. Le Rouic, Jean-Francois, Becquet Frank, Ducournau, Didier. Does 23 gauge sutureless vitrectomy modify the risk of postoperative retinal detachment after macular surgery?: A comparison with 20 gauge vitrectomy. Retina. 2011;31(5):902–8.
38. Misra A, Ho-Yen G, Burton RL. 23 gauge sutureless vitrectomy and 20 gauge vitrectomy: A case series comparison Eye. 2009;23,1187–91.
39. Tan CSH, Wong H-K, Yang FP, Lee J-J. Outcome of 23 gauge sutureless transconjunctival vitrectomy for endophthalmitis. Eye. 2008;22:150–1.

CHAPTER

7

27 Gauge Vitrectomy System

Yusuke Oshima

Transconjunctival microincision vitrectomy surgery (MIVS) with 25 or 23 gauge instrumentation has evolved radically during the past several years.[1-6] This system has no doubt simplified the vitrectomy procedure and offers numerous potential advantages over traditional 20 gauge surgery. Several arguments in the early years of MIVS have been settled by the recent innovations and improvements, e.g. using recently-refined stiffer instruments and wide-angle viewing system eliminating the frustration with tool fragility, powerful light source combined with chandelier system improving the endoilluminating brightness through a small gauge optic fiber, and the new generation vitrectomy machine dramatically improving the vitrectomy performance of small gauge vitrectomy probe. More surgeons will be shifting from 23 gauge system to 25 gauge shortly and can easily imagine 27 gauge or much smaller gauge instruments as the next generation of MIVS. Prior to the introduction of MIVS, smaller gauge instruments have been used for postoperative management of vitrectomized eyes. For example, we have performed transconjunctival fluid-fluid exchange and fluid-air exchange through a 27 gauge needle for many years, and there are no reports of serious complications related to wound integrity with a 27 gauge needle. Therefore, 27 gauge (0.40 mm), if it is practical, may be the best-suited technology for the perfectly sutureless MIVS. This chapter introduces the current status and future perspectives of 27 gauge instrumentations for transconjunctival 27 gauge MIVS.

27 GAUGE ILLUMINATION SYSTEM (LIGHT SOURCE AND FIBERS)

When developing a smaller gauge vitrectomy system, one of the most crucial concerns may be the reduced endoillumination through a small gauge optic fiber. The recent introduction of more powerful light sources using xenon light and mercury vapor light has enabled us to develop smaller-gauge illumination tools.

Light source

Xenon illuminator

To overcome the insufficient illumination of conventional light sources for these surgical procedures, brighter illuminators, e.g. xenon light source, have been developed (Table 7.1 and Figures 7.1A to C). The increased power of xenon lights is substantial even with 25 gauge (0.50 mm) light pipe and several types of newly developed 27 gauge (0.40 mm) chandelier light fiber, and the intraocular illumination is equal to or brighter than the illumination achievable with 20 gauge probes with conventional halogen or metal halide light bulbs.[7]

Mercury vapor illuminator

Although the new xenon illuminators are useful and have an integrated filter system to improve safety by cutting off high levels of ultraviolet (UV) illumination, no commercially available light sources, including xenon lights, are safe for long periods of exposure with respect to photochemical retinal damage.

To obtain a more powerful illumination source with minimal phototoxicity to the retina, a mercury vapor illuminator (Photon II, Synergetics Inc.

TABLE 7.1: Xenon light source

Photon™	Synergetics Inc.
Accurus Xenon Illuminator	Alcon Laboratories Inc.
Bright Star	DORC Inc.

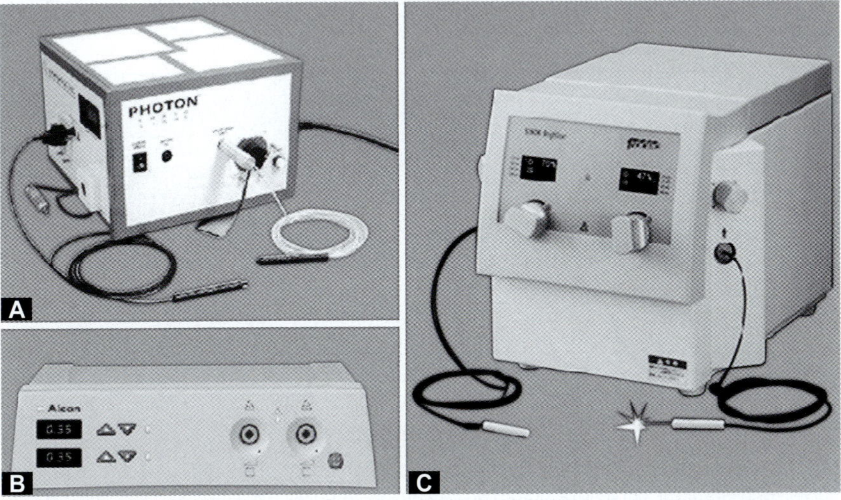

Figs 7.1A to C: Photograph of xenon illuminator. (A) Photon (Synergetics Inc.); (B) Accurus xenon illuminator (Alcon Laboratories Inc.); (C) Bright Star (DORC)

St Charles, Missouri) has been newly developed (Figure 7.2).[8] The luminous efficacy of the mercury vapor illuminator reaches 402 lumens/watt of optical power, which is brighter than any commercially available xenon light illuminators (ranging from 277 to 355 lumens/watt). The actual output level of the mercury vapor illuminator can be enhanced to 56 lumens through a 25 gauge chandelier fiber, which is approximately twice as bright as that of the xenon light source that maximally enhances only up to 29 lumens through the same chandelier fiber (Courtesy of Synergetics, Inc.). After passing through a 435 nm cut-off filter, the output of the mercury vapor illuminator has only two spectral output peaks at 550 and 580 nm, and the entire spectral output curve is mostly confined within the range of the photopic spectral system (Figure 7.3). Therefore, the spectral distribution of the mercury vapor bulb reduces phototoxicity with higher hazard efficiency. The hazard efficacy is 2200 lumens/hazard watt in the mercury vapor illuminator, which is much higher than the hazard efficacy measured in a xenon or halogen light source, ranging from 1150 to 1900 lumens/hazard watt. The illumination generated by the

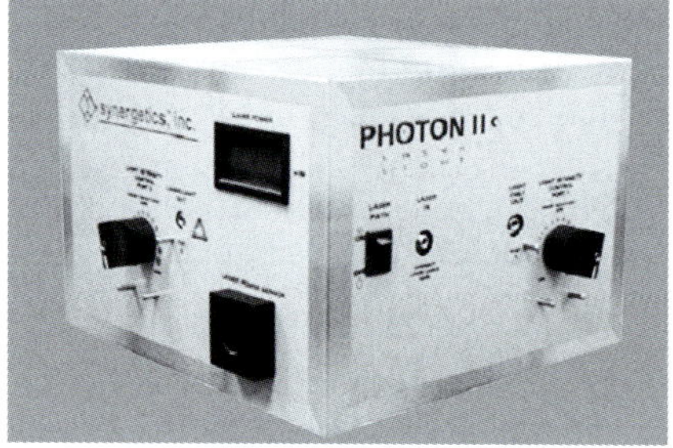

Fig. 7.2: Photograph of mercury vapor illuminator; Photon II (Synergetics Inc.)

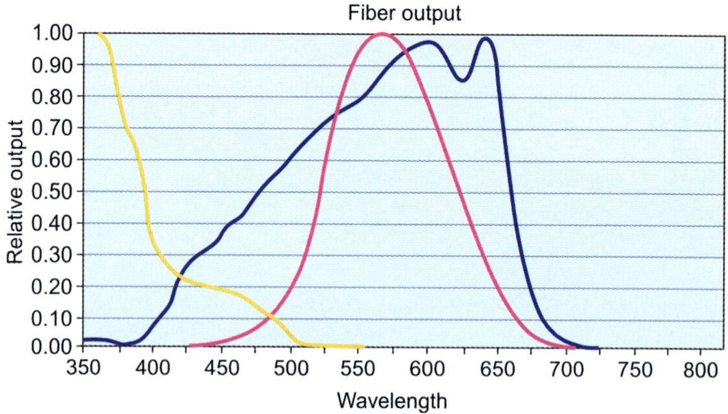

Fig. 7.3: Spectral output curve of a mercury vapor light, normal photopic spectral sensitivity curve, and spectral curve of phototoxic hazard in aphakic eyes are shown. The relative output of the mercury vapor lamp is filtered by an integrated 435 nm filter, resulting in an output curve mostly confined within the photopic spectral sensitivity of humans

mercury vapor light source has a green-yellowish hue which is comfortable to surgeons' eyes.

Small Gauge Optic Light Fibers

27/29 gauge chandelier fiber

Currently, two types of 27 gauge chandelier fiber are commercially available (Figures 7.4A and B): one is a standard type of 27 gauge chandelier (Synergetics Inc.) and another is the 27 gauge twin-light chandelier developed by Dr. Eckardt (DORC, Zuidland, Holland).[9] Both chandelier fibers provide sufficient endoillumination during vitrectomy when connecting to a xenon light source (Photon or BrightStar).

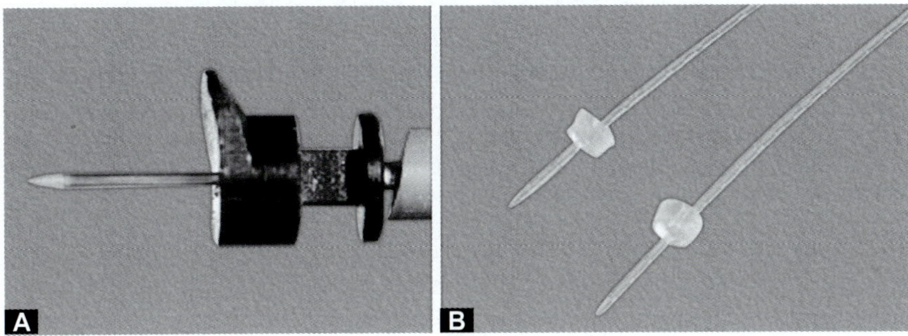

Figs 7.4A and B: Photograph of 27 gauge chandelier illumination fiber. (A) 27 gauge Awh/Tano chandelier™ (Synergetics); (B) 27 gauge Eckardt twinlight™ chandelier (DORC)

27/29 gauge one-step illumination fiber

Because of the higher illumination capabilities of the mercury vapor illuminator than any other commercially available light source, high levels of endoillumination are possible through a 29 gauge (0.32 mm) light fiber (Microfiber, Synergetics Inc.). Two types of 27/29 gauge illumination probe compatible with the mercury vapor illuminator have been newly developed.

27/29 gauge one-step, self-retaining chandelier illumination fiber

A new chandelier illumination fiber consists of a retractable 27 gauge thin-walled needle socket and a 29 gauge (0.32 mm) inner light fiber has been developed (Figures 7.5A and B).[8] Because of its hands-free and self-retaining nature, bimanual manipulation is possible. Insertion through a 27 gauge sclerotomy facilitates surgical entry and closure, and conjunctival peritomy and suture placement are not needed. In addition to the self-retaining, reliable sutureless, and hands-free nature, this probe is convenient for single-step transconjunctival insertion without the need for a preincision using a needle or an MVR blade. After inserting the 27 gauge needle socket transconjunctivally, the tip of the 29 gauge light fiber can be easily exposed by retracting the outer needle socket. The retracted needle wall then serves as a heat shield to prevent thermal burns on the sclera. The maximum illumination of the 29 gauge light

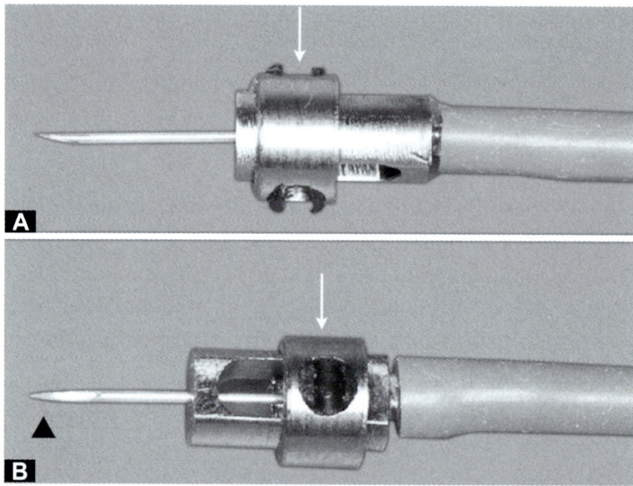

Figs 7.5A and B: View of the 27/29 gauge one-step, self-retaining chandelier illumination fiber; (A) The device consists of a retractable 27 gauge needle socket (white arrow) through which the 29 gauge light fiber passes; (B) The tip of the 29 gauge light fiber (arrowhead) can be exposed easily by fully retracting the outer needle wall (white arrow)

fiber with mercury vapor illuminator is sufficiently bright to obtain a clear, homogeneous and wide-angle endoillumination, making it suitable for use in combination with a panoramic-viewing system.

27/29 gauge one-step, wide-field illumination light pipe

A 27/29 gauge wide-field illumination light pipe is newly designed also. This light pipe consists of a 27 gauge thin-walled needle and a 29 gauge (0.32 mm) inner light fiber (Microfiber) with the fiber tip fixed at the top of the needle (Figure 7.6). The side-cutting design of the needle wall serves as an optical shield to minimize the reflected glare from the tip to the surgeon's eyes. After one-step insertion of the 27 gauge needle transconjunctivally, the probe of the light pipe can be introduced only about 10–13 mm into the vitreous cavity because of the short total length (13 mm) of the needle. Therefore, the structure can eliminate potentially dangerous localized bright spots that may occur by using conventional light pipes.

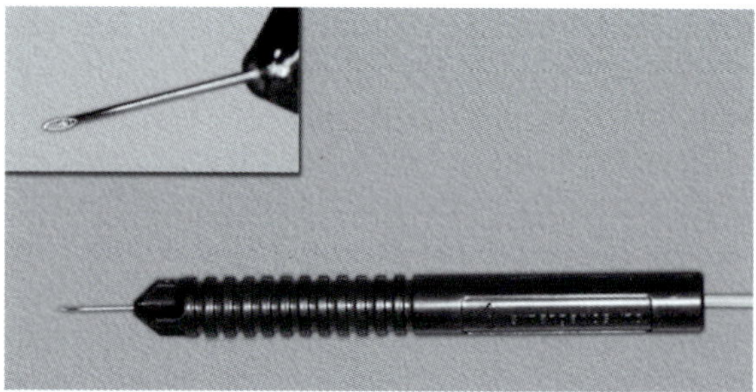

Fig. 7.6: View of the 27/29 gauge one-step, wide-field illumination light pipe. This light pipe consists of a 27 gauge thin-walled needle and a 29 gauge inner light fiber with the fiber tip fixed at the top of the needle

27 GAUGE VITREOUS CUTTER

Development of a practical 27 gauge vitreous cutter was the key step for establishing a 27 gauge vitrectomy system. A pneumatic 27 gauge cutter with its maximum cutting rate reaching to 2,500 cutting per minute (cpm) has been developed in collaboration with DORC.[10] A shorter shaft length (25 mm) provides rigidity similar to a conventional 25 gauge cutter. Using a high-speed camera, we evaluated the 27 gauge cutter's duty cycle. The duty cycle of the 27 gauge cutter is approximately 60% at 1,000 cpm and 40% at 1,500 cpm, which is equal to or slightly better than that of a standard 25 gauge cutter. Based on the duty cycle evaluation and infusion flow rate measurements, we found that the pressure of the vented gas forced infusion system (Accurus, Alcon Laboratories, Inc.) can be set within a normal range of 20 to 30 mm Hg, providing safe control of intraocular pressure (IOP) during vitrectomy. This might suggest the the 27 gauge vitrectomy can be performed within a normal range of IOP during vitreous cutting. Although the vitrectomy performance (cutting efficiency and flow volume) of the current 27 gauge vitrectomy probe dose not exceed that of 23 or 25 gauge systems and is approximately 70% as compared with that of the standard 25 gauge vitreous cutter, the performance of 27 gauge vitrectomy is feasible and sufficient to be clinically applied for macular surgery and other simple cases.

27 GAUGE SURGICAL INSTRUMENTS

To enhance the advantages of microincision vitrectomy surgery, several 27 gauge accessories, such as microforceps, membrane spatula, diathermy, and endolaser probe, have been developed and commercially available from several manufactures for expanding the surgical indications of 27 gauge vitrectomy.

27 Gauge Microforceps

Two types of 27 gauge membrane forceps are currently available for proliferative epiretinal tissue or internal limiting membrane removal.

27 gauge asymmetrical microforceps

The size of the shaft is substantially thinner, i.e. 0.40 mm in diameter, and the length of the shaft (32 mm) is the same as that of a standard 20 gauge microforceps. The shape of the grasping end is asymmetric, which is similar to that of the 20 gauge instrument, but much sharper and thus suitable for transconjunctival insertion and easy visualization of target tissue. Although the grasping end of the 27 gauge microforceps is very compact, the distance between the two tips of the grasping end is wide enough to grasp both thin and thick proliferative epiretinal tissue.[11]

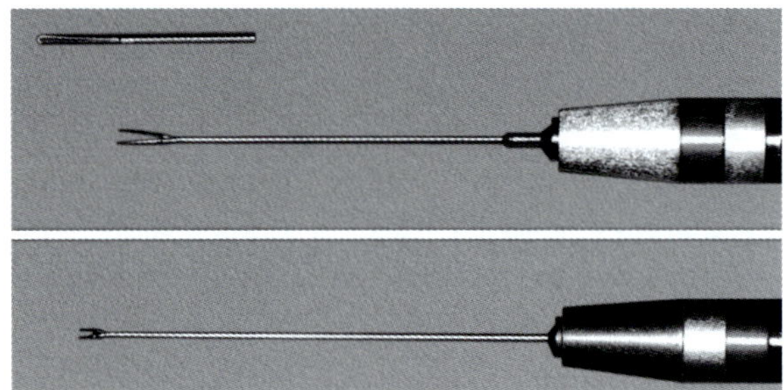

Fig. 7.7: View of the 27 gauge end-gripping microforceps (top) and the standard 25 gauge forceps (bottom)

27 gauge end-gripping microforceps

A 27 gauge end-gripping microforceps was developed by DORC (Zuidland, Holland) (Figure 7.7). The length of the shaft is substantially shortened to 28 mm to strengthen the stiffness of the thinner shaft. The end-gripping design is suitable for grasping much tough and thick proliferative epiretinal tissue.

Other 27 Gauge Instruments

A 27 gauge membrane spatula with side bevel (DORC and ASICO, Westmont, IL) was developed to separate proliferative membranes from the retinal surface and to create a posterior vitreous separation from the retinal surface at the disk margin during diabetic vitrectomy or macular hole surgery. A 27 gauge curved endophotocoagulation probe (DORC and Synergetics Inc.) with a 200 µm inner laser fiber can be used for one-step entry. A 27 gauge trocar-cannula system (DORC and MANI Inc. Tochigi, Japan) consisting of a 27 gauge steel or polyamide cannula and a microvitreoretinal blade trocar for better one-step entry. Although this trocar-cannula system is unnecessary for every 27 gauge vitrectomy, it is helpful to avoid missing the 27 gauge entry site for instrument insertion in complex cases sometimes requiring frequent instrument exchanges during surgery. A 27 gauge diathermy was also developed by DORC for 27 gauge diabetic vitrectomy.

Surgical Techniques, Indications and Limitations of Current 27 Gauge System

The most distinguished characteristic of 27 gauge system superior to the larger gauge MIVS systems is the simplicity for creating rigid self-sealing wounds. As expected, the size of 27 gauge (0.4 mm) is ideal and easy for wound self-sealing. Procedures for 27 gauge system seem to be much easier than those of current 23 or 25 gauge system because no special techniques are necessary. The sclerotomies created by a one-step perpendicular insertion of the 27 gauge trocar-cannula can be self-sealed after simple removal of the 27 gauge cannula at the end of surgery. The rigidity of 27 gauge vitrectomy cutter, one of the major concern about 27 gauge instrument, has been improved stiff enough by

TABLE 7.2: Current indications for 27 gauge vitrectomy

• Macular diseases
— Epiretinal membrane proliferation
— Idiopathic or secondary macular hole
— Macular traction syndrome
— Macular edema associated with
– diabetic retinopathy
– retinal vein occlusion
– uveitis
— Persistent pseudophakic cystoid macular edema
— Subinternal limiting membrane hemorrhage
• Simple vitreous hemorrhage
• Vitreous biopsy
• Primary rhegmatogenous retinal detachment
• Moderate proliferative diabetic retinopathy with or without focal tractional retinal detachment

shortening the shaft length to 25 mm. The length of 25 mm is enough to reach the posterior retina if the axial length of the operated eye is under 28 mm. This means the current 27 gauge system can be used for most cases except high myopic cases with longer axial length at present. Current indications for transconjunctival 27 gauge vitrectomy are listed in Table 7.2. Similar to the early years of the introduction of 25 gauge system, the primary indications for 27 gauge system may be macular diseases and simple vitreous hemorrhage and more recently it is feasible for treating primary retinal detachment and moderately severe diabetic cases.

Currently, all intraocular manipulations can be performed with 27 gauge instruments and the procedures are simple and similar to those with conventional 23 gauge or 25 gauge system. Posterior vitreous separation from the retina can be simply created by a gentle suction with 27 gauge vitrectomy probe (Figures 7.8A to D). Otherwise, a 27 gauge membrane pick (available form DORC or ASCICO) was used for separating the vitreous membrane strongly adherent to the retina for example in cases with asteroid hyalosis. Not only the epiretinal membrane but also the internal limiting membrane can be clearly observed with the 27 gauge endoillumination and easily peeled by use of a 27 gauge microforceps, the shaft of which has been refined rigid enough to grasp both tough and fragile membrane tissues. Some surgeons may argue the fragility of 27 gauge cutter for peripheral vitreous shaving. However, peripheral vitreous shaving is feasible to accomplish either by the conventional method with scleral depression (Figures 7.9A to F) or by the use of wide-angle system without scleral depression. As most surgeons acknowledged, vitrectomy under the wide-angle viewing will have less chance to move the eye ball to see the peripheral regions, a 27 gauge peripheral vitrectomy will

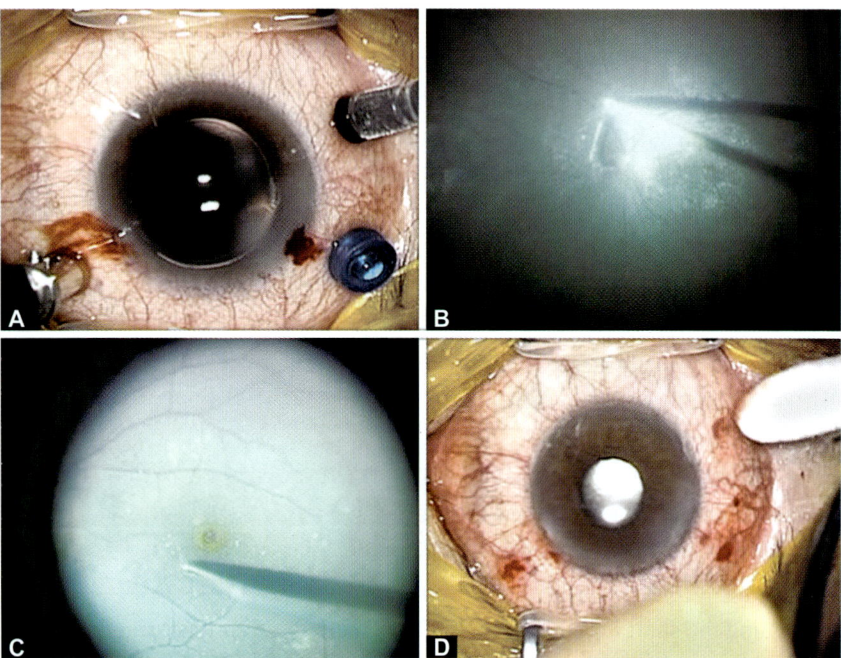

Figs 7.8A to D: (A) Standard setting for 27 gauge macular hole surgery. Only one port set by a trocar-cannula system for instrument exchanges. The other two ports were set by one-step entry instruments (sharp-tipped infusion line and 27/29 gauge one-step chandelier optic fiber); (B) Suction from the 27 gauge vitreous cutter is sufficient to create a posterior vitreous membrane separation from the retina. The Weiss ring can be well visualized by intravitreal injection of triamcinolone acetonide; (C) Internal limiting membrane (arrowheads) was carefully peeled by use of 27 gauge Eckardt type end-gripping microforceps; (D) At the end of surgery, the sclerotomies can easily and completely self-seal by simple removal of the 27 gauge instruments

practically be more comfortable and surgeons may almost feel no differences in fragility between the 27 gauge and other larger gauges if the wide-angle viewing system was used.

Several previous literature have reported the efficacy of using small gauge instruments for diabetic vitrectomy, we have found the 27 gauge vitrectomy system may be equal to or somewhat more advantageous to the current small gauge (23 or 25 gauge) for diabetic vitrectomy. Because of its small size, the 27 gauge cutter can play several roles concurrently during surgery (i.e. as a cutter, aspirator, peeling forceps, and membrane scissors). In eyes with diabetic traction retinal detachment, bimanual techniques simply using a forceps and a cutter is also very useful with 27 gauge system (Figures 7.10A to D). The much smaller blunt tip of the 27 gauge cutter probe can be much easier to insert into the spaces between the detached retina and the adherent fibrovascular membrane. The fibrovascular tissues were cut and removed using the 27 gauge cutter instead of the conventional use of scissors. Even if the fibrovascular membranes were extensively and strongly adherent to the detached retina,

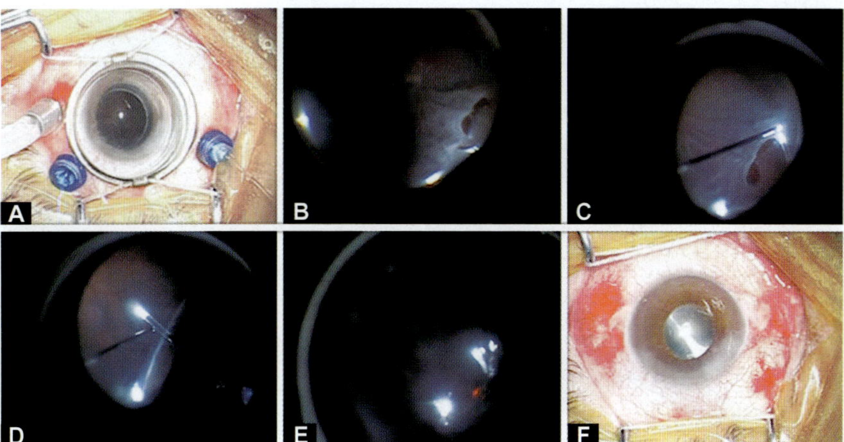

Figs 7.9A to F: (A) Standard 27 gauge vitrectomy setting for primary rhegmatigenous retinal detachment. A 27 gauge twin-light chanderlier was used with one optic fiber passing through the closure valve attached cannula; (B) Panoramic fundus view under the 27 gauge twin-light chandelier endoillumination with xenon light source; (C) The retinal break and vitreous traction were clearly visualized under the chandelier illumination. The shaft of the 27 gauge cutter is rigid enough for peripheral vitreous shaving; (D) Combined with scleral depression technique, the vitreous shaving can be performed reaching to the ora serrata as usual even by the 27 gauge cutter; (E) A 27 gauge endo-laser photocoagulation was applied around the retinal breaks following fluid-air exchange; (F) At the end of surgery, all sclerotomies completely self-sealed by simple removal of the 27 gauge instruments despite extensive peripheral vitreous shaving performed

membrane separation and dissection from the retina can be performed using a membrane spatula. The less chance for instrument exchanges and less chance to encounter iatrogenic breaks with blunt-tipped instruments may facilitate time-saving surgery even in these challenging cases. The only drawback of the current 27 gauge system is the lower cutting performance. Therefore, it will no doubt take much longer time for treating the cases requiring extensive vitrectomy such as retinal detachment vitrectomy surgery. However, the smaller port area of the 27 gauge cutter combined with high-speed cutting is very beneficial to avoid creating inadvertent retinal breaks during the peripheral vitreous shaving. This may be helpful contributing to lower the intraoperative complication and lower vitreous incarceration with less traction to the retina.

CLINICAL EXPERIENCES WITH 27 GAUGE SYSTEM

Based on our clinical experiences over 100 cases with the 27 gauge system, this system is no doubt feasible to supersede the current 25 and 23 gauge systems at least for treating macular diseases and simple vitreous hemorrhage. More recently, we have extended the indication to primary rhegmatogenous retinal detachment and moderately severe proliferative diabetic retinopathy and obtained overall favorable surgical outcomes as well. We did neither experienced any eyes required conversion to larger-gauge instrumentation

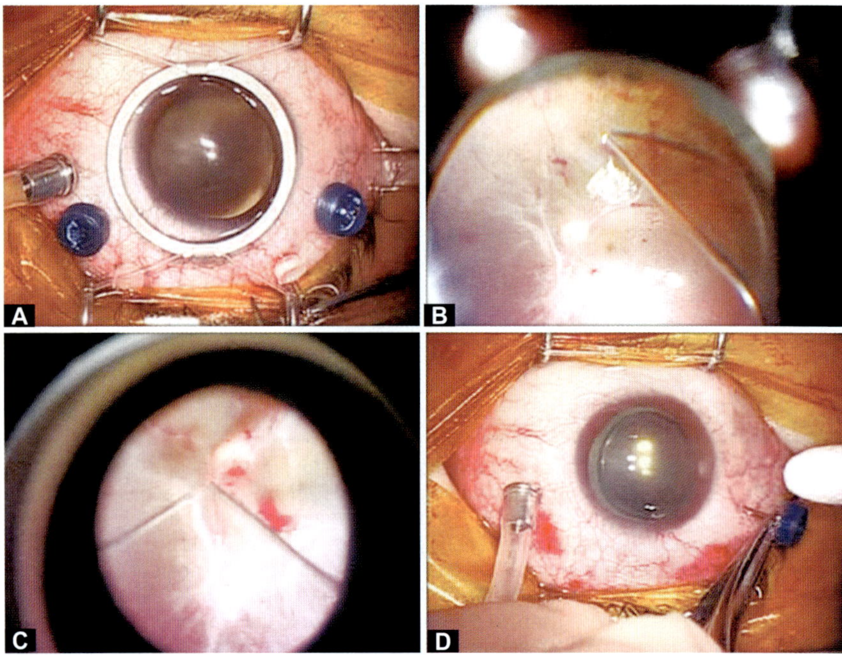

Figs 7.10A to D: (A) Standard setting of 27 gauge vitrectomy for treating diabetic traction retinal detachment. An one-step entry infusion line and two closure valve attached cannulas were set for bimanual intraocular manipulation. The 27 gauge twin-light chandelier fibers were transconjunctivally inserted passing through the sclera at 1 and 11 o'clock after a pre-incision using a 27 gauge guidance needle; (B) Panoramic fundus view under the 27 gauge chandelier endoillumination with xenon light source. Sufficient illumination and wide-angle view of the fundus are obtained for peripheral vitrectomy by 27 gauge vitreous cutter; (C) Bimanual technique with 27 gauge instruments for fibro vascular membrane dissection; (D) Less subconjunctival bleeding and scaring and well-preserved conjunctiva can be obtained with perfect would self-sealing in 27 gauge vitrectomy system. This may provide advantages for diabetic vitrectomy because repeated surgeries and/or subsequent filtering surgery may required for these patients

during surgery nor any eyes having serious intra or postoperative complications attributed to 27 gauge system during follow-up. The 27 gauge vitrectomy can begin immediately after simply creation of sclerotomies at the pars plana by one-step vertical insertion, complex techniques for creating a self-sealing wound, such as angled-insertion technique or two-step entry method, are no longer required. In addition, a 27 gauge trocar-cannula system is available but not necessary for all cases such as simple vitreous biopsy because the small gauge eliminates concerns about extensive vitreous incarceration in the small sclerotomy. Using the 27 gauge system, opening and closing procedures can be simplified, and this may contribute to saving total operating time with this system. In addition, because of the small size and multifunctionalities of the 27 gauge cutter, reducing the use of various instruments for manipulation in complex cases will eliminate time wasted in instrument exchanges and, as a result, also contribute to saving total operating time. After simple removal of all instruments, surgery can be closed at once and all sclerotomies self-sealed completely without the need for suturing in any cases, even in the case with thin sclera or after extensive peripheral vitreous shaving or multiple surgeries. Surgeons will no longer need for caring about the wound-sealing related complications if 27 gauge system is used.

FUTURE PESPECTIVE

Minimally invasive vitrectomy surgery is another abbreviation of "MIVS." The final goal of transconjunctival surgery would be to achieve perfect self-sealing wounds with stable postoperative IOP from one day after surgery, tiny changes on the ocular surface with limited subconjunctival hemorrhage and scar, acceptable operating time with minimal intra and postoperative complications, favorable anatomic success and early visual rehabilitation. The 27 gauge system may have one-step advanced (OR: near) to this final goal as compared with current 23 and 25 gauge system. Although the development of 27 gauge vitrectomy is still an ongoing project and has not yet been established as a widely accepted system, the feasibility and safety of 27 gauge vitrectomy in selected cases have been demonstrated and confirmed. Highly efficient 27 gauge cutters may not be just a dream. New generation machines no longer use spring coil cutters but a dual-actuation technology that allows for ultra-high cutting rate with duty cycle control. If this technology was applied to 27 gauge, we would be able to achieve a much higher performance. Similar to the recent evolution in 23 and 25 gauge systems, further development and refinement of the 27 gauge instruments' functionality is underway and will continue over the coming years allowing us to establish this system as an ultra-minimally invasive surgery for the full spectrum of vitreoretinal pathologies in the future.

REFERENCES

1. Fujii GY, De Juan E Jr, Humayun MS, et al. A new 25 gauge instrument system for transconjunctival sutureless vitrectomy surgery. Ophthalmol. 2002;109:1807–12.
2. Lakhanpal RR, Humayun MS, de Juan E Jr, et al. Outcomes of 140 consecutive cases of 25 gauge transconjunctival surgery for posterior disease. Ophthalmol. 2005;112:817–24.
3. Ibarra MS, Hermel M, Prenner JL, Hassan TS. Longer term outcomes of transconjunctival sutureless 25 gauge vitrectomy. Am J Ophthalmol. 2005;139:831–36.
4. Eckardt C. Transconjunctival sutureless 23 gauge vitrectomy. Retina. 2005;25:208–11.
5. Fine HF, Iranmanesh R, Iturralde D, Spaide RF. Outcomes of 77 consecutive cases of 23 gauge transconjunctival vitrectomy surgery for posterior segment disease. Ophthalmol. 2007;114:1197–200.
6. Rizzo S, Genovesi-Ebert F, Vento A, et al. Modified incision in 25 gauge vitrectomy in the creation of a tunneled airtight sclerotomy: An ultrabiomicroscopic study. Graefes Arch Clin Exp Ophthalmol. 2007;245:1281–8.

7. Oshima Y, Awh CC, Tano Y. Self-retaining 27 gauge transconjunctival chandelier endoillumination for panoramic viewing during vitreous surgery. Am J Ophthalmol. 2007;143:166–7.
8. Oshima Y, Chow DR, Awh CC, et al. Novel mercury vapor illuminator combined with a 27/29 gauge chandelier light fiber for vitreous surgery. Retina. 2008;28:171–3.
9. Eckardt C, Eckert T, Eckardt U. 27 gauge Twinlight chandelier illumination system for bimanual transconjunctival vitrectomy. Retina. 2008;28:518–9.
10. Oshima Y, Wakabayashi T, Sato T, Ohji M, Tano Y. A 27 gauge instrument system for transconjunctival sutureless microincision vitrectomy surgery. Ophthalmol. 2010;117:93–102.
11. Sakaguchi H, Oshima Y, Tano Y. 27 gauge transconjunctival nonvitrectomizing vitreous surgery for epiretinal membrane removal. Retina. 2007;27:1131–2.

CHAPTER

8

MIVS in Macular Hole

SN Jha

INTRODUCTION

Macular Hole represents a full thickness defect or dehiscence in the central retina at the umbo.[1] By definition, it is a tear or defect of foveal retina involving its full thickness from internal limiting membrane to outer segment of photoreceptor layer. Lamellar holes involve only a portion of the retinal layers.

With the better understanding of this disease pathogenesis and improvement in vitreoretinal surgical technique and instrumentation, excellent visual outcomes can be achieved. The prevalence rate of macular hole in India has been found to be 0.17%.[2]

CLINICAL FEATURES AND WORK UP

The disease affects women more often than men and usually it occurs in the seventh decade. The reported ratio is 2–3: 1.[3,4]

Risk of fellow eye getting affected with macular hole is from 3–29%.[5]

Patients with smaller macular hole may have no symptoms and are diagnosed on routine ophthalmoscopic evaluation. If they do have symptoms, they usually complain of blurred vision and metamorphopsia. Those with larger holes will complain of scotoma or a defect in central vision and metamorphopsia.

SIGNS

Visual acuity of the affected eye may vary according to the size, duration, location and associated subretinal cuff of fluid. In smaller holes it may vary from 20/25–20/40 while in larger holes it may be 20/80 to 20/400.

Patient can be given Amsler Grid in which, they appreciate bending/ waviness of lines and scotomas.

On direct ophthalmoscopy, macular hole can be seen as well-defined excavation at the macula and choroidal reflex can be seen through it. In some cases, few yellowish deposits can be seen at the base of the hole suggestive of lipofuscin-laden macrophages.

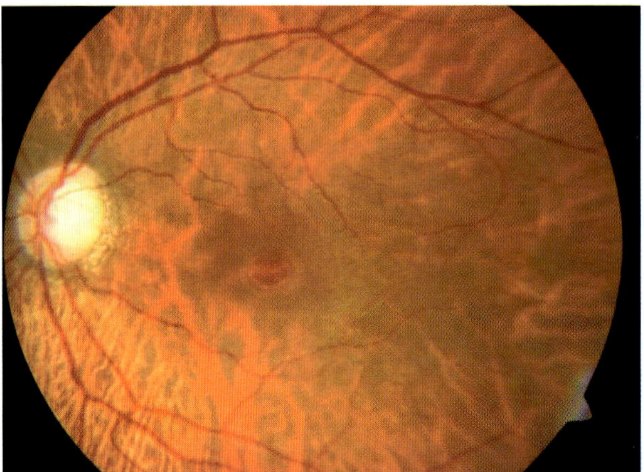

Fig. 8.1: Full thickness macular hole

Slit lamp biomicroscopy will also reveals same findings. Additionally, surrounding subretinal fluid can be appreciated, if present.

The Watzke-Allen test can be performed on slit lamp. Herein, a thin narrow vertical beam of light is projected onto the macula with a contact lens in place and the patient is asked to observe the light carefully and is asked to draw it on a paper later. In a full thickness macular hole, the line drawn is broken. Narrowing or thinning is suggestive of small macular hole, partial thickness macular hole or other differential diagnosis. A simple test using Maddox rod also reveals broken line suggestive of full thickness macular hole.

The laser aiming beam test also is performed similarly, but this time a small 50 µm spot size laser-aiming beam is placed within the lesion. A positive test is obtained when the patient fails to detect the aiming beam when it is placed within the lesion but is able to detect it once it is placed onto normal retina. This test is useful in detection of small macular hole where Watzke-Allen sign is negative.

INVESTIGATIONS

Fundus Fluorescein Angiography (FFA)

Fluorescein angiography of fundus reveals window defect at the area of macular hole (Figure 8.2).

Optical Coherence Tomography

Optical coherence tomography (OCT) has made a great impact on the diagnosis, management and follow-up of macular pathologies, in particular macular holes. Figure 8.3 shows a typical macular hole, with attached hyaloid and cystoid spaces.

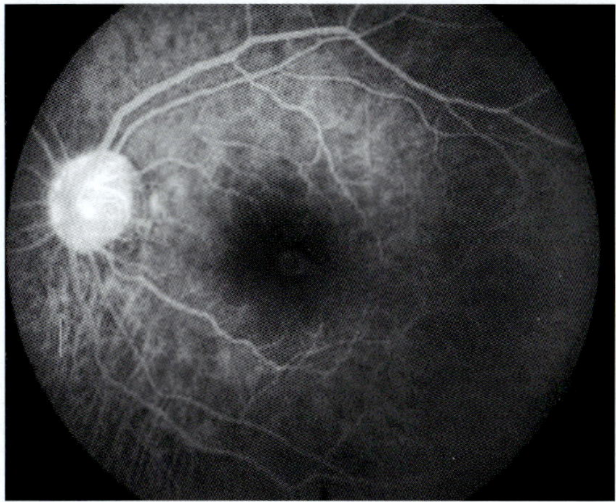

Fig. 8.2: Late AV phase of FFA showing window defect

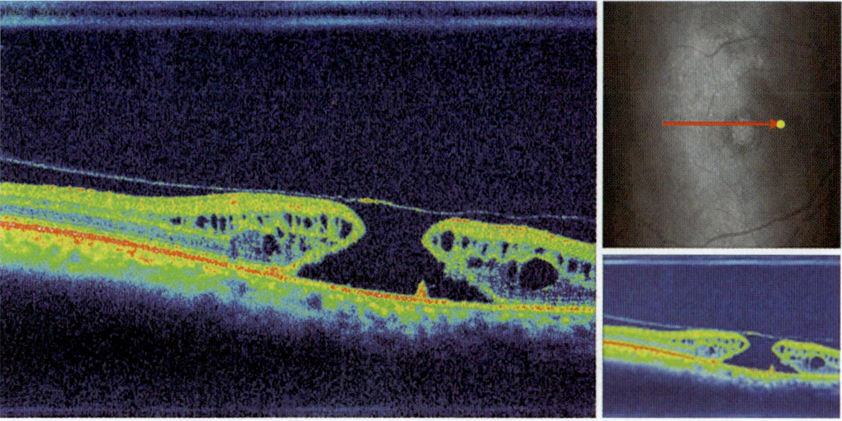

Fig. 8.3: Stage III—Full thickness macular hole without PVD
(*Courtesy:* Dr RK Akhaury and Dr Ranjana Kumar)

NATURAL HISTORY

Up to 50% of the stage 1 holes close spontaneously while others may progress to become larger sized holes. Most stage 2 and above macular holes will have increase in size to become larger stage 3 macular holes. This progression takes weeks to months to occur. Some stage 2 holes remain stable for years without progression. Some of these eyes have vitreous opacity in front of fovea and present as central scotoma.[6]

TYPES OF MACULAR HOLE

Primary—No known cause, hence called idiopathic.

Secondary—Associated with risk factors are as follows:

1. Trauma
2. Proliferative diabetic retinopathy
3. Severe hypertensive retinopathy

4. Optic disk coloboma
5. CNVM
6. CME
7. Macular pucker
8. Lightening
9. Electrocution, welding
10. Retinal detachment
11. Accidental Nd-YAG laser
12. Vitrectomy of ERM.

PATHOGENESIS

The pathogenesis is incompletely understood.[7,8] A number of theories have been put forward to explain the pathogenesis.

Knapp 1869 Macular hole due to ocular trauma
Noyes 1871 Full thickness defect in retinal tissue due to trauma
Fuchs and Coats 1901,1907 Cystoid degeneration
Lister 1924 Anteroposterior traction
Morgan and Schatz 1986 Involutional thinning and vascular theory
Gass 1995 Tangential traction forces
Tornambe 2003 Hydration theory

The major milestone in understanding of pathogenesis of macular hole was classification by Gass.[1,9,10]

Gass argued that other theories could not explain the biomicroscopic changes that are evident in eyes with macular hole. This includes development of foveolar spot and loss of foveolar depression. According to Gass points against anteroposterior traction were absence of foveolar–retinal tenting, rarity of macular tears with flaps and infrequency of posterior vitreous detachment after macular hole formation. Chronic low-grade traction due to ocular rotation stimulates cellular proliferation of Müller cells, astrocytes and retinal pigment epithelium realigning vitreous fibers and redirecting the tractional force in tangential direction.[11]

STAGES OF DEVELOPMENT OF SENILE MACULAR HOLE BY GASS[9]

Stage I	Ia (yellow spot): Shallow foveolar detachment. It measures 100–200 micron
	Ib (yellow ring): Perifoveolar vitreous contraction. It leads to foveal detachment
Stage II	FTMH noted clinically with defect < 400 micron
Stage III	FTMH>400 micron with surrounding cuff of edema with or without pseudo-operculum
Stage IV	FTMH>400 micron with anterior displacement of pseudo-operculum and complete PVD
FTMH	Full thickness macular hole
PVD	Posterior vitreous detachment

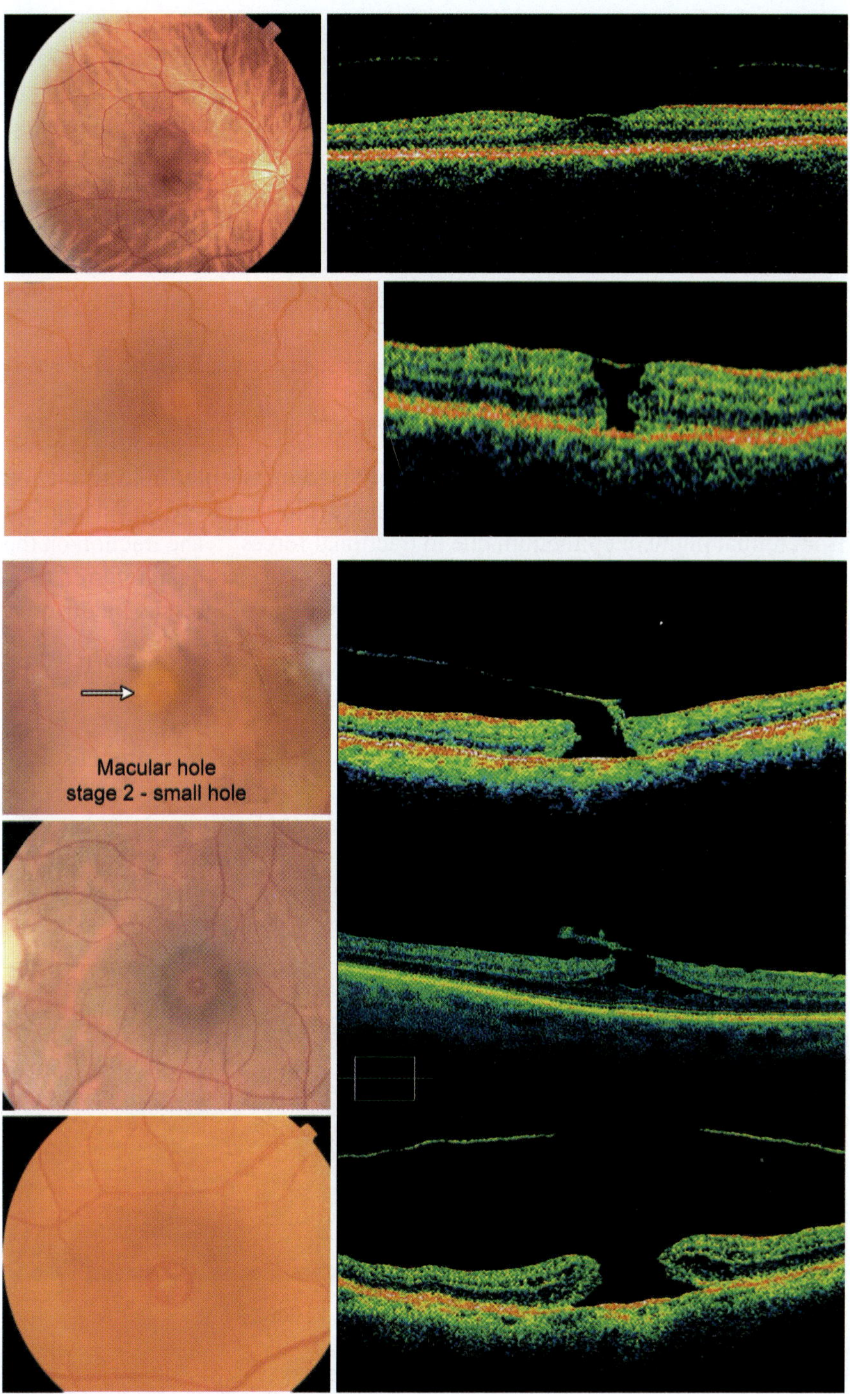

Fig. 8.4: OCT based classification
(*Courtesy:* Online Journal of Ophthalmology and e-ophthalmology)

The advent of Optical Coherence Tomography has helped to further elaborate the stages of macular hole formation. Ezra published an OCT documented study suggesting that failure of normal age-related separation of cortical vitreous from posterior pole as a result of an abnormally tenacious attachment to the fovea leads to macular hole formation.[12]

Stage I A	Cystic space in the inner part of fovea
B	Cystic space in both inner and outer parts of fovea with perifoveal vitreous detachment but a persistent attachment at the fovea
Stage II	Full thickness hole due to dehiscence in the foveal psuedocyst. The hyaloid is attached to the fovea
Stage III	Hyaloid has separated from the fovea, pseudo-operculum is seen suspended on posterior hyaloid
Stage IV	Complete posterior vitreous detachment

With the latest spectral OCT the initial stage of macular hole formation starts as a triangular elevation of outer photoreceptor layer and its detachment from retinal pigment epithelium due to tractional forces.[13] The traction on the fovea occurring prior to anatomic changes to the fovea has been referred to as Stage 0. This clinical appearance may resolve without progression in 40–50% of patients.

OCT BASED PROGNOSIS

A factor called hole form factor (HFF) is calculated on OCT to prognosticate the behavior of hole after surgery. It is defined as the ratio of the sum of the lengths of the two sides of macular hole to the base diameter. HFF between 0.9–1 has been correlated with better anatomical outcome and greater improvement in visual acuity after ILM peeling in macular hole surgery whereas HFF less than 0.5 is found to have poor prognosis (Figure 8.5).[14]

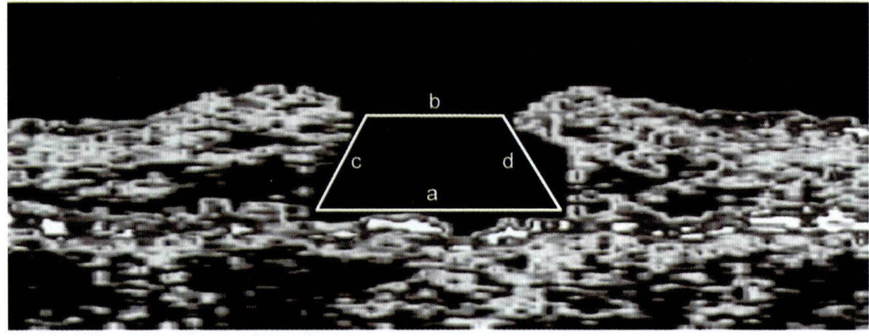

Fig. 8.5: Hole Form Factor BJO 2002

$$\text{Hole Form Factor (HFF)} = \frac{c + d}{a}$$

a = base diameter
b = minimum diameter
c = left arm length
d = right arm length

Differential Diagnosis

A true macular hole can clinically be described as a round, well defined, punched out lesion, reddish in color, surrounded by a cuff of subretinal fluid due to a neurosensory detachment with yellow deposits in the crater. Gass first described lamellar macular hole in 1975 as macular lesion that resulted from cystoid macular edema.[15] This term describes an abortive process in full thickness macular hole formation. The varied presentation of lamellar macular defect may mimic a macular hole. OCT provides insight into the underlying etiology and pathogenesis of vitreomacular interface abnormality including macular hole, lamellar hole, macular pseudohole, epiretinal membrane and vitreomacular traction. Only 28% of lamellar holes diagnosed on OCT examination were detected clinically on fundus examination.[16] Therefore, OCT is an important diagnostic tool, which also helps in classification of different subtypes of lamellar macular defects.

Lamellar macular defects were categorised into three different subtypes based on their OCT appearance: Lamellar macular holes (LMH), macular pseudoholes (MPH), and foveal pseudocysts (FP).[17]

OCT studies have also demonstrated that lamellar holes have thin fovea resulting from avulsion of inner layer of macula. The ultra high resolution OCT based criteria for diagnosis of lamellar macular hole is as follows:[18]

1. An irregular foveal contour
2. A break in the inner fovea
3. Separation of the inner from the outer foveal retinal layers, leading to an intraretinal split
4. Absence of a full thickness foveal defect with intact photoreceptors posterior to the area of foveal dehiscence.

A macular pseudohole is said to result from the centripetal contraction of an ERM that subsequently leads to verticalization of the foveal slopes and a sharply punched out defect.[19]

Foveal pseudocyst is described as a precursor to macular hole or lamellar macular hole formation due to direct vitreomacular traction.[16] ERM can also result in avulsion forces leading to the formation of pseudocyst which can progress to a lamellar macular defect due to deroofing.[20]

Various parameters as measured by OCT: Base diameter, defect depth, central foveal thickness and perifoveal thickness has helped to prognosticate the subtypes of lamellar macular hole. It has been found that macular pseudoholes have smaller diameter and thicker central foveal tissue, therefore, they have better visual acuity than LMH and FP whereas both LMH and FP are shown to have deeper and wider intraretinal split and also thin central foveal tissue.[17]

Although the visual prognosis for patients with a lamellar hole is known to be excellent,[21] some patients have poor visual acuity. Vitrectomy with gas tamponade (SF6) may be an effective method for a lamellar macular hole with poor visual acuity[22] and OCT showed an anatomical restoration of the fovea without intraretinal split.

MACULAR HOLE SURGERY

Full thickness macular hole were once considered untreatable and surgery was indicated once extensive retinal detachment occurred.[23, 24] Then came the era of prophylactic surgery wherein pars plana vitrectomy (PPV) was suggested for patients with impending macular hole to release the tangential forces. PPV alone was found to prevent macular hole development in 80% of in patients who were at risk of developing FTMH. In 1991, Kelly and Wendel[25] first demonstrated a surgical procedure to close idiopathic macular hole that was accompanied by improvement in visual acuity. With the advances in vitreoretinal surgical techniques focus on prophylactic therapies to prevent macular hole formation became less important.

Without surgery macular hole development leads to loss of central vision that stabilizes at 20/200 to 20/400 level.[26] But peripheral vision is maintained.

Macular hole surgery continues to undergo evolution. Therefore, the indication of surgery currently stands as follows; full thickness macular hole with stage II and above (i.e. III and IV) have to be treated. Patients with stage III and IV have moderate to large holes with visual acuity of 6/18 or below (20/60 to 20/400) following surgery, these patients readily gain two or more line improvement after surgery. The benefit to risk ratio is lower with early stages. Stage II macular holes are small and the visual acuity ranges from 6/12 to 6/18 (20/40–20/60). These eyes also present with shorter duration of symptoms. These patients will have better preoperative visual acuity and end up with better postoperative visual acuity. An unsuccessful surgery may result in larger hole size and thus worse postoperative visual acuity. FTMH with visual acuity of > 6/12 presenting with minimum symptoms such as metamorphopsia and smaller hole size rarely requires surgery. Spontaneous closure of macular hole is known though rare. Freeman et al[27] observed spontaneous regression in 4% of all cases. Therefore, these patients can be followed-up.

A standard treatment involves 3 port pars plana vitrectomy, removal of cortical vitreous, removal of epiretinal membrane (ERM) with or without ILM peeling, filling of gas for endotamponade and face down position for variable duration. Adjuncts were once used to improve surgical closure. These included TGF–B, autologous platelet concentrate, bovine thrombus.[28] Photocoagulation was also tried.[29] Improved surgical rate were possible without them so these methods were discontinued.

SURGICAL TECHNIQUE

Conventional pars plana vitrectomy technique includes a three-port system; separate continuous infusion cannula, fiberoptics endoilluminator light probe and vitrectomy cutting probe. Earlier, 20 gauge system and currently 25 gauge and 23 gauge systems have been employed and shown good results.[30]

After the removal of central vitreous, posterior cortical vitreous must be identified and separated. In stage IV FTMH a PVD is already present and can be identified by the presence of Weiss ring. If there is no posterior vitreous seperation then it can be identified using a soft tipped silicone suction cannula. The cannula can be lightly applied close to the retinal surface and when there is occlusion of its orifice by cortical vitreous, the cannula flexes. This has been called as "fish strike sign' or "divining rod sign".

The cortical vitreous can also be visualized with the help of staining with dye such as ICG, trypan blue and more commonly triamcinolone, its particles adhere to the cortical vitreous. One to two drops of triamcinolone acetonide aqueous suspension (40 mg/mL) can be injected with the help of 20 to 25 gauge cannula into the midvitreous. The creation of posterior vitreous detachment can also be conducted with vitrectomy probe with active aspiration and a vacuum of 200-300 mm Hg keeping the probe nasal to the disk. Bottle height should be raised to maintain high IOP and prevent collapsing of globe. Once the PVD is visualized as a floating membrane, vitrectomy is then completed. With the help of the latest wide-angle system the periphery must be screened for iatrogenic retinal breaks. The incidence of retinal break formation during macular hole surgery is 5.5%[31] after PVD induction. At this point of surgery epiretinal membrane can be removed alone or along with ILM peeling. To stain ERM and ILM various dyes can be used. There are many studies with ICG. It is available as 25 mg powder and reconstituted with sterile water for injection to make it 0.5% or 0.25 %. It is injected into midvitreous and kept for 1 min. It should be consumed within 10 hours. Studies have shown safety [32] and toxicity with ICG.[33] Clinical reports have attributed complications like RPE damage, optic nerve atrophy or visual field defects.[33,34] Novel dyes like brilliant blue (0.25 mg/mL) have been found to be safe.[35] This dye can be used in fluid filled eye. Studies have reported excellent hole closure rate even without use of any dye.[36] But use of dyes lowers the risk of inadvertent trauma to the retina.

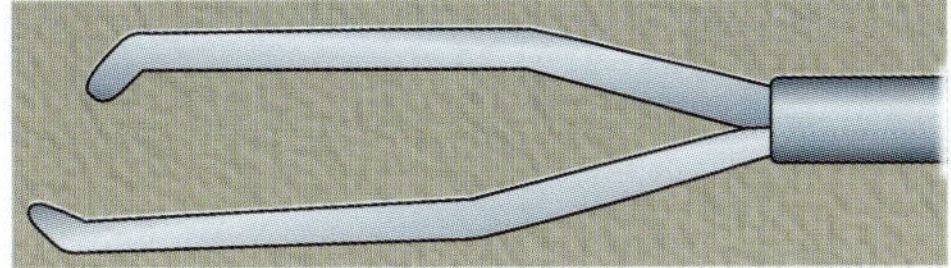

Fig. 8.6: ILM peeling forceps

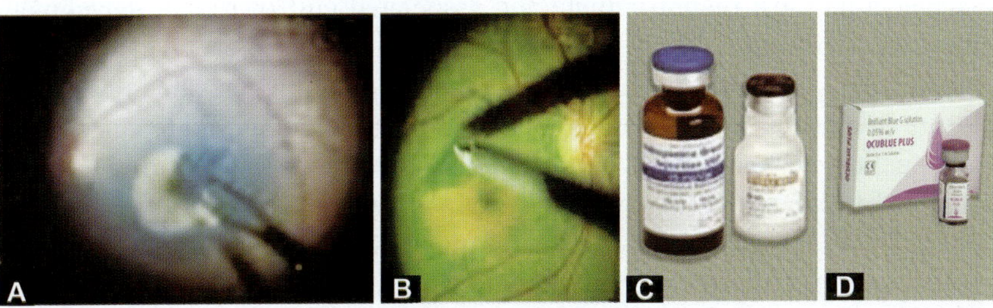

Figs 8.7A to D: (A) ILM peeling with brilliant blue; (B) ILM peeling with ICG; (C) ICG vial; (D) Brilliant Blue vial

The ILM is subsequently peeled in a circular fashion about one disk diameter away from hole and within the temporal arcade. Extra fine forceps, the ILM peeling forceps now available in 23 gauge and 25 gauge systems are helpful. One useful tip about lifting of ILM is by silicone tipped cannula that is convenient and less traumatic. Air fluid exchange is then performed. Fluid is removed just anterior to the optic nerve with passive aspiration. Drainage through the macular hole should be avoided.

MIVS AND CHANGING PARADIGM IN MACULAR HOLE SURGERY

The maximum impact that MIVS has in vitreous surgery is on macular hole surgery due to straight line approach without any digression.The handicap quoted for MIVS in other indications do not apply for macular hole though with new generation vitreous surgery machines and xenon light source, handicap hardly exists. MIVS cuts down morbidity and with 25 gauge the eye is as quiet as topical phacoemulsification for cataract. With 23 and 25 gauge systems tunnelled sclerotomies are shown to be air tight in UBM studies.[37] Transconjunctival sutureless vitrectomy have benefits of halving the surgical time with minimum trauma to the eye.[38] Only problem about instrumentation has been taken care of by availability of disposable instruments. It is way better than the maintainence of costly reusable forceps.

Surgical Objective of Macular Hole Surgery

Surgical objective of macular hole surgery is two-fold. First surgery intends to relieve tractional forces; second it activates reparative healing mechanism.[39, 40] Several studies have suggested that removal of internal limiting membrane is a useful adjunct for patients undergoing macular hole repair. The internal limiting membrane peeling removes the template upon which the glial cells proliferates and contracts and thus enlarges the macular hole. Peeling removes the tangential traction. Removal of ILM injures the muller cell footplates and trigger reparative gliosis. ILM peeling serves to increase macular hole edge mobility and reduce macular hole diameter.[40] The future of closure of MH also depends on chorioretinal adhesion between the edges of neurosensory retina and between the retina and retinal pigment epithelium.[41] The edges of macular hole must reapproximate and associated cuff of retinal detachment must reattach[42] and also if cystoid macular edema is present then it must reabsorb.[43] Additionally, ILM peeling has shown higher rate of primary closure of macular hole as compared with eyes undergoing MH repair without ILM peeling, 92% and 82% respectively.[44] Late reopening of hole was also found to be higher in no ILM peeling group when compared with ILM peeling group (7% vs 0.6%).[44] ILM peeling eliminates all tractional forces and ERM can be meticulously removed along with ILM peeling.

POSTOPERATIVE POSTURING

Face down posturing is thought to aid hole closure by allowing the buoyant force of intraocular gas bubble, which is maximal at the apex of the bubble to be in contact with the macula.[45] The gas bubble keeps the edges of macular hole dry and prevents entry of vitreous into the hole and provides scaffold for glial cell proliferation.[43,46] Also surface tension is constant around the bubble's interface with the retina so as long as volume of intraocular gas is sufficient, i.e. 2/3rd to 3/4th of vitreous cavity.[47]

The greatest perioperative morbidity associated with macular hole surgery is strict postoperative face down positioning (FDP) for at least a week.[25] Few studies recommend posturing as long as 4 weeks.[48]

There is still controversy as to whether face down positioning following macular hole is necessary or not. Peeling of ILM removes all tangential force, therefore, patients should not need FDP. The successful report of Tornamby Pilot study[49] wherein all patients had membrane peeling and nil FDP supports the approach avoiding FDP. Various other studies favor no FDP or a minimum of one day FDP[50] and show 90% anatomical and 95% functional success rate.[49]

Posturing is essential to the success of the procedure is controversial. Another question that follows is what is the optimal duration to keep the macula dry and to allow the healing to occur? The optical coherence tomography studies have demonstrated that retinal flattening, reabsorption of fluid from the intraretinal cysts and reapproximation of retinal dehiscence can occur as early as first postoperative day.[51]

Endotamponading Agents

In original description of macular hole surgery, use of nonexpansible gas of SF6 with 1 week FDP was indicated.[25] The long-term tamponade with silicone oil has also been suggested but its removal requires another surgery. Persisting macular hole after reoperation with silicone is also high. Anatomical closure is found to be only 65% as compared with C3F8 gas 91%.[52] C3F8 and densiron 68[53] share advantage of having longer effect and both do not require positioning. Densiron 68 is a mixture of silicone oil and amphiphilic perfluorohexyloctane, which facilitates better contact with the retina compared with standard silicone oil. Vitrectomy and air tamponade combined with 1 to 3 day face down positioning produced an excellent rate of macular hole closure.[54]

With the use of gas there are more chances of early cataract formation. The cataract progression following macular hole surgery is found to be 64% within first year. Therefore, these days it is advocated to undergo combined macular hole and cataract surgery. Lens extraction also allows a more complete vitrectomy.[55]

REFERENCES

1. Gass JD. Reappraisal of biomicroscopic classification of stages of development of a macular hole. Am J Opthalmol. 1995;119:752–9.
2. Sen P, Bhargava A, Vijaya L, George R. Prevalence of idiopathic macular hole in adult rural and urban south Indian population. Clin Experiment Ophthalmol. 2008;36:257–60.
3. Aaberg TM. Macular holes: A review. Surv Ophthalmol. 1970;15:139–62
4. Aaberg TM, Blair CJ, Gass JD. Macular holes. AM J Ophthalmol. 1970; 69:555–62.
5. Bronstein MA, Trempe CL, Freeman HM. Fellow of eyes with macular holes. Am J Ophthalmol. 1981;92:757–61.
6. Gass JD, Van Newkirk M. Xanthic scotoma and yellow foveolar shadow caused by a pseudooperculum after vitreofoveolar separation. Retina. 1992;12:242–44.
7. Watzke RC. Atypical presentations of macular holes. Arch Ophthalmol. 1994;112:446.
8. Kakehashi A, Schepens CL, Trempe CL. Vitreomacular observations. II. Data on the pathogenesis of idiopathic macular breaks. Graefes Arch Clin Exp Ophthalmol. 1996;234:425–33.
9. Gass JD. Idiopathic senile macular holes: Its early stages and pathogenesis. Arch Ophthalmol. 1988;106:629–39.
10. Johnson RN, Gass JD. Idiopathic macular holes: observations, stages of formation, and implications for surgical intervention. Ophthalmol. 1998;95:917–24.
11. Green WR. The macular hole. Histopathological studies. Arch Ophthalmol. 2006;124:317–21.
12. Ezra E. Idiopathic full thickness macular hole: Natural history and pathogenesis. Br J Ophthalmol. 2001;85:102–9.
13. Zofia Michalewska, Janusz Michalewski, et al. A study of macular hole formation by serial spectral optical coherence tomography. Clinical and Experimental Ophthalmol. 2009;37:373–83.
14. Ullrich S, Haritoglou C, et al. Macular hole size as a prognostic factor in macular hole surgery. Br J Ophthalmol. 2002;86:390–3.
15. Gass JD. Lamellar macular hole: A complication of cystoid macular edema after cataract extraction: A clinicopathologic case report. Trans. Am Opthalmol Soc. 1975;73:230–50.
16. Haouchine B, Massin P, Gaudric A. Foveal pseudocyst as the first step in macular hole formation: A prospective study by optical coherence tomography. Ophthalmol. 2001;108:15–22.
17. Chen JC, Lee LR. Clinical spectrum of lamellar macular defects including pseudoholes and pseudocysts defined by optical coherence tomography. Br J Ophthalmol. 2008; 92:1342–6.
18. Andre J. Witkin, BS Tony, et al. Redefining lamellar holes and the vitreomacular interface: An ultrahigh-resolution optical coherence tomography study. Ophthalmol. 2006;113(3):388–97.
19. Allen AW, Gass JD. Contraction of a perifoveal epiretinal membrane simulating a macular hole. Am J Ophthalmol. 1976;82:684–91.
20. Haouchine B, Massin P, Tadayoni R, et al. Diagnosis of macular pseudoholes and lamellar macular holes by optical coherence tomography. Am J Ophthalmol. 2004;138:732–9.
21. Gass JDM. Vitreofoveal separation and lamellar hole formation. In: Gass JDM, editor. Stereoscopic atlas of macular diseases: Diagnosis and treatment. 4th ed. St Louis: CV Mosby, 1997:926–27.

22. Hirakawa M, Uemura A, Nakano T, Sakamoto T. Pars plana vitrectomy with gas tamponade for lamellar macular holes. Am J Ophthalmol. 2005;140:1154–55.
23. Gonvers M, Machemer R. A new approach to treating retinal detachment with macular hole. Am J Ophthalmol. 1982;94:468–72.
24. Margherio RR, Schepens CL. Macular Holes II. Management. Am J Ophthalmol. 1972;74:233–40.
25. Kelly NE, Wendel RT. Vitreous surgery for idiopathic macular holes. Arch Ophthalmol. 1991;109:654–59.
26. Casuso LA, Scott IU, Flynn HW, et al. Long-term follow-up of unoperated macular holes. Ophthalmology. 2001;108:1150–55.
27. Freeman WR, Azen SP, Kim JW, Elhaig W, Mishell DR, Bailey I. Vitrectomy for the treatment of full-thickness stage 3 or 4 macular holes–results of a multicentred randomized clinical trial. Arch Ophthalmol. 1997:115:11–21.
28. Ezra E, Aylward WG, Gregor ZJ. Membranectomy and autologous serum for the retreatment of full-thickness macular holes. Arch Ophthalmol. 1997;115:1276–80.
29. Makabe R. Krypton laser coagulation in idiopathic holes. Klin Monatsbl Augenheilkd 1990;196:202–4.
30. Rizzo S, Belting C, Creasti F, Genovesi-Ebert F. Sutureless 25 gauge vitrectomy for idiopathic macular hole repair. Graefes Arch Clin Exp Ophthalmol. 2007;245:1437–40.
31. Sjaarrda RN, Glaser BM, et al. Distribution of iatrogenic retinal break in macular hole surgery. Ophthalmol. 1995;102:1387–92.
32. Da Mata AP, Burk SE, Foster RE, et al. Long-term follow-up of indocyanine green-assisted peeling of the retinal internal limiting membrane during vitrectomy surgery for idiopathic macular hole repair. Ophthalmol. 2004;111:2246–53.
33. Engelbrecht NE, Freeman J, Sternberg P Jr, et al. Retinal pigment epithelial changes after macular hole surgery with indocyanine green-assisted internal limiting membrane peeling. Am J Ophthalmol. 2002;133:89–94.
34. Kanda S, Uemura A, Yamashita T, Kita H, Yamakiri K, Sakamoto T. Visual field defects after intravitreous administration of indocyanine green in macular hole surgery. Arch Ophthalmol. 2004;122:1447–51.
35. Mochizuki Y, Enaida H, et al. The internal limiting membrane peeling with brilliant blue G staining for retinal detachment due to macular hole in high myopia. Br J Ophthalmol. 2008;92:7.
36. Kazuyuki Kumagai, Mariko Furukawa, et al. Long-term outcomes of internal limiting membrane peeling with and without indocyanine green in macular hole surgery. Retina. 2006;26:613–17.
37. Rizzo S, Genovesi-Ebert F, Vento A, et al. Modified incision in 25 gauge vitrectomy in the creation of a tunneled airtight sclerotomy: An ultrabiomicroscopic study. Graefes Arch Clin Exp Ophthalmol. 2007;245:1281–88.
38. Rizzo S, Genovesi-Ebert F, Murri S, et al. 25 gauge sutureless vitrectomy and standard 20 gauge pars plana vitrectomy in idiopathic epiretinal membrane surgery: A comparative pilot study. Graefes Arch Clin Exp Ophthalmol. 2006;244:472–9.
39. Smiddy WE, Feuer W, Cordahi G. Internal limiting membrane peeling in macular hole surgery. Ophthalmol. 2001;108:1471–78.
40. Brooks HL Jr. Macular hole surgery with and without internal limiting membrane peeling. Ophthalmol. 2000;107:1939–48.
41. Thompson JT, Smiddy WE, Glaser BM, Sjaarda RN, Flynn HW. Intraocular tamponade duration and success of macular hole surgery. Retina. 1996;16:373–82.

42. Fekrat S, Wendel RT, Cruz Z, Green RW. Clinicopathological correlation of an epiretinal membrane associated with a recurrent macular hole. Retina. 1995;15:53–7.
43. Madreperla S, Geiger GL, Funata M, Cruz Z, Green RW. Clinicopathologic correlation of macular hole treated by cortical vitreous peeling and gas tamponade. Ophthalmol. 1994;101:682–6.
44. Kumagai K, Furukawa M, Ogino N, Uemura A, Demizu S, Larson E. Vitreous surgery with and without internal limiting membrane peeling for macular hole repair. Retina. 2004;24:721–7.
45. Thompson JT, Smiddy WE, Glaser BM, Sjaarda RN, Flynn HW. Intraocular tamponade duration and success of macular hole surgery. Retina. 1996; 16:373–82.
46. Dhawahir-Scala FE, Maino A, Saha K, et al. To posture or not to posture after macular hole surgery. Retina. 2008;28:60–5.
47. Isomae T, Sato Y, Shimada H. Shortening the duration of prone positioning after macular hole surgery-comparison between 1 week and 1 day prone positioning. Jpn J Ophthalmol. 2002;46:84–8
48. Dori D, Thoelen AM, Akalp F, et al. Anatomic and functional results of vitrectomy and long-term intraocular tamponade for stage 2 macular holes. Retina. 2003;23:57–63.
49. Tornambe PE, Poliner LS, Grote K. Macular hole surgery without face down posturing. A pilot study. Retina. 1997;17:179–85.
50. Simcock PR, Scalia S. Phacovitrectomy without prone posture for full thickness macular holes. Br J Ophthalmol. 2001;85:1316–19.
51. Michel JJ, Gallemore RP, McCuen BW, Toth CA. Features of macular hole closure in the early postoperative period using optical coherence tomography. Retina. 2000;20:232–37.
52. Lai JC, Stinnett SS, McCuen BW. Comparison of silicone oil versus gas tamponade in the treatment of idiopathic fullthickness macular hole. Ophthalmol. 2003;110: 1170–74.
53. Alexandra Lappas, Andreas Michael, et al. Use of heavy silicone oil Densiron 68 in the treatment of persistent macular holes. Acta Ophthalmologica. 2009;87:866–70.
54. Macular hole surgery with air tamponade and optical coherence tomography-based duration of facedown positioning. Retina. 2008;28;8:1087–96.
55. Duker JS, Wendel R, Patel AC, et al. Late reopening of macular holes after initially successful treatment with vitreous surgery. Ophthalmol. 1994;101:1373–8.

CHAPTER

9

MIVS for Vitreoretinal Interface Disorders

Alay S Banker, Rohan Chauhan

Idiopathic macular hole, epiretinal membrane (ERM), and vitreomacular traction syndrome (VMTS) are macular surface disorders that may result in visual morbidity, especially in the elderly. All three conditions have been associated with pathological vitreomacular adhesions.[1] Although they share some similarities, these conditions are distinct from one another based on histology, surgical anatomy, clinical characteristics and differing natural courses. Still, diagnosis is sometimes confusing, as there may be overlap in both subjective and objective findings.

VITREORETINAL MACULAR TRACTION SYNDROME

Vitreoretinal macular traction syndrome, the least common of these three disorders, is characterized by an incomplete posterior vitreous detachment, in which the vitreous remains attached to the macular area. This results in retinal traction and the development of increased macular thickness and cystoid changes. Patients may experience decreased vision, metamorphopsia, photopsia, and micropsia.[2,3]

Some individuals have an unusually strong attachment between the posterior vitreous cortex, macula, and peripapillary retina.[4-7] One theory is that, pre-existing cell migration on the inner retina may cause an unusually strong vitreoretinal adhesion, preventing completion of the subsequent PVD.[8] So, individuals with such anomalous adhesions might be at higher risk for developing VMTS during normal age-related vitreal changes.

Two distinct clinicopathological features of VMTS suggest different forms of epiretinal fibrocellular proliferation, namely epiretinal membranes interposed in native vitreous collagen, and those composed of single cells or a cellular monolayer proliferating directly on the internal limiting membrane (ILM). Remnants of the cortical vitreous that remain attached to the ILM following posterior vitreous separation may determine the clinicopathological features of the disease. The predominance of myofibroblasts may help explain the increased prevalence of CME and the progressive vitreomacular traction that characterizes VMTS.[9]

VMTS, ERM and impending macular hole syndrome may present very similarly, particularly in regard to foveal appearance. Differences include substantial distortion of the retinal vessels, which is more common in macular pucker, and the cystic changes that are more common in VMTS. There may be symptomatic overlap in patients who have VMTS and ERM. Patients who have either condition often suffer from vision loss and metamorphopsia. In contrast, patients who have impending macular hole syndrome typically have nonspecific symptoms and less vision loss. There are some histological differences between the disorders as well. A thickened layer of epiretinal tissue can be dissected and removed from the macular area in both VMTS and ERM. The predominant ultrastructural feature of tissue specimens in VMTS is the presence of fibrous astrocytes; notably absent are retinal pigment epithelial cells, which dominate the cellular features of ERM cases. VMTS and impending macular hole are associated with anomalous vitreous detachment, but VMTS is rarely associated with progression to a full-thickness macular hole. This difference in the natural course between idiopathic macular hole and VMTS is not fully understood.[8]

OCT can play a critical role in diagnosing VMTS and appears more sensitive than slit lamp biomicroscopy in identifying vitreoretinal adhesions. In one study, such adhesions were identified only 8% of the time using biomicroscopy vs. 30% of the time with OCT. OCT can help confirm the diagnosis of VMTS when clinically invisible. It can also help explain the pathogenesis of the disease and objectively assess anatomical improvement of secondary macular changes following surgery. On OCT, VMTS is characterized by the appearance of a perifoveal vitreous detachment with focal adhesion to the fovea; it is often associated with cystoid macular edema (CME).[10-13]

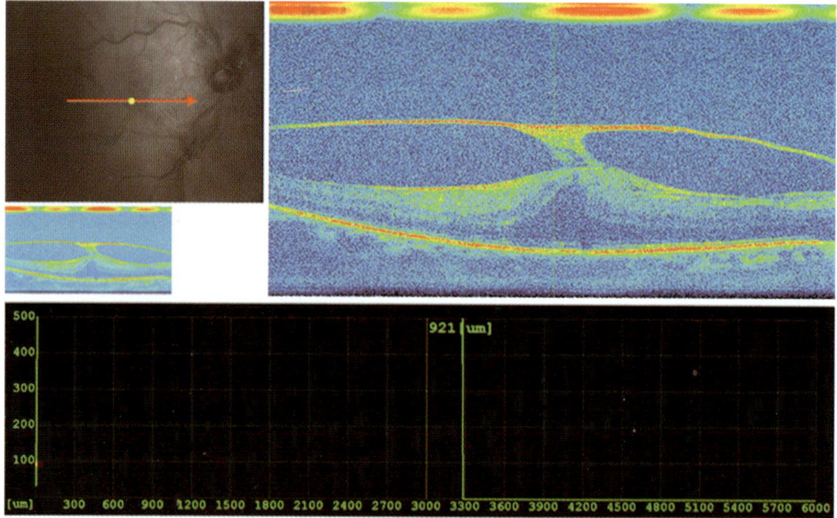

Fig. 9.1A: A Vitreomacular traction syndrome with cystoid macular edema (*Courtesy:* Dr RK Akhaury and Dr Ranjana Kumar)

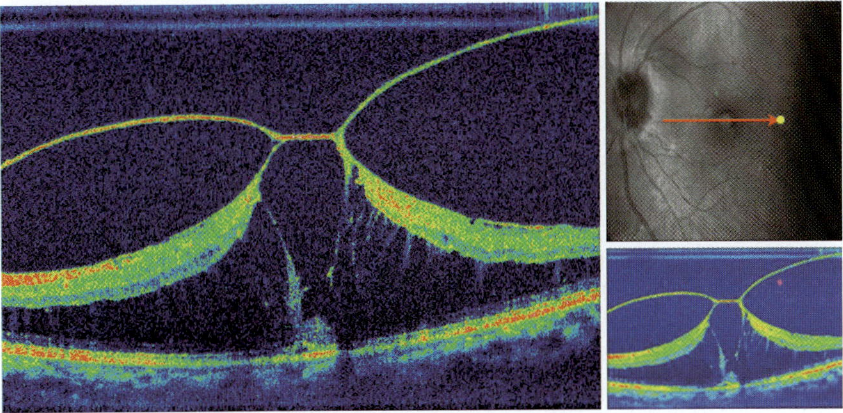

Fig. 9.1B: Severe VMTS with tractional retinal detachment
(*Courtesy:* Dr RK Akhaury and Dr Ranjana Kumar)

Vitrectomy effectively resolves traction in VMTS syndrome and improves visual acuity in most cases.[1,11,14-19] This is demonstrable with OCT, which reveals release of traction and reduction in macular thickness postoperatively.[11,14,15] It is the treatment of choice to prevent deterioration of visual function before irreversible damage occurs to the retina.[18,19] However, approximately 10% of VMTS patients will experience spontaneous resolution of cystoid macular changes following posterior vitreous detachment, making surgery unnecessary.[20] For this reason, some have suggested it is prudent to wait several months before attempting vitrectomy.[21]

Factors that limit visual improvement include accelerated development of nuclear sclerotic cataracts, recurrence of epiretinal membrane, persistent macular edema and macular hole development.[15-17,22] Of note, one study differentiated between two types of incomplete PVD; one type appeared as a V-shaped detachment, the other as a partial detachment temporal to the fovea but attached nasally. Patients treated in the former group had a much more favorable postsurgical outcome than those in the latter.[22] Such prognostic differences further illuminate the importance of careful evaluation with OCT in caring for patients with VMTS.

The rationale for vitrectomy is supported by a study of the natural course of VMTS; patients with symptomatic VMTS experienced worsening of visual acuity during the course of the study unless spontaneous, complete PVD occurred.[23]

There are many similarities and differences among VMTS, impending macular hole and ERM. Specific risk factors and pathogenic features of these conditions are not entirely understood. Recognizing each disorders distinguishing features allows for a more precise diagnosis, more appropriate prognostic patient counseling and appropriate referral for surgical intervention, when indicated.

EPIRETINAL MEMBRANE

This ocular pathology was first described by Iwanoff in 1865, and it has been shown to be a relatively common entity, occurring in about 7% of the population. EMMs have been called a variety of names, including epiretinal membranes, cellophane maculopathy, preretinal macular gliosis, preretinal macular fibrosis, macular pucker, preretinal vitreous membranes, epiretinal astrocytic membranes, surface wrinkling maculopathy, internoretinal fibrosis, and silk-screen retinopathy; all of which pertain to clinicoanatomic descriptions of pathologic findings produced by EMMs of varying severity and differing morphologic characteristics.

EMMs can be associated with a variety of ocular conditions, such as posterior vitreous detachments (PVD), retinal tears, retinal detachments, retinal vascular occlusive diseases, ocular inflammatory diseases, and vitreous hemorrhage. However, a large proportion does not occur in the context of any associated disease or known history and therefore are classified as idiopathic epimacular membranes (IEMM).[24-27]

- The usual symptoms caused by EMMs run the spectrum from no symptoms at all to severe visual dysfunction.
  - Early on, EMMs cause little or no visual disturbance.
  - As the membrane progresses, the visual disturbance is often vague and difficult for the patient to describe.
  - Mild distortion or blurring is the most common symptom.
  - Vision better than 20/50 is present in 78–85% of cases, while 56–67% have vision better than 20/30. Only 2–5% have vision poorer than 20/200.
  - In more advanced cases, metamorphopsia, micropsia, or Amsler Grid abnormalities may be present.
  - In contrast, vision is markedly reduced in patients with EMMs associated with retinal detachment. Vision is 20/60 or better in only 7% of cases and 56% have vision poorer than 20/200 after successful retinal reattachment surgery.

Physical Properties

The clinical findings in EMMs vary according to the degree of severity of the membrane. Gass formulated a classification system based on the appearance of the membrane and the underlying retinal tissue and vessels.

- Grade 0 membranes
  - Grade 0 EMMs are translucent membranes not associated with any retinal distortion.
  - These EMMs also are known as cellophane maculopathy owing to the cellophane like sheen coming from the inner retinal surface as it is seen ophthalmoscopically.

- Grade 1 membranes
  - Membranes causing an irregular wrinkling of the inner retinal surface are classified as grade 1 EMMs.
  - The crinkled cellophane appearance is caused by the gathering of the inner retinal layers into folds following the contraction of the overlying membrane.
  - Fine, superficial, radiating folds extend outward from the margins of the contracted membrane.
  - Wrinkling may be sufficient to produce tortuosity of the paramacular vessels pulling them toward the fovea.
  - Cystoid macular edema, retinal hemorrhage, exudates, and RPE disturbances are typically absent.
- Grade 2 membranes
  - Membranes, especially those that develop after retinal detachment surgery, have an opaque, thick appearance.
  - Gross, full-thickness puckering of the macula may be present along with retinal edema, small hemorrhages, cotton-wool spots, and, infrequently, a localized detachment of the retina.
  - These membranes are labeled macular puckers or grade 2 membranes.

Pseudomacular Holes

ERMs are likely to develop following the transient vitreomacular traction that occurs during posterior vitreous detachment. Dehiscence in the internal limiting membrane occurs, allowing migration and proliferation of glial cells on the inner retinal surface.[27,28-30]

Imaging Studies

Fluorescein Angiography

Performing an angiogram in cases of EMMs does not contribute anything significant in its diagnosis since the clinical picture is often specific enough. In less advanced cases, the angiographic picture is basically unremarkable. More significant findings, such as vessel tortuosity and macular edema, may be seen in more advanced cases.

- Perform fluorescein angiography to rule out other lesions that may mimic EMMs.
- Macular holes typically show early background fluorescence through the hole that disappears in the later phases.
- EMMs with pseudoholes typically do not exhibit this fluorescence since normal retinal tissue exists in the area.
- An exudative macular degeneration also may mimic the appearance of an EMM, but its angiographic picture of early fluorescence and leakage is easily distinguishable from EMMs.

Fluorescein angiograms of EMMs can reveal subtle leakage of the perifoveal capillaries or evidence of ischemia due to capillary dropout, which can assist with counseling for postoperative expectations.

Ocular Coherence Tomography

- Ocular coherence tomography (OCT) can elucidate the presence or absence of an EMM.
- OCT can objectively measure other effects of the EMM on the retina, such as macular thickening, presence or absence of macular edema (e.g. cystoid macular edema), and any associated vitreous traction on the retina (Figure 9.2).

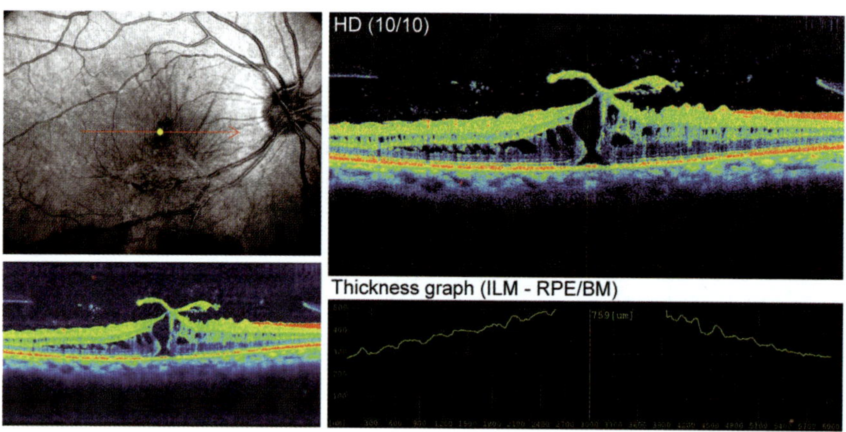

Fig. 9.2: Epiretinal membrane with surface wrinking. Note radiating lines seen on the redfree SLO image (*Courtesy:* Dr Subhash Prasad)

- OCT allows the monitoring of the postoperative return of the normal retinal architecture as well as the presence of persistent traction or folds of the retina (Figure 9.3).

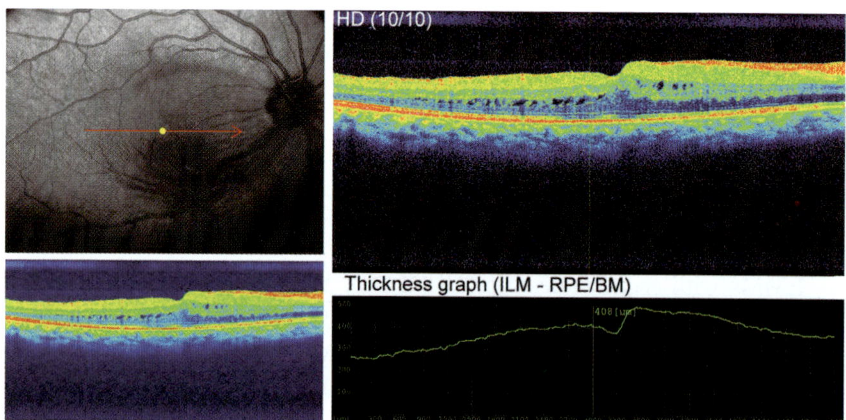

Fig. 9.3: Postoperative OCT of the same patient after 1 week wherein patient underwent 23 gauge vitrectomy with triamcinolone assisted PVD and ILM peeling (*Courtesy:* Dr Subhash Prasad)

Treatment

Isolate EMM as the main cause of a patient's visual impairment prior to planning a corrective procedure. Evaluate the patient carefully to rule out other pathologic conditions, such as macular holes, subfoveal choroidal neovascular membranes, cystoid macular edema, or retinal vascular occlusive disease, that may mimic the appearance of a true membrane.

Surgical treatment of EMM is usually not an emergency procedure. Only when there is macular edema does it become a more urgent procedure.

Several surgical techniques exist for the treatment of EMM. However, 3 basic stages of treatment exist.

Vitrectomy

- Pars plana vitrectomy is performed to excise the posterior and central vitreous in phakic patients and the remainder of the anterior vitreous in aphakic and pseudophakic patients. This step is especially important in cases where marked adherence of the vitreous to the macula is present.
- Lately, questions have been raised regarding the need for vitrectomy in EMM peeling, especially in those cases where no significant PVR exists.
- The main advantages of doing a vitrectomy are the prevention of vitreous contraction and elimination of vitreous traction on the macula. In addition, removal of the vitreous is believed by many to increase the safety of the mechanical aspects of the membrane removal.
- The main disadvantages of vitrectomy include cataractogenesis and increased possibility of creating iatrogenic retinal breaks. Vitrectomy has been shown to increase the rate of cataract formation through unclear mechanisms.
- Studies have shown that a three-fold increase in the rate of significant cataract formation exists in patients that have undergone vitrectomy after a follow-up period of only 6 months.
- Some surgeons feel that the effectiveness of membrane peeling is negated significantly by the cataract formation such that they have foregone vitrectomy in selected cases, opting to perform noninfusion/nonvitrectomy membrane peelings. The main disadvantage of this technique is the persistence of floaters postoperatively, which may be very bothersome to some patients. Furthermore, some surgeons have seen no significant difference in either cataractogenesis or development of retinal breaks/detachments in their series comparing vitrectomizing and nonvitrectomizing techniques.
- While the vitrectomy can be performed using the standard 20 gauge system, surgeons are also using smaller gauge vitrectomy systems (e.g. 23 gauge, 25 gauge) for surgical management of EMM.[4,5] These systems are transconjunctival with the potential to create self-sealing wounds. Complications appear low while affording the potential for more rapid surgical and visual recovery.

Epiretinal Membrane Peeling

- From the time Machamer developed the concept of membrane peeling in the mid 1970s, several variations and refinements in both technique and instrumentation have been developed.
- This procedure basically involves identifying the outer edge of the membrane and creating a dissection plane with the use of a blunt-tipped pick or a bent needle.
- Once the edge of the membrane is seen, it may be gently lifted off the retinal surface with the use of a pick or fine forceps.
- The membrane should be lifted in a tangential rather than an anteroposterior fashion so as not to pull on the underlying retina and create tears. This maneuver is relatively straightforward if the edge of the membrane is visible.
- Charles developed a maneuver that approaches the membrane from inside out in cases where the edge is difficult to identify.[6] It involves creating a slit on the thickest part of the membrane with a straight microvitreoretinal blade and using this opening as the edge with which to start the peeling. The peeling is performed moving the forceps in a circular fashion similar to capsulorrhexis. The freed membrane should be removed either by pulling it out with the forceps through the sclerotomy or by using the vitreous cutter.

Internal Limiting Membrane (ILM) Peeling

- Removal of the ILM at the time of EMM peeling is a current controversy.
- Vital stains, such as indocyanine green (ICG) dye and Trypan blue dye, have been used to assist ILM and EMM peeling. Dyes that stain the ILM highlight foci of EMM and potentially reduce the risk of recurrence or the persistence of symptoms.
- Similar to its use in macular hole surgery, the use of ICG has proponents and detractors on the basis of its potential toxic effects. Haritoglou et al suggested that ICG-assisted ILM peeling may adversely affect the functional outcome of surgery for EMM.[7]

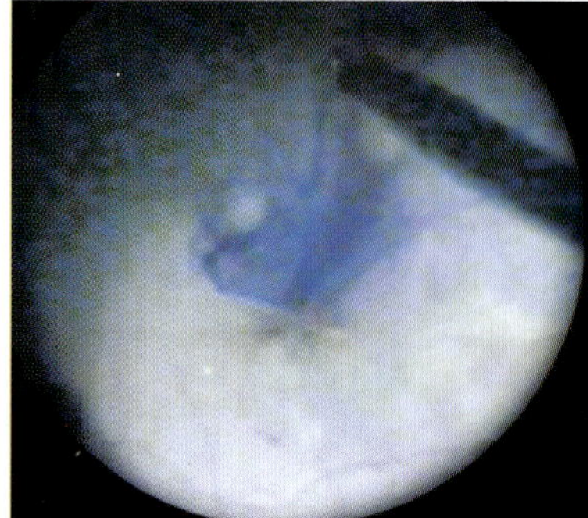

Fig. 9.4: Staining of ILM using brilliant blue

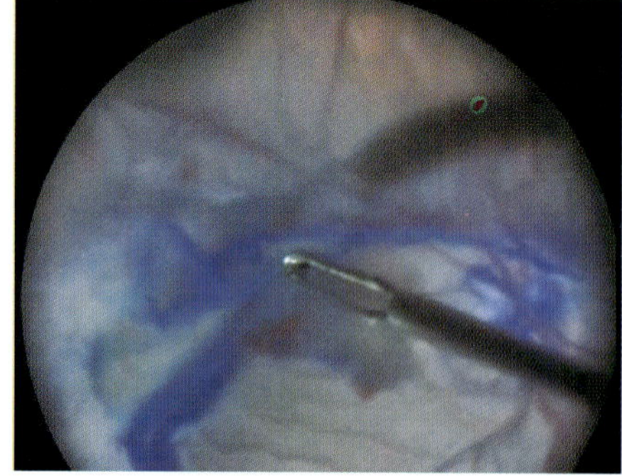

Fig. 9.5: ILM peeling using Alcon DSP ILM forceps

- Hillenkamp et al prospectively evaluated the effect of ICG dye in the setting of EMM surgery.[8] No difference or evidence of ICG toxicity was observed. Both visual function and macular morphology improved in patients with and without ICG dye use.
- However, Garweg et al suggested that ILM peeling with ICG dye, but not with trypan blue dye, may result in loss of the central visual field over time.[9] No difference in visual acuity was noted. This study suggests that the ICG dye, not necessarily the ILM peeling, may have an adverse effect following EMM surgery.

Management of Retinal Breaks

- Once the membrane is removed, it is imperative for the surgeon to look for any breaks in the retina, both in the posterior pole and in the periphery.
- Any maneuvers completed to remove the membranes, no matter how elegant, become irrelevant if the retina detaches because of missed breaks.
- Careful scleral depression of the anterior retina combined with indirect ophthalmoscopy should be performed to detect breaks in the periphery.
- Breaks without subretinal fluid accumulation can be treated by laser retinopexy or cryoretinopexy.

The presence of significant amounts of subretinal fluid necessitates internal drainage under air, retinopexy, and gas tamponade.

Prognosis

- Numerous studies have addressed the potential benefit of surgery to remove the EMMs. These studies have looked at the quantification of the postoperative visual acuity improvement as well as the subjective improvements through postoperative quality of life questionnaires. They have also looked at other prognostic factors that may influence visual outcomes.
- Surgical removal of clinically significant EMMs usually results in improvement in both visual acuity and biomicroscopic appearance of the retina. Studies have shown that, postoperatively, 78–87% of patients with IEMM and 63–100% of patients with postdetachment membranes improved at least 2 Snellen lines. Patients with poorer preoperative vision tended to improve the most, but those patients with better preoperative vision obtained the best final results.
- Visual acuity has also been evaluated through the use of postoperative questionnaires. A large-scale study showed that surgery improved the symptom of distortion the most, with moderate-to-severe symptoms most improved. Improvement was also seen in other daily tasks, such as reading small print.
- Sometimes, however, the metamorphopsia may persist despite improvement in visual acuity. This is seen mostly in cases where there is incomplete peeling of the membrane. On the other hand, there are cases wherein the

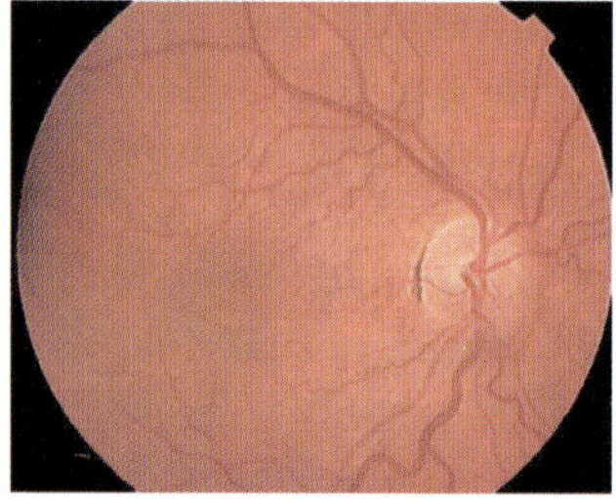

Fig. 9.6: Fundus picture showing only subtle thickening of the fovea with faint ERM

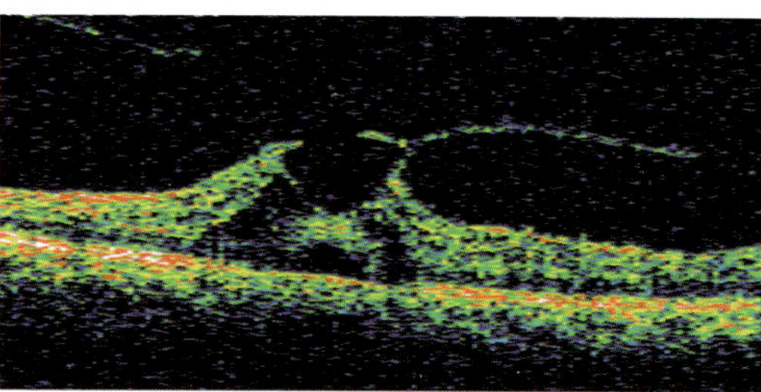

Fig. 9.7: OCT showing incomplete V-shaped posterior vitreous detachment and a tractional retinal detachment at the fovea

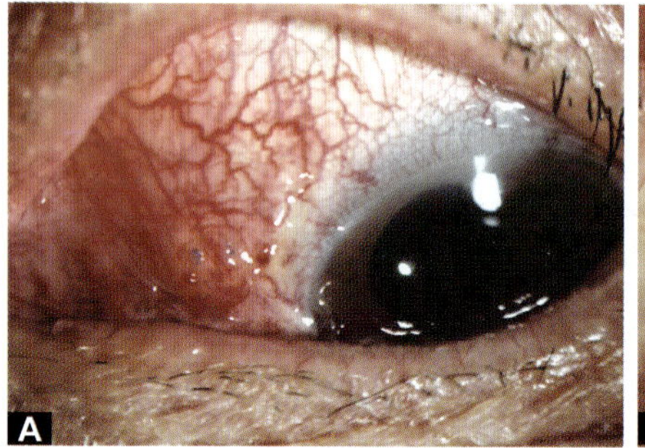

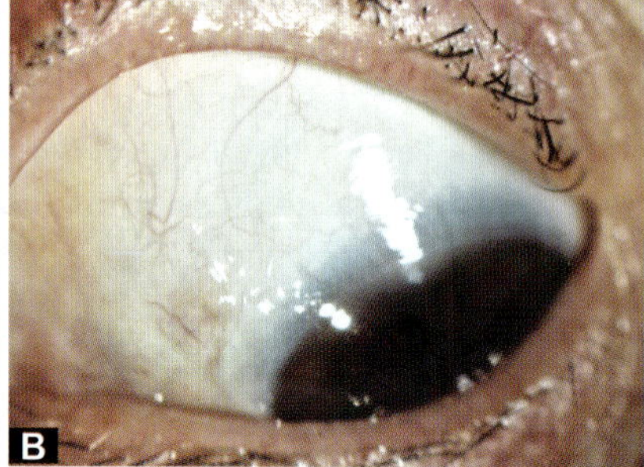

Figs 9.8A and B: Anterior segment photography of eyes after performing 20 gauge standard vitrectomy (A: postoperative 1 week, B: postoperative 6 weeks)

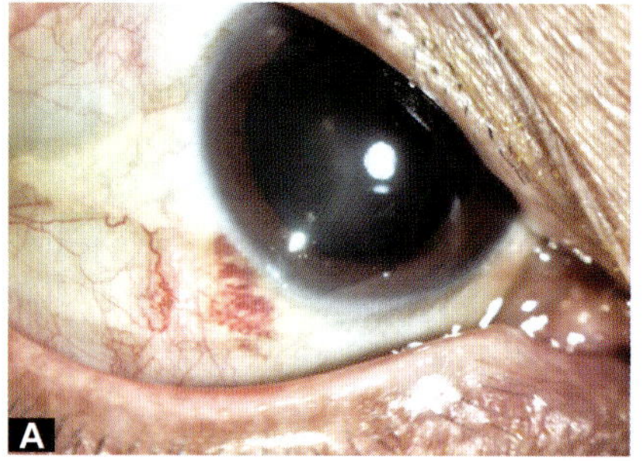

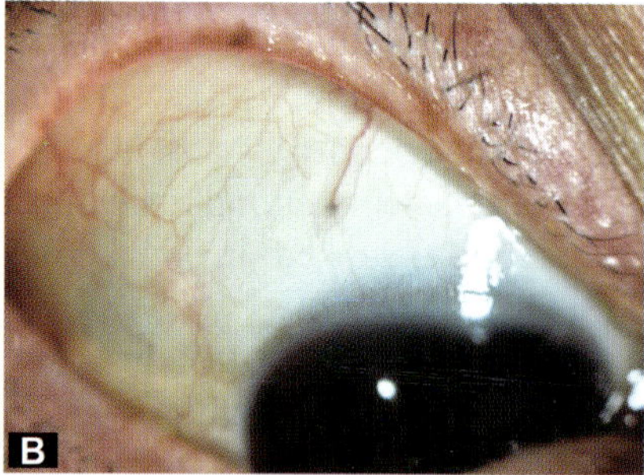

Figs 9.9A and B: 23 gauge transconjunctival sutureless vitrectomy (A: postoperative 1 week, B: postoperative 6 weeks)

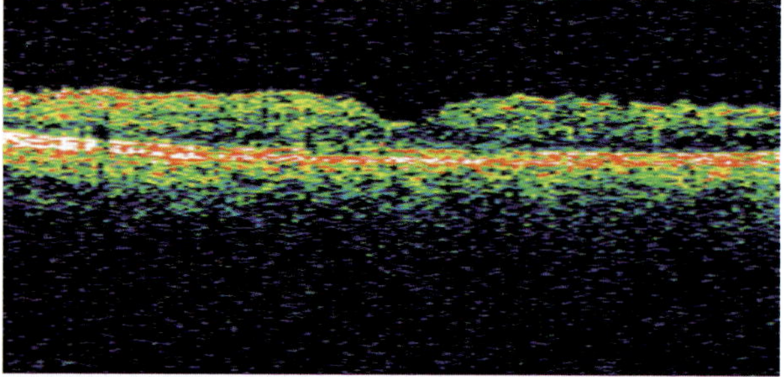

Fig. 9.10: Postoperative OCT showing resolution of retinal edema after release of the traction and restoration of normal foveal dip

distortion is improved but the Snellen acuity remains unchanged. This mainly is encountered in cases where there is long-standing macular edema.

The presence of new or accelerated cataract formation has been shown to occur in the surgical treatment of EMMs.

Clinical Case

A 61-year-old white male presented complaining of floating spots and sparkly things in the center of his right eye for the past month. His ocular history was significant for a subconjunctival hemorrhage in his left eye due to blunt trauma by vegetative matter; this occurred one year earlier. He denied any trauma history involving the right eye. His medical history was significant for hypertension and hyperlipidemia. He underwent aortic bifemoral bypass in 2001. Medications included lisinopril 20 mg qd, metoprolol 100 mg q12h, simvastatin 40 mg qd and prophylactic baby aspirin 81 mg qd.

Diagnostic Data

Best-corrected visual acuity was 20/150 O.D. and 20/20 O.S. Biomicroscopy revealed a normal cornea, iris, anterior chamber and lens O.U. Pupils, motilities and IOP all appeared normal. Dilated fundus exam revealed a subtle epiretinal membrane (ERM) with associated traction lines and an unusual elevated appearance in the foveal area of the right eye. There was an incomplete posterior vitreous separation and a subtle area of thickened posterior hyaloid overlying the macula (Figure 9.6). The macula in the left eye was flat and unremarkable.

REFERENCES

1. Koerner F, Garweg J. Diseases of the vitreomacular interface. Klin Monatsbl Augenheilkd. 1999;214(5):305–10.
2. Maumenee AE. Further advances in the study of the macula. Arch Ophthalmol. 1967;78(2):151–65.
3. Gass JD. Macular dysfunction caused by vitreous and vitreoretinal interface abnormalities: Vitreous traction maculopathies. In: Gass JD. Stereoscopic Atlas of Macular Diseases: Diagnosis and Treatment, 3rd ed. Vol. 2. St Louis: Mosby-Year Book, 1987:676–93.
4. Sebag J. Age–related differences in the human vitreoretinal interface. Arch Ophthalmol. 1991;109(7):966–71.
5. Sebag J. Anatomy and pathology of the vitreoretinal interface. Eye. 1992;6(6): 541–52.
6. Foos RY, Wheeler NC. Vitreoretinal juncture. Synchysis senilis and posterior vitreous detachment. Ophthalmol. 1982;89(12):1502–12.
7. Smiddy WE, Green WR, Michels RG, de la Cruz Z. Ultrastructural studies of vitreomacular traction syndrome. Am J Ophthalmol. 1989;15;107(2):177–85.
8. Smiddy WE, Michels RG, Green WR. Morphology, pathology, and surgery of idiopathic vitreoretinal macular disorders. A review. Retina. 1990;10(4):288–96.
9. Gandorfer A, Rohleder M, Kampik A. Epiretinal pathology of vitreomacular traction syndrome. Br J Ophthalmol. 2002;86(8):902–9.

10. Gallemore RP, Jumper JM, McCuen BW 2nd, et al. Diagnosis of vitreoretinal adhesions in macular disease with optical coherence tomography. Retina. 2000; 20(2):115–20.
11. Johnson MW. Tractional cystoid macular edema: A subtle variant of the vitreomacular traction syndrome. Am J Ophthalmol. 2005;140(2):184–92.
12. Munuera JM, Garcia-Layana A, Maldonado MJ, et al. Optical coherence tomography in successful surgery of vitreomacular traction syndrome. Arch Ophthalmol. 1998; 116(10):1388–9.
13. Schuman JS, Puliafito CA, Fujimoto JG. Optical Coherence Tomography of Ocular Diseases. 2nd ed. Thorofare, NJ: Slack Inc.; 2004:58.
14. Larsson J. Vitrectomy in vitreomacular traction syndrome evaluated by ocular coherence tomography (OCT) retinal mapping. Acta Ophthalmol Scand. 2004;82(6): 691–4.
15. Petropoulos IK, Stangos AA, Brozou CG, et al. Vitrectomy for vitreomacular traction syndrome. Klin Monatsbl Augenheilkd 2003;220(3):122–6.
16. Gribomont AC. Surgical prognosis in idiopathic vitreomacular syndrome and epiretinal membrane. J Fr Ophthalmol. 2005;28(7):739–42.
17. Jiang YR, Ma Y, Li XX. Analysis of the effect of surgical management on vitreomacular traction syndrome. Zhonghua Yan Ke Za Zhi 2004;40(10):670–3.
18. Smiddy WE, Michels RG, Glaser BM, de Bustros S. Vitrectomy for macular traction caused by incomplete vitreous separation. Arch Ophthalmol. 1988;106(5):624–8.
19. McDonald HR, Johnson RN, Schatz H. Surgical results in the vitreomacular traction syndrome. Ophthalmol. 1994;101(8):1397–403.
20. Kusaka S, Saito Y, Okada AA, et al. Optical coherence tomography in spontaneously resolving vitreomacular traction syndrome. Ophthalmologica. 2001;215(2):139–41.
21. Rodriguez A, Infante R, Rodriguez FJ, Valencia M. Spontaneous separation in idiopathic vitreomacular traction syndrome associated with contralateral full–thickness macular hole. Eur J Ophthalmol. 2006;16(5):733–40.
22. Yamada N, Kishi S. Tomographic features and surgical outcomes of vitreomacular traction syndrome. Am J Ophthalmol. 2005;139(1):112–7.
23. Hikichi T, Yoshida A, Trempe CL. Course of vitreomacular traction syndrome. Am J Ophthalmol. 1995;119(1):55–61.
24. Wise GN. Relationship of idiopathic preretinal macular fibrosis to posterior vitreous detachment. Am J Ophthalmol. 1975;79(3):358–62.
25. Wiznia RA. Posterior vitreous detachment and idiopathic preretinal macular gliosis. Am J Ophthalmol. 1986;15;102(2):196–8.
26. Hirokawa H, Jalkh AE, Takahashi M, et al. Role of the vitreous in idiopathic preretinal macular fibrosis. Am J Ophthalmol. 1986;15;101(2):166–9.
27. Roth AM, Foos RY. Surface wrinkling retinopathy in eyes enucleated at autopsy. Trans Am Acad Ophthalmol Otolaryngol. 1971;75(5):1047–58.
28. Smiddy WE, Maguire AM, Green WR, et al. Idiopathic epiretinal membranes. Ultrastructural characteristics and clinicopathologic correlation. Ophthalmol. 1989; 96(6):811–21.
29. Appiah AP, Hirose T, Kado M. A review of 324 cases of idiopathic premacular gliosis. Am J Ophthalmol. 1988;106(5):533–5.
30. Ciulla TA, Pesavento RD. Epiretinal fibrosis. Ophthalmic Surg Lasers. 1997;28(8):670–9.

CHAPTER

10

Microincision Vitrectomy System in PDR

Cyrus Shroff, Charu Gupta

Conventional 20 gauge vitrectomy was the gold standard for simple and complicated vitrectomies for proliferative diabetic retinopathy.[1,2] However, with increasing comfort of vitreoretinal surgeons with the 23 gauge and 25 gauge systems, refinement in small gauge instrumentation, advent of brighter light sources and wider acceptance of the wide-angle viewing system the trend is towards microincision vitrectomy system (MIVS).

SMALL GAUGE VITRECTOMY

Smaller incisions facilitate faster wound healing, decrease astigmatism, improve patient comfort and decrease postoperative inflammation, thereby enabling early visual recovery.[3]

There has been a change in vitrectomy technique with the advent of MIVS and newer vitrectomy machines. There is great interest in the concept of 'port-based flow limiting' a term pioneered by Steve Charles which aims at increasing surgical safety. Cutting speed, diameter of the vitrectomy probe and more recently duty cycle are parameters which affect 'port-based flow'. Faster cutting speed leads to a decrease in the volume of each individual 'bite', thereby increasing fluidic resistance at the port (Figure 10.1). Increased

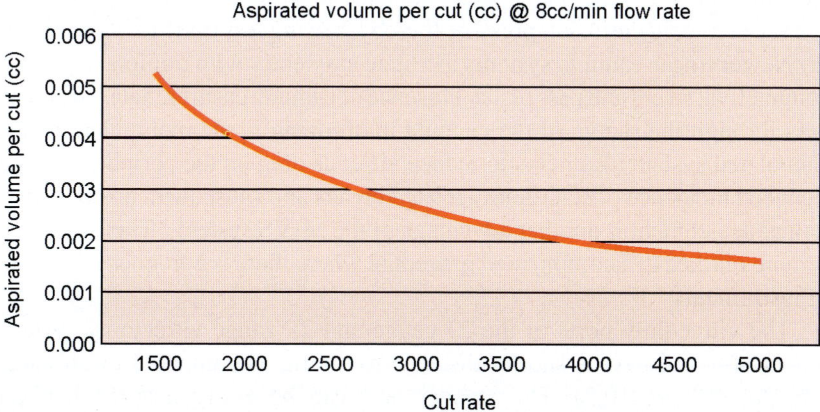

Fig. 10.1: Graph showing relationship between cutting speed and aspirated volume per cut

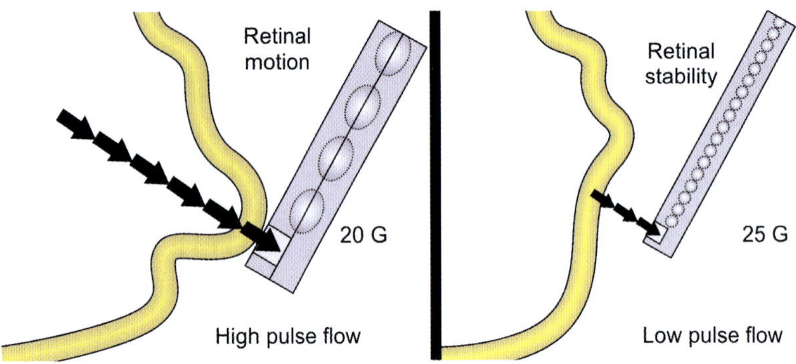

Fig. 10.2: Increased retinal stability with small gauge vitrectomy as compared to 20 gauge vitrectomy

fluidic resistance translates to better fluidic stability which in turn decreases vitreoretinal traction and the incidence of iatrogenic retinal breaks. By using small gauge cutters greater fluidic resistance is achieved at the port as resistance is proportional to the fourth power of the diameter of the probe. Therefore, better fluidic and retinal stability can be achieved with small gauge vitrectomy (Figure 10.2). The opening and closing cycle of the vitrector port is called the duty cycle. With standard pneumatic cutter the port opening time decreases as cutting rate increases. In the newer vitrectomy system (Constellation) it is possible to achieve beneficial port-based flow by altering the duty cycle of the vitrectomy cutter. There are 3 duty cycle settings: 'Core'-open bias cutting, 'Shave'- closed bias setting, 50-50. Settings can be changed so as to perform the safest possible vitrectomy.[4]

Another advantage of the newer vitrectomy system in diabetic vitrectomy is the ability to control intraocular pressure during surgery. A sensor embedded in the cassette measures infusion flow and calculates pressure drop through the infusion line. This enables maintenance of the pressure within 2 mm Hg the whole time. This is especially useful in diabetics as there is a lower risk of bleeding due to intraocular pressure fluctuation and it is also possible to work at a lower average infusion pressure thereby causing less optic nerve damage[4].

Newer trocar-cannula systems facilitate easy entry with minimal trauma to conjunctiva, sclera and pars plana. Presence of cannula ensures that instruments pass through the sleeve of the cannula minimizing tissue manipulation. The cannulated system also helps to reduce vitreous drag on the peripheral retina. Reduced incidence of sclerotomy related breaks and subsequent postoperative retinal detachment is another advantage of the MIVS system.[3] This advantage is more marked in a complicated procedure where there is a frequent exchange of instruments.

The vitrectomy ports of the 23 gauge and 25 gauge vitrectomy systems are smaller and have a shorter distance to the tip as compared to 20 gauge vitrector (Figure 10.3). The smaller port can be easily inserted between

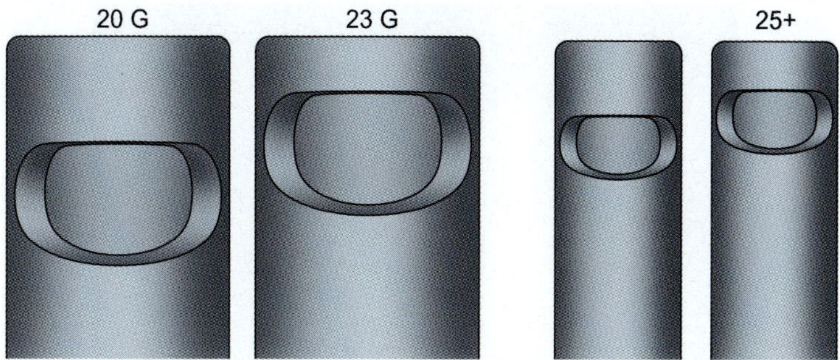

Fig. 10.3: Placement of the port closer to tip in small gauge vitrectors enhances the ability to dissect membranes

the fibrovascular membrane and retina allowing successful membrane segmentation. In complicated cases, where bimanual membrane surgery is required, the small gauge vitrectomy probe, being finer can also be used as a scissors for blunt dissection. This not only decreases incidence of iatrogenic retinal break formation but also limits the instrument exchanges. This maneuverability of the vitrectomy probe is also useful in peripheral dissection when there is minimal posterior hyaloid separation till the periphery.[3,5-7] Smaller diameter of the MIVS vitrectomy probe also enables its usage as a haem stopper (Figures 10.4 to 10.7).

Thorough base excision is essential to prevent some of the most dreaded postoperative complications of diabetic vitrectomy. However, a thorough base excision with scleral depression may be a limitation in some eyes undergoing transconjunctival MIVS especially if they have shallow fornices and in cases with extensive membranes extending to the periphery. A 360° peritomy can be done in these cases with transscleral insertion of the cannulas (Figure 10.8).

In MIVS there is also an option of being able to interchange the infusion site (making it superonasal or superotemporal) thereby approaching the membrane sitting temporally.

Another significant advantage of transconjunctival MIVS over conventional 20 gauge vitrectomy in surgery for PDR is preservation of conjunctiva which allows for repeated vitrectomy and filtering surgery in patients with diabetes complicated with NVG even after vitrectomy.

25 gauge vitrectomy has some limitations in complex TRD's due to lack of instrument rigidity, slower vitreous cutting ability and suboptimal fluidics due to the reduced caliber of the instruments. The newer 25 gauge plus system has overcome some of these disadvantages. For simple diabetic vitrectomies the choice between 23 gauge system and 25 gauge system depends on the comfort level of operating surgeon. However, the 23 gauge vitrectomy system is ideal for complicated cases as it combines the advantages of smaller incision with the sturdier instrumentation and fluidics as in 20 gauge system.

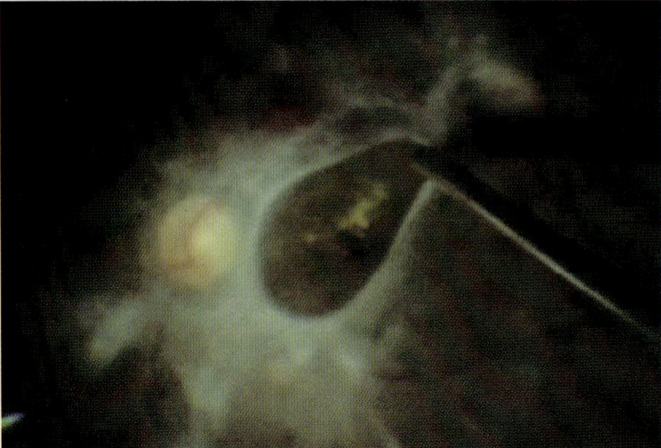

Fig. 10.4: Dissection of membrane close to retina with a 23 gauge vitrector

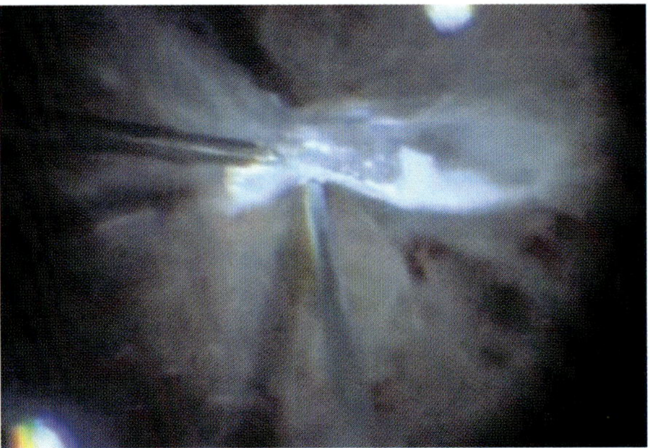

Fig. 10.5: Blunt dissection with 23 gauge vitrector

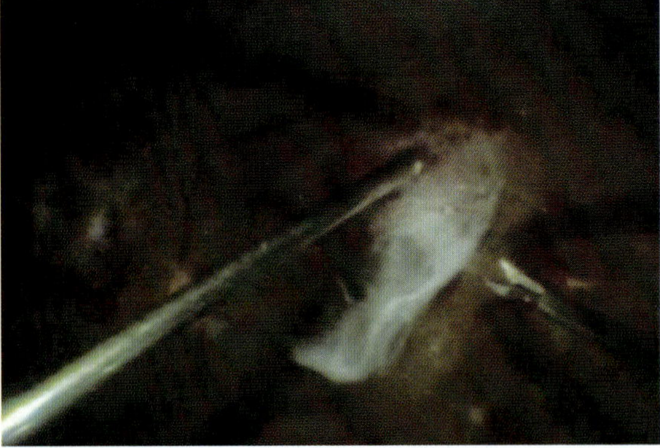

Fig. 10.6: Bimanual dissection using suction with 23 gauge vitrector and scissors

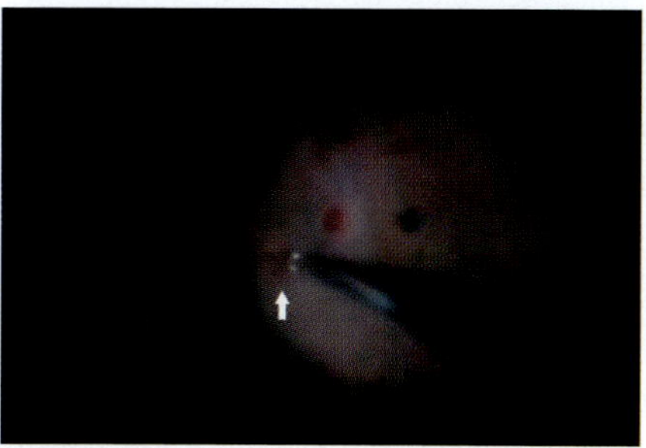

Fig. 10.7: Fine tip of 23 gauge vitrector used as a blunt instrument to stop bleeder

ENDOILLUMINATION

Evolution of endoillumination is driven by the need for a brighter, wider and more even field of illumination. With advent of small gauge vitrectomy and wide-angle viewing systems brighter and safe illumination is of paramount importance.

Xenon light source which is now replacing the conventional tungsten halogen or metal halide bulbs gives a much brighter illumination. Conventional light sources had a maximum illumination of 10 lumens which was halved when used in lighted instruments, wide-angle probes and chandelier systems. The illumination obtained with xenon light source and 25 gauge/27 gauge probes is brighter than that achieved with 20 gauge probe and conventional light source. To reduce phototoxicity, xenon illuminators have an integrated filter system which cuts off high levels of ultraviolet illumination.[8]

The development of self-retaining endoillumination—chandelier lighting system has revolutionized the safety and efficacy of bimanual surgery[8] for complicated diabetic vitrectomies. The Chandelier system provides wide field illumination with a low risk of macular phototoxicity due to the significant distance between the light source and the posterior pole. Tornambe Torpedo (Insight Instruments, Buffalo, NY), Awh Chandelier (Synergetics),[9,10] DORC Neptune Dual Chandelier (Kingston, NH) are some of the options available.[11]

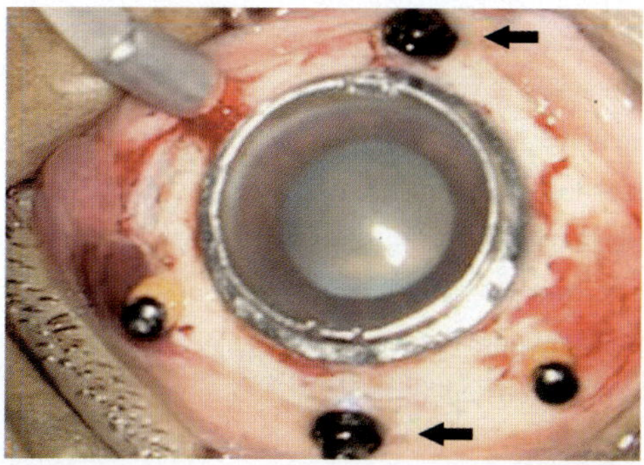

Fig. 10.8: 23 gauge transscleral sclerotomies with self-retaining endoillumination (Tornambe Torpedo) at 12 o'clock and 6 o'clock (blue arrows)

DORC Neptune Dual Chandelier consists of two 25 gauge fibers attached to a common footplate. Twin fibers at 11o'clock and 1o'clock provide shadow free illumination and the footplate ensures stability of the fibers so that the light stays directed to the posterior pole Another method to obtain a shadow free illumination is by using 2 fibers at 12 o'clock and 6 o'clock (Figure 10.8).

VIEWING SYSTEM

Wide-angle viewing systems are important to the wider acceptance of MIVS. A thorough base excision is essential especially in complicated vitrectomies. With the earlier 25 gauge system, there was an inability to do a good base excision. 23 gauge system and wide-angle viewing have helped to overcome this disadvantage, thereby making it possible to tackle all cases, simple and complicated by MIVS.

Wide-angle viewing system can be contact or noncontact. Ideally, sutures for lens stabilization should be avoided in keeping with the concept of minimal trauma. Newer contact lenses are lighter, have a smaller diameter and have flanges for stabilization. Noncontact wide-angle systems (BIOM) have the advantage of causing less trauma to corneal epithelium and easier scleral depression. The disadvantage is that the image resolution and stereopsis is inferior to the contact lens system.

INDICATIONS FOR SURGERY

With improved surgical techniques and better understanding of disease process, the indications of vitrectomy in diabetic retinopathy have, over the years, expanded[12] (Table 10.1).

1. Clearing of media opacities: Removing nonresolving vitreous hemorrhage was one of the earliest indications for vitrectomy in diabetic retinopathy

TABLE 10.1: Indications of vitrectomy in diabetic retinopathy

Indications
• Clearing media opacities
– Nonresolving vitreous hemorrhage
– Neovascularization of anterior segment
– 'Ghost cell glaucoma'
• Release traction and traction-related complications
– Tractional retinal detachment involving macula
– Combined tractional rhegmatogenous retinal detachment
– Progressive fibrovascular proliferation
– Dense premacular hemorrhage
– Macular edema with a 'taut hyaloid'
• Improve oxygen diffusion
– Recalcitrant macular edema

(Figure 10.9). Pan retinal photocoagulation is the only lasting treatment to counter retinal ischemia, which leads to elimination of growth factors responsible for new vessel formation and breakdown of blood-ocular barrier. Vitrectomy to clear media opacities enables completion of photocoagulation. In presence of neovascularization of anterior segment or 'ghost cell glaucoma' early vitrectomy is indicated.

2. Release traction and traction related complications: With widespread use of photocoagulation for PDR, prevalence of nonresolving vitreous hemorrhage decreased. Tractional retinal detachment involving macula and combined retinal detachment subsequently were the more common indications for vitrectomy. An understanding of the concept of vitreoschisis, bimanual surgery and recently MIVS has improved the surgical results. Surgeries for dense premacular hemorrhage, macular edema with a taut PHF, progressive fibrovascular proliferation are some of the newer indications which have benefited with the advent of MIVS (Figures 10.10 and 10.11). Relatively atraumatic surgery, early postoperative recovery and good surgical results have increased confidence levels of surgeon and patient.
3. Improved oxygen diffusion: Induction of PVD with removal of ILM from the posterior pole relieves vitreoretinal traction and changes the molecular flux across the vitreoretinal interface improving oxygen supply to retina.[13] Recalcitrant macular edema is one of the newer indications of vitrectomy based on the above hypothesis (Figures 10.12A and B). Removal of ILM has become easier technically but carries a potential risk of retinal damage. In future , enzymatic vitreolysis which provides a complete PVD with no remnants of cortical vitreous on ILM may be the least traumatic option.

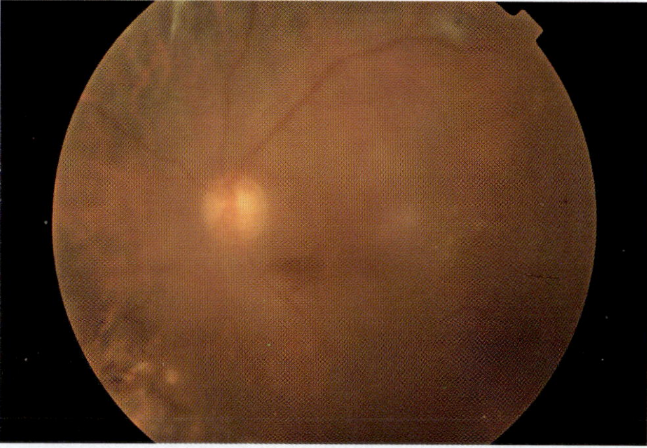

Fig. 10.9: Lasered proliferative diabetic retinopathy with recurrent vitreous hemorrhage

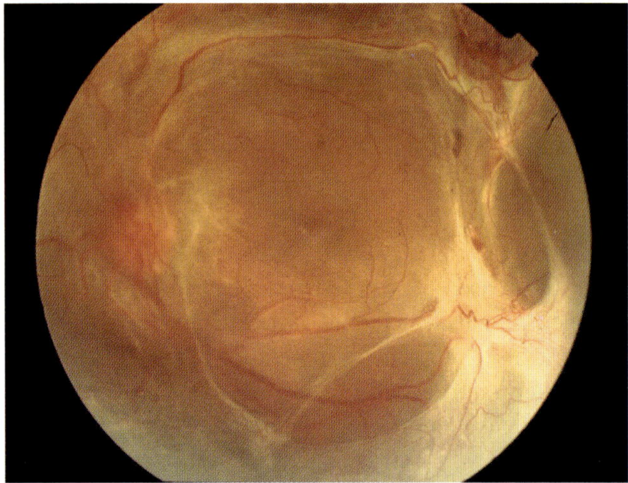

Fig. 10.10: Diabetic retinopathy with tractional retinal detachment involving macula

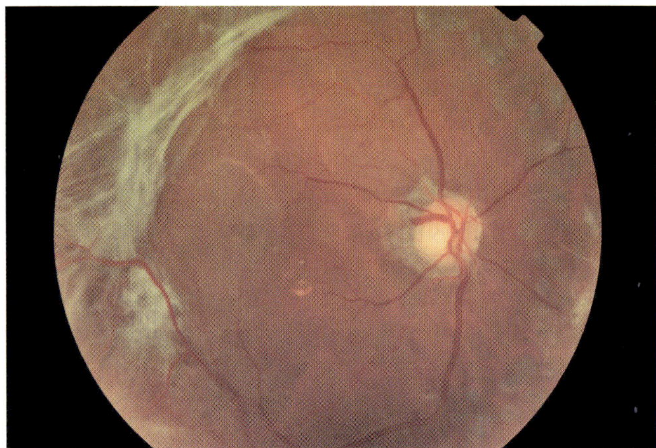

Fig. 10.11: Diabetic retinopathy with tractional retinal detachment and macular hole

SURGICAL TECHNIQUE

Preoperative Assessment

Systemic

A complete evaluation by physician and attending anesthetist is advocated. Close monitoring of blood sugar levels, hypertension and assessment of kidney status in diabetics is important. Blood thinning agents like Asprin, Clopidogrel, etc. should be stopped 3–7 days prior to surgery. Local anesthesia is preferred as most of the patients are diabetics and have associated systemic problems. A preanesthetic evaluation to assess the cooperation of the patient for a long surgery under local anesthesia is done. If cooperation is doubtful general anesthesia may be administered.

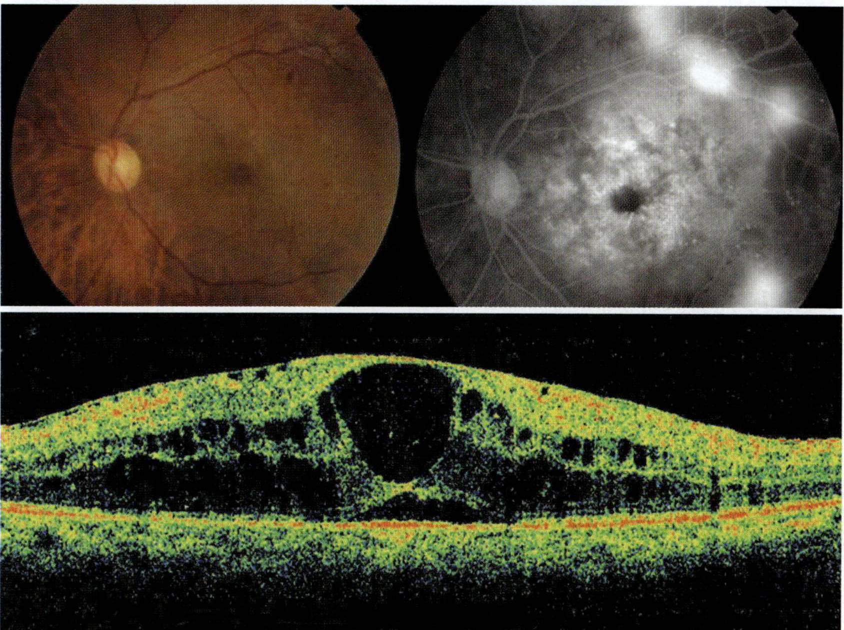

Fig. 10.12A: Preoperative color photo, FFA and OCT of a case of proliferative diabetic retinopathy with epiretinal membrane at macula and cystoid macular edema

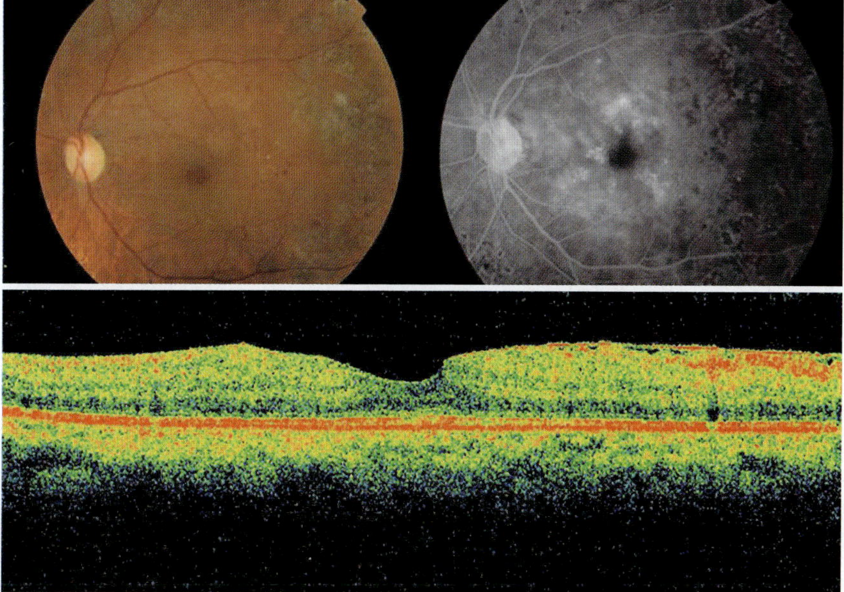

Fig. 10.12B: Postoperative color photo, FFA and OCT showing resolution of neovascularization, macular edema and restoration of foveal contour

Ocular

A detailed history including the duration of vision loss, other eye status, previous laser treatment, previous steroid or anti-VEGF therapy is important to prognosticate. (Table 10.2, Figure 10.13).

TABLE 10.2: Ocular examination

• Visual acuity
• Intraocular pressure
• Slit lamp examination
– Corneal status
– Pupillary dilation
– Iris neovascularization (NVI)
– Lens status
– Slit lamp biomicroscopy—macular status
• Indirect ophthalmoscopy
• FFA and OCT
• Ultrasonography

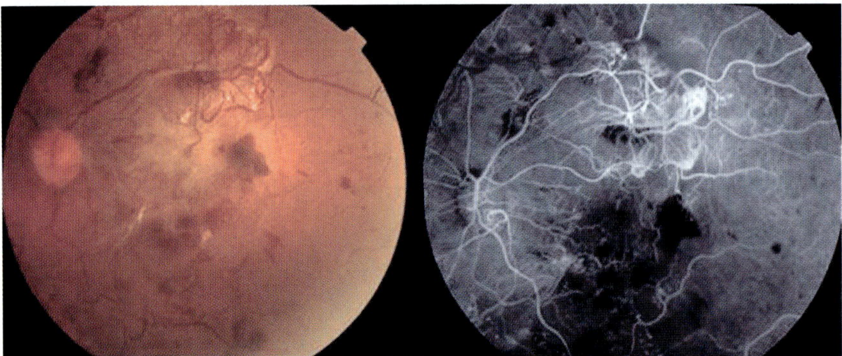

Fig. 10.13: Case of progressive fibrovascular proliferation. FFA shows macular ischemia

Preoperative Avastin

Retinal ischemia in diabetes and other vascular disorders stimulates production of VEGF, a key molecule responsible for ocular neovascularizatio.[14] Bevacizumab (Avastin), an anti-VEGF agent has been advocated for use in a variety of neovascular diseases like PDR, vascular occlusions, rubeosis iridis and corneal neovascularization. Pharmacologic involution of retinal neovascularization by administering intravitreal Avastin preoperatively decreases intraoperative complications.[15,16] It reduces intraoperative bleeding and facilitates membrane dissection. A relatively bloodless surgical field enables precise separation of the proliferative tissue from the retina and helps avoid accidental vessel damage and iatrogenic break formation. Less intraoperative bleeding decreases need for frequent instrument exchanges, use of endodiathermy and surgical time.[3,17,18]

Avastin besides causing involution of vessels also causes contraction of the proliferative tissue. This makes point adhesions between the membrane and retina more visible and creates a safer space for instrument manipulation during delamination. This aggravation of fibrosis could lead to a rapid development or progression of TRD.[19] Oshima et al reported that presence of ring shaped fibrovascular membrane formation and absence of laser photocoagulation were risk factors for progression of TRD after intravitreal Avastin administration.[3]

Caution should therefore be exercised in the timing of vitreous surgery after intravitreal Avastin administration. There is a lesser incidence of complications due to enhanced contraction of fibrous tissue if vitrectomy is performed within a week of intravitreal Avastin administration.

Pretreatment with Avastin is still not standard of care and the decision to pretreat is at the surgeon's discretion. Younger, poorly managed diabetic patients who are more likely to be phakic, have greater severity of retinopathy and presence of extensive vascular membranes are definite indications for pre-treatment. Care should be taken in cases with severe ischemia and occluded vessels. We normally administer intravitreal bevacizumab 3–5 days prior to surgery. The patient should be ascertained fit for surgery and the date of surgery scheduled before administering bevacizumab.

LENS STATUS

The most common complication of pars plana vitrectomy is development of nuclear sclerotic cataract. The incidence of cataract after PPV has been reported between 17% and 100%, with an increase in incidence with the use of tamponading agents especially silicone oil.[20,21] Besides the inevitable need of a subsequent cataract surgery which delays visual recovery, the presence of a crystalline lens during vitrectomy serves as an anatomic impediment to intraoperative surgical maneuvers especially a thorough vitreous base excision and access to epiretinal proliferation especially if it is extensive and extends to the periphery.

Most surgeons now prefer to do a combined cataract surgery with vitrectomy even if there are minimal lenticular changes. In young diabetics it may be better to leave them phakic if surgical objectives can be achieved. The earlier problem of increased anterior segment neovascularization after a combined approach has been taken care of by aggressive intraocular laser photocoagulation and advent of phacoemulsification with in the bag intraocular lens implantation. The disadvantages of concurrent cataract extraction are optic/lens capture and posterior synechiae which are more pronounced in diabetic eyes possibly due to an exaggerated fibrin response.[22-24] A 2 stage approach where the cataract surgery is performed few weeks before vitrectomy and suturing the cataract wound helps in overcoming this problem. Closure of the cataract wound with 10-0 nylon is done in all cases to decrease chances of wound leakage and anterior chamber fluctuation at the time of insertion of trocar-cannula, scleral depression and gas exchange. The corneoscleral sutures can be removed or retained at the end of vitrectomy depending on the comfort level of the operating surgeon. Some surgeons prefer to make 23 gauge/25 gauge entry prior to cataract surgery to minimize distortion of the corneal wound.

SCLEROTOMIES

Earlier, standard 20 gauge sclerotomies were made with the infusion cannula inferotemporally and the active ports superotemporally and superonasally. In MIVS, position of sclerotomies is same as in 20 gauge vitrectomy. For most cases sclerotomies are made transconjunctivally. However, we use a modified approach in the more difficult cases especially those with extensive membranes. After a 360° peritomy the 23 gauge sclerotomies are made transsclerally. The advantages of this modification are, ease in entry of chandelier illumination, thorough base dissection and easier access to membranes extending anteriorly. The disadvantage is in the need to suture the sclerotomies in a larger number of cases especially if gas is not used. For complicated vitrectomies self-retaining endoilluminators are placed at 12 o'clock and 6 o'clock to give a diffuse shadow free illumination. The endoilluminator should be taped such that the direction of light is towards the posterior pole.

VITRECTOMY

A core vitrectomy is done using a noncontact wide-angle system. For initial vitrectomy, the settings would vary from 2,000 to 5,000 cuts/min with suction at 300 to 600 mm Hg depending on the gauge of vitrectomy and the vitrectomy machine being used. An advantage of the Alcon Constellation vitrectomy system is the ability to work at a lower infusion pressure without globe collapse. In cases with proliferative membranes with or without TRD, after the vitreous hemorrhage has been cleared and the anterior vitreous cut in the line of sclerotomies, an attempt is made to identify the posterior hyaloid/vitreoschisis in the midperiphery. In most cases it is easier to identify this layer temporally as the separation from the retina is more marked here. After an opening is made it is extended circumferentially. As the subhyaloid space is opened up it may be important to clear up the subhyaloid hemorrhage before enlarging the can opener opening. As eyes with extensive membrane have incomplete vitreous separation it may not be possible to separate the membrane all over the periphery. In cases where a 360° separation from the periphery is obtained a base excision with scleral depression is done. A thorough base excision is an important step as it improves peripheral visualization enabling easier detection of retinal breaks and more complete laser treatment. Close vitreous shaving also decreases chance of immediate postoperative bleed and incidence of anterior hyaloidal proliferation. In cases where there is hardly any vitreous separation it is useful to use a bimanual approach with forceps and cutter to create an opening in the posterior hyaloid. This is a distinct advantage gained with small gauge vitrectomy.

MEMBRANE DISSECTION

Bimanual membrane delamination or modified en bloc dissection is the procedure of choice.[2,25] With the self-retaining endoillumination in place, membrane dissection is started from an area where the membrane is isolated from the periphery. In most situations it is easier to start dissection superiorly and progress inferiorly. When starting dissection it is important to keep the concept of vitreoschisis in mind so as to identify the correct surgical plane at the outset. This makes the dissection easier and atraumatic.[26,27] At the edge of TRD, the anterior edge of the membrane is held with a forceps and with a scissors a thin elastic membrane is invariably teased out which is the true hyaloid (Figure 10.14). Finding this plane improves visualization of the vascular epicenters. Raising the membrane with forceps close to these epicenters makes dissection with the scissors precise and avoids inadvertent damage to retinal vessels. Contraction or fibrosis of the membranes by preoperative Avastin also expedites dissection as discussed earlier.[3] A 23 gauge cutter is used for blunt dissection of fine attachments between the membrane and the retina. Large areas of separation can be obtained by holding the membrane with forceps and using the tip of cutter. The cutter can also trim the membrane, be used to apply pressure to bleeders to achieve hemostasis and also aspirate blood before it clots. Multiple uses of the vitrectomy probe enables lesser instrument exchanges thereby decreasing surgical time. The wide-angle system enables us to detect any undue traction especially in cases where a 360° separation from the periphery cannot be obtained. As the dissection proceeds the hyaloid gets separated and simultaneous relief of traction avoids intraoperative break formation. Iatrogenic breaks are more often seen in long-standing TRD where the retina is thin. If an intraoperative break occurs it is important to relieve all traction around the break and mark it to enable identification at time of laser treatment. Another problem encountered in extensive TRD's especially

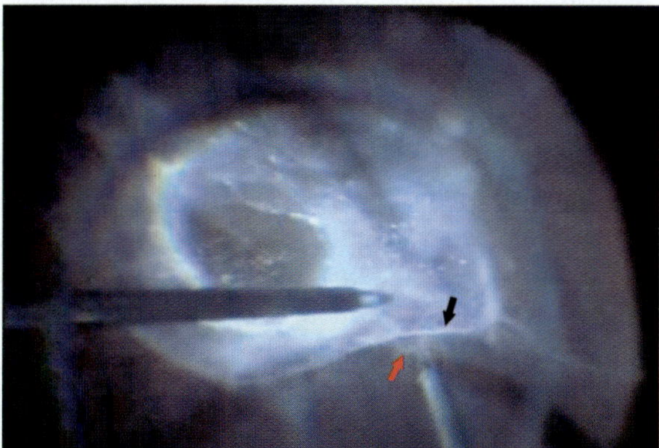

Fig. 10.14: Plane of dissection. Black arrow denotes the vitreoschisis plane. Red arrow depicts the correct plane of dissection

in combined retinal detachment is the tendency of the retina to get bullous as dissection progresses. PFCL may be used to stabilize the retina in absence of a posterior break.

With modern wide-angle viewing systems and small gauge instrumentation a complete membrane dissection is obtained in nearly all cases. In the rare situation when the posterior hyaloid does not separate till the periphery or there is residual traction a belt buckle or scleral buckle may be used.

While dissecting vascular epicenters special care is taken along the major vessels and the optic disk. Along the major vessel if a clear separation between the membrane and retina is not visible it may be safer to isolate and coagulate the attachment. It should be ensured that it is not a broad attachment holding retina and if such is the case a careful segmentation is done. Fibrovascular tissue overlying the disk is often removed with forceps. If adhesion to disk is very firm it may be preferable to trim the proliferative tissue as removal may cause hemorrhage from the fine papillary blood vessels or in extreme cases even avulse the retina at the disk. We prefer to remove the stalk in most cases. Bleeding is controlled by raising bottle height. Removing the stalk relieves peripapillary traction, decreases chance of postoperative bleeding and there has been no unfavorable visual outcome despite the reported presence of axons in histopathology specimens of optic disk stalk.[28]

HEMOSTASIS

It is important to ensure hemostasis peroperatively and at the end of surgery. In cases of nonresolving vitreous hemorrhage with no membranes it is important to search for any subtle bleeder or flat NVE. These simple cases often have a higher incidence of postoperative rebleed.

Continuing with dissection in presence of blood decreases visualization and increases chances of inadvertent damage to vessels and iatrogenic break formation. Any bleeding that occurs during dissection should be tackled immediately or else the clot that forms tends to take up the shape of the membrane as adhesions reform at the vascular epicenters. If that happens the ensuing dissection can be more difficult and traumatic than of the original membrane. Usually the clot can be removed with a soft tipped cannula by stripping it gently from the retina. In some cases when a strong adhesion has formed a bimanual dissection may be required. The bimanual technique is also helpful to control active bleeding, a soft tipped cannula removes the blood and an endodiathermy in the other hand coagulates the bleeder. Most bleeders can also be controlled by raising bottle temporarily. Direct pressure by a blunt instrument (23 gauge vitrector) works well especially on bleeders over the optic disk and major vessels where coagulation is avoided. Adrenaline is routinely used in infusion fluid.

A thorough examination of the retina for any active bleeder after lowering the infusion bottle is a must before fluid-air exchange or at the end of surgery.

TAMPONADE

Tamponade is often indicated in cases undergoing bimanual surgery for extensive TRD's . However, in absence of a retinal break and if it is a localized TRD not involving macula no tamponade is given. There has been a decrease in incidence in peripheral retinal break formation and use of tamponade with MIVS possibly due to lesser vitreous drag with the cannulated system.

Silicone oil tamponade is preferred in combined rhegmatogenous tractional RD as there is an incomplete relief of peripheral traction and often an element of PVR coexisting.[29] In all other cases long acting gas, C3F8, is used. It has been postulated that gas has a hemostatic effect by mechanically tamponading the fragile vessels and by the biochemical effect of antifibrinolytic substances compartmentalized close to the bleeding sites.[30,31] It may take 2–3 weeks for restabilizing the integrity of the injured blood vessels, so a long acting gas C3F8 is preferred to a short acting gas SF6. Another advantage of gas tamponade compared to use of silicone oil is a lesser tendency to have large bleeds in the immediate postoperative period. If bleeding does occur it does not clot over the posterior pole and therefore, there is a lesser incidence of reproliferation of membranes.[32] Long acting gas has also been found to be effective in displacing subretinal hemorrhage often seen in chronic TRD. Disadvantage of long acting gas is delayed visual recovery, increased incidence of cataract in phakic patients and excessive fibrin formation.

PHOTOCOAGULATION/CRYOTHERAPY

Aim of photocoagulation is to achieve regression of neovascular proliferation and to create chorioretinal adhesion around retinal breaks. Laser photocoagulation in pan retinal pattern, around pre-existing/iatrogenic breaks and 360° close to the ora serrata is helpful in decreasing the postoperative complications. Fill in laser photocoagulation is applied in presence of pre-existing PRP. Wide-angle viewing system has made endophotocoagulation till the periphery easier and safer. A LIO system can also be used to ensure complete peripheral laser treatment. Cryotherapy of the anterior retina and sclerotomy sites has been found to decrease the incidence of recurrent vitreous hemorrhage.[33] Meticulous base excision with a broad laser close to the ora may achieve the same purpose. The disadvantage of cryotherapy is that it causes increased postoperative inflammation and incites reproliferation. Its role is limited to cases with NVI and some surgeons use it to prevent fibrovascular ingrowth at sclerotomy site.

CLOSURE

In MIVS, closure involves removal of the cannulas. The cannulas should be removed slowly, in a tangential direction and pressure is applied with a blunt instrument. To avoid vitreous wick the eyewall should be supported while removing the cannula, cannula is removed slowly and avoid massaging the sclerotomy site. The sclerotomy site should be carefully checked for leakage and sutured in case of slightest doubt. Postoperative hypotony and risk of bleeding should be avoided. In cases where tamponade has not been used many surgeons administer Avastin at the end of surgery.

COMPLICATIONS

Complications are an inevitable though avoidable part of any surgical procedure. With improved instrumentation and surgical expertize the intraoperative and postoperative complications have reduced over the years (Table 10.3).

TABLE 10.3: Postoperative complications

• Persistent epithelial defect
• Anterior chamber inflammation
• High intraocular pressure
• Shallow anterior chamber
• Malpositioning of intraocular lens
• Cataract
• Vitreous hemorrhage
• Retinal detachement
– Tractional
– Rhegmatogenous
• Rubeosis iridis and neovascular glaucoma
• Anterior hyaloidal fibrovascular proliferation

POSTOPERATIVE HYPOTONY

Special care should be taken in diabetic vitrectomy to avoid postoperative hypotony. It is advisable to err on the side of caution and suture the scleral incision in case of the slightest doubt. Postoperative hypotony not only predisposes to postoperative vitreous hemorrhage but also choroidal detachment which is difficult to manage in the labile systemic condition of most diabetic patients.

POSTOPERATIVE VITREOUS HEMORRHAGE

Recurrent vitreous hemorrhage is one of the commonest complications after diabetic vitrectomy.[2] The incidence varies from 29% to 75%. Postoperative vitreous hemorrhage can be broadly classified into early and late.

Early postoperative hemorrhage is often due to residual blood on retinal surface which was not cleared intraoperatively or was present in the peripheral vitreous skirt. Other causes could be inadvertent intraoperative trauma to retinal vessels, residual fibrovascular tissue and persistent retinal traction. In MIVS it is often due to postoperative hypotony as mentioned earlier.

Late vitreous hemorrhage is most commonly seen due to neovascularization at sclerotomy site. Recalcitrant fibrovascular proliferation, persistent neovascularization due to inadequate laser photocoagulation, incomplete removal of fibrovascular proliferation, retinal break formation, iris or angle neovascularization are other causes of late postoperative vitreous hemorrhage.

Preoperative and in some cases postoperative Avastin, complete bimanual membrane delamination, complete laser photocoagulation (panretinal and peripheral), long acting gas tamponade, careful wound closure help in decreasing the incidence of postoperative vitreous hemorrhage, rubeosis iridis and anterior hyaloidal proliferation (AHFVP).

POSTOPERATIVE RETINAL DETACHMENT

Postoperative retinal detachment could be tractional or rhegmatogenous. Reproliferation of membranes is the commonest cause. Membrane dissection in the correct plane, complete removal of all membranes and tamponade with gas helps to decrease reproliferation.

Rhegmatogenous retinal detachment could be due to a posterior or a peripheral break. To avoid missing of a posterior retinal break during laser photocoagulation the break should be marked during the course of surgery and all traction around the hole should be relieved. As mentioned earlier the cannulated system in MIVS and a thorough base excision decreases incidence of peripheral retinal break formation.

REFERENCES

1. Aaberg TM, Abrams GW. Changing indications and techniques for vitrectomy in management of complications of diabetic retinopathy. Ophthalmol. 1987;94:775–9.
2. Eliott D, Lee MS, Abrams GS. Proliferative diabetic retinopathy: Principles and techniques of surgical treatment. In: Ryan SJ, Hinton DR, Schachat AP, Wilkinson P, eds. Retina. Vol. 3. Surgical Retina. 4th ed. Philadelphia: Elsevier Mosby; 2006:2413–5.
3. Oshima Y, Shima C, Wakabayashi T, et al. Microincision vitrectomy surgery and intravitreal bevacizumab as a surgical adjunct to treat diabetic traction retinal detachment. Ophthalmol. 2009;116:927–38.
4. Kaiser PK. Advanced vitreous cutter offers duty cycle control. Retinal Physician. 2009;15–17.
5. Ibarra MS, Hermel M, Prenner JL, Hassan TS. Longer-term outcomes of transconjunctival sutureless 25 gauge vitrectomy. Am J Ophthalmol. 2005;139(5): 831–6.
6. Eckardt C. Transconjunctival sutureless 23 gauge vitrectomy. Retina. 2005;25:208 –11.
7. Fine HF, Iranmanesh R, Iturralde D, Spaide RF. Outcomes of 77 consecutive cases of 23 gauge transconjunctival vitrectomy surgery for posterior segment disease. Ophthalmol. 2007;114:1197–2000.
8. Endo internet.
9. Tornambe PE. Vitrectomy surgery illumination using #26 Torpedo Mini Lights. Video presented at The Fourth Annual Vitreous Society Film Festival; San Fransisco; 2002.

10. Oshima Y, Awh CC, Tano Y. Self-retaining 27 gauge transconjunctival chandelier illumination for panoramic viewing during vitreous surgery. Am J Ophthalmol. 2007; 43:166–7.
11. Eckardt C. Twin lights: A new chandelier illumination for bimanual surgery. Retina. 2003;23:893–4.
12. Joussen AM, Joeres S. Benefits and limitations in vitreoretinal surgery for proliferative diabetic retinopathy and macular edema. Developments in Ophthalmol. 2007;39:69–87.
13. Gandorfer A, Messmer EM, Ulbig MW. Resolution of macular edema after surgical removal of the posterior hyaloid and the internal limiting membrane. Retina. 2000; 20:126–33.
14. Adamis AP, Miller JW, Bernal MT, et al. Increased vascular endothelial growth factor levels in the vitreous of eyes with proliferative diabetic retinopathy. Am J Ophthalmol. 1994;118:445–50.
15. Avery RL, Pearlman J, Pieramici DJ, et al. Intravitreal bevacizumab (Avastin) in the treatment of proliferative diabetic retinopathy. Ophthalmol. 2006;113:1695–705.
16. Spaide RF, Fisher YL. Intravitreal bevacizumab (Avastin) treatment of proliferative diabetic retinopathy complicated by vitreous hemorrhage. Retina. 2006;26: 275–8.
17. Chen E, Park CH. Use of intravitreal bevacizumab as a preoperative adjunct for tractional retinal detachment repair in severe proliferative diabetic retinopathy. Retina. 2006;26:699–700.
18. Rizzo S, Genovesi-Ebert F, Di Bartolo E, et al. Injection of intravitreal bevacizumab (Avastin) as a preoperative adjunct before vitrectomy surgery in the treatment of severe proliferative diabetic retinopathy (PDR). Graefes Arch Clin Exp Ophthalmol. 2008;246:837–42.
19. Arevalo JF, Maia M, Flynn HW Jr, et al. Tractional retinal detachment following intravitreal bevacizumab (Avastin) in patients with severe proliferative diabetic retinopathy. Br J Ophthalmol. 2008;92:213–6.
20. Schiff WM, Barile GR, Hwang JC, et al. Diabetic vitrectomy: Influence of lens status upon anatomic and visual outcomes. Ophthalmol. 2007;114:544–50.
21. Federman JL, Schubert HD. Complications associated with the use of silicone oil in 150 eyes after retina-vitreous surgery. Ophthalmology. 1988;95(7):870–6.
22. Schachat AP, Oyakawa RT, Michels RG, Rice TA. Complications of vitreous surgery for diabetic retinopathy: Postoperative complications. Ophthalmol. 1983;90:522–9.
23. Lahey JM, Francis RR, Kearney JJ. Combining phacoemulsification with pars plana vitrectomy in patients with proliferative diabetic retinopathy: A series of 223 cases. Ophthalmol. 2003;110:1335–9.
24. Honjo M, Ogura Y. Surgical results of pars plana vitrectomy combined with phacoemulsification and intraocular lens implantation for complications of proliferative diabetic retinopathy. Ophthalmic Surg Lasers. 1998;29:99–105.
25. Han DP, Murphy ML, Mieler WF. A modified en bloc excision technique during vitrectomy for diabetic traction retinal detachment: Results and complications. Ophthalmol. 1994;101:803–8.
26. Schwartz SD, Alexander R, Hiscott P, et al. Recognition of vitreoschisis in proliferative diabetic retinopathy. Ophthalmol. 1996;103:323–8.
27. Chu TG, Lopez PF, Cano MR, et al. Posterior vitreoschisis. Ophthalmol. 1996;103: 315–22.
28. Pendergast SD, Martin DF, Proia Ad, et al. Removal of optic disc stalks during diabetic vitrectomy. Retina. 1995;15:25–8.

29. Riedel KG, Gabel VP, Neubauer L, et al. Intravitreal silicone oil injection: Complications and treatment of 415 consecutive patients. Graefes Arch Clin Exp Ophthalmol. 1990;228:19.
30. Yang CM, Yeh PT, Yang CH. Intravitreal long-acting gas in the prevention of early postoperative vitreous hemorrhage in diabetic vitrectomy. Ophthalmol. 2007;114:710–5.
31. Koutsandrea CN, Apostolopoulos MN, Chatzoulis DZ, et al. Hemostatic effects of SF6 after diabetic vitrectomy for vitreous hemorrhage. Acta Ophthalmol Scand. 2001;79:34–8.
32. Chow DR, Bustros S. Control of perioperative bleeding in vitreoretinal surgery. In: Ryan SJ, Hinton DR, Schachat AP, Wilkinson P, eds. Retina. Vol. 3. Surgical Retina. 4th ed. Philadelphia: Elsevier Mosby; 2006:2413–5.
33. Yeh PT, Yang CM, Yang CH, Huang JS. Cryotherapy of the anterior retina and sclerotomy sites in diabetic vitrectomy to prevent recurrent vitreous hemorrhage: An ultrasound biomicroscopy study. Ophthalmol. 2005;112:2095–102.

CHAPTER

11

Small Gauge Vitrectomy in Endophthalmitis

(It is better than Conventional 20 Gauge Vitrectomy for Endophthalmitis)

Gopal S Pillai, Lalit Verma

Small gauge vitreous surgery is a recent advance, idea borrowed from anterior segment colleagues. There have been concerns regarding increased incidence of infectious endophthalmitis after small gauge vitreous surgery—But after refinements in wound construction, conjunctival displacement, single step entry with better and sharper instrumentation, taking steps to prevent post-operative leaks, incidence of endophthalmitis seems to be no higher than conventional surgery. Infact, more and more surgeons are employing small gauge vitreous surgery in the management of postoperative endophthalmitis. Some of the challenges which one may face during vitrectomy for endophthalmitis include:

1. Corneal, limbal and scleral involvement and melt
2. Cheese wiring of sutures
3. Poor visibility due to corneal haziness
4. Poor visibility due to papillary fibrin
5. Lens management in post-traumatic and endogenous endophthalmitis
6. IOL dislocation when anterior segment is cleaned
7. Cases which may need IOL removal
8. Infusion placement in the presence of choroidal edema and exudates
9. Shift of infusion or active ports from one side to other
10. Poor flow as infusion can get blocked with exudates
11. Absence of PVD, especially in post-traumatic endophthalmitis
12. Fragile retina and PVD induction can cause RD
13. Dialysis at the active port
14. Peripheral retinal tears during vitrectomy
15. Chances of bleed high as tissues are hyperemic.

Now let us see, how small gauge vitrectomy would fare in the presence of these challenges.

Corneal, Limbal and Scleral Involvement and Melt

Corneal and limbal as well as scleral involvement is not infrequent in endophthalmitis. It may spread out from the region of the surgical wound or the area of trauma. The sclera and cornea may start sloughing out and may even need tectonic support to save the globe. Small gauge vitrectomy will help us in this stage as we can easily go in through the nonnecrotic areas and without any sutures take the instruments out of the eye. In an ordinary 20 gauge vitrectomy, the scleral port sutures may be difficult to be placed through sloughed sclera.

Cheese Wiring of Sutures

Again, since the sutures may cheese wire through the sclera and cornea, it may be always better to consider doing sutureless procedures in vitrectomy for endophthalmitis. With large openings of 20 gauge surgery chances of cheese wiring will increase.

Poor Visibility due to Corneal Haziness or Pupillary Fibrin

No gross difference between 20 gauge or small gauge vitrectomy in media haze. However, if the media haziness is secondary to anterior or posterior capsular opacification or fibrin, then the small gauge probe can help us remove the opacification or fibrin through a small paracentesis or through the port in a more controlled fashion than with a 20 gauge probe.

Lens Management in Post-traumatic and Endogenous Endophthalmitis

If one has to do a lensectomy or phacofragmentation to remove the crystalline lens, the advantage of sutureless vitrectomy is lost because there is no small gauge phacofragmentor and lensectomy with small gauge probe may be more time consuming. However, the improved fluidics of small gauge vitrectomy including lesser turbulence can be of value in managing the surgery. Lesser fluid turbulence can help in reducing endothelial loss in anterior segment management of endophthalmitis surgery.

IOL Dislocation or Intended Removal of IOL

In cases where there is a dislocated IOL or where there is a need to remove the IOL, then we may have to enlarge the limbal incision and here too, the advantage of sutureless incision is lost. However, more fluidic stability and less turbulence may help in reducing endothelial loss during such surgeries which also requires an IOL removal.

Infusion Cannula Placement in the Presence of Choroidal Edema or Exudates

Infusion cannula placement in endophthalmitis is a very critical step. In many cases, there will be choroidal edema and thickening and exudates are very close to the insertion of the port that a blunt MVR blade or a blunt trocar/cannula system can cause a dialysis and the tip of the cannula can become suprachoroidal or subretinal. It is more common in small gauge vitrectomy system because the sharp edge of the trocar is followed by the blunt tubing of the port. Another reason is that the cannula is about 4 mm only in small gauge. We routinely use 6 mm infusion cannulas in endophthalmitis so that this complication does not arise. However, in 25 or 23 gauge systems, we do not at this point of time have a 6 mm infusion cannula.

Shift of Infusion or Active Port from One Port to Another

During the course of vitrectomy, one may need to change the active port from one port to another or need to change the infusion cannula from one port to another. This is easily achieved in a small gauge vitrectomy system as one can easily pluck out the infusion cannula from one port and insert it onto another port to suit our need and necessity for the active port. This can help us in virtually having the active instrument through any of the three ports including the infusion port.

Poor Flow as Infusion can get Blocked with Exudates

The rate of flow through a small gauge 25 gauge system is much lesser than that through a classical 20 gauge system and because of this and the narrow bore of the 25 gauge system, the small gauge probe gets blocked very quickly with exudates. Even though at the beginning of surgery, the tip of the port is visualized, during the course of surgery, since the flow of fluid is small, it may easily be blocked by the thick exudates of endophthalmitis. Once the cannula is blocked, it may give rise to sudden hypotony and its complications.

Absence of PVD

Posterior vitreous detachment may be absent in many cases with endophthalmitis. In most cases, we can very carefully induce a PVD, and a more controlled induction may be possible with a small gauge system. In cases where PVD is difficult to be induced, we may use the probe to go as close to the retina as possible to shave the exudates. In such a scenario, it is always better to have the small probe, with its tip very close to the edge of the probe.

PVD Induction in Fragile Retina causing Retinal Tear

If the PVD is not easily inducible, and if we continue pulling on the vitreous to induce a PVD, it could cause tears in fragile and inflamed retina. The incidence will be lesser with a small gauge probe as there will be more fluidic control for the same.

Retinal Dialysis of the Active Port

When there are a lot of exudates around the sleeve of the port and when blunt instruments go in and out of the port, there can be chances of retinal dialysis.

The chances of such dialysis are lesser in a port with a sleeve as in small gauge surgery as the instrument always passes in and out of the eye through the sleeve. However, in a large gauge probe, the entries are risky in terms of retinal dialysis.

Peripheral Tears during Vitrectomy

The incidence of peripheral tears during vitrectomy may be the same with both small gauge and large gauge systems. But in the management of such a tear, closer shaving and relief of vitreous traction on the tear may be more efficient with a small gauge vitrectomy system than a classical 20 gauge system.

Conclusion

Small gauge vitreous biopsy also offers tissue diagnosis through a very small opening without risk of vitreous pull or hypotony in contrast to a 20 gauge vitreous biopsy. Thus, the small gauge system offers many surgical advantages over the classical 20 gauge system in the surgical management of endophthalmitis. This is in addition to the fact that small gauge systems are less painful and lesser inflammatory than the classical 20 gauge systems in the management of endophthalmitis.

CHAPTER

12

MIVS for Vitreous Hemorrhage

Sourav Sinha

The evolution of modern vitreoretinal surgery has produced significant advancements since its first description in 1971 by Machemer et al.[1] His original 17 gauge multifunctional instrument began a wave of ingenuity that would dramatically change the way we treat ocular disease.

Since then, improvements in technology, surgeon experience, and our understanding of pathophysiology have led to increasingly safer and effective vitrectomy. Following Machemer's initiative, numerous investigators have sought to develop a smaller, sutureless vitrectomy system to minimize iatrogenic insult to eyes with posterior segment pathology. These efforts led to the development of the 23 and 25 gauge transconjunctival sutureless vitrectomy system by de Juan and coworkers, first described by Fujii et al in 2002.[2,3]

The development of small incision vitrectomy allows for smaller construction and less traumatic operations that may result in less post-operative inflammation, less patient morbidity, and faster patient recovery. Improvements in small gauge surgical techniques and instrumentation have led to more efficient vitreous removal, and they have helped to expand the surgical indications.

VITREOUS HEMORRHAGE

The causes for vitreous hemorrhage are multiple, but the commonest in our setting are due to proliferative diabetic retinopathy, venous occlusions, trauma and Eales'.

Most surgeons would take up all cases of vitreous hemorrhage today with the 23 gauge system. The availability of different instrumentation, improved quality of light source and ease of procedures such as silicone oil injection have made things much easier.[4] The cutting port is nearly 50% closer to the tip of the probe in 23 and 25 gauge systems as compared to 20 gauge system. Since the high cutting rate limits the movement of the retina, membrane removal can often be achieved by this instrument alone. This is particularly useful in tractional retinal detachment cases with limited vitreoretinal attachment.

In cases with more extensive attachments bimanual membrane dissection may be done.

Basic steps of visualizing the cannula prior to starting vitrectomy which should be followed by all beginners. Need to remove the anterior vitreous before proceeding to midvitreous cavity will help in better visualization throughout the surgery.[5] Proceeding from the periphery to the center helps in most cases. It is also not a good idea to use suction to try to induce PVD as one would do in a case of retinal detachment. Presence of underlying membranes can lead to retinal tears.

Using of triamcinolone acetonide (TA) to stain the vitreous is of immense help in some cases where one is not able to visualize the vitreous very well.[6] The timing of injecting the TA is also important. It should be done after debulking the vitreous. Upon completing vitrectomy one should trim the vitreous skirt as short as possible so as to prevent trickling down of the hem postopertively. It is also important to prevent an inadvertent lens touch by not trying to perform vitrectomy in the diagonally opposite area in the far periphery. It is better to change hands and do vitrectomy on the same side. Checking posterior to sclerotomy sites after completion of surgery should be done routinely. Tears posterior to sclerotomy sites with the 23 and 25 gauge systems are far less common than with 20 gauge system.

PROLIFERATIVE DIABETIC RETINOPATHY

Surgical indications for PDR have evolved over the past 3 decades toward earlier intervention as techniques and instrumentation improve. Surgeons gain more experience, and procedures become safer with fewer complications. Currently, the most common indications for 23 gauge vitrectomy in PDR are severe premacular subhyaloid hemorrhage, nonclearing vitreous hemorrhage (VH), and tractional retinal detachment.[7] In all surgical cases of PDR complications, the relationship between the posterior hyaloid and the retina is one of the most important factors associated with the severity of disease. To precisely plan a surgical repair, it is crucial for a surgeon to understand the variety of vitreoretinal adhesions in diabetic eyes.

Nonclearing VH is the most common proliferative diabetic indication for 23 gauge sutureless vitrectomy. Though the Diabetic Retinopathy Vitrectomy Study suggested that acute intervention at 6 months is better than intervention at 1 year, most surgeons currently do not wait nearly as long to perform vitrectomy given the increased safety and ease of surgery, particularly with 23 and 25 gauge instrumentation. Most now wait 6 to 8 weeks from presentation to allow spontaneous clearing of the hemorrhage, and generally prefer to follow parameters such as the amount and pace of improvement, need to apply laser in the face of anterior segment neovascularization, status of the other eye, and patient employment and lifestyle issues. Some surgeons proceed with surgery even sooner if the hemorrhage is located in the premacular space due to its potential retinal toxicity and promotion of surface wrinkling.

Ghost-cell glaucoma may complicate cases of very severe VH if degenerated nonclearing red blood cells (ghost cells) reduce or block aqueous outflow through the trabecular meshwork. 23 gauge vitrectomy is an ideal surgical option if the intraocular pressure is uncontrollably elevated despite medical intervention. Aphakic eyes offer easy access for 23 gauge instruments to the anterior chamber. In pseudophakic eyes, an opening can be made in the posterior capsule with a 23 gauge vitrector to allow access to the accumulated ghost cells.

Contraction of fibrovascular proliferation along the retinal surface can lead to tractional retinal detachments, potentially affecting the macula. In such cases, the posterior hyaloid is generally attached to the retina, epiretinal fibrous tissue, and sometimes the vitreous base. Vitrectomy can relieve the traction between these structures thereby restoring the anatomy and improving VA. Extramacular tractional retinal detachments, particularly when nasally located, are infrequently approached surgically as they do not often progress into visually significant regions.[8] However, some may induce macular retinal folds if they are broadly attached to the macula by a taut posterior hyaloid.

Retinal breaks may form if progressive fibrous contraction occurs at epicenters or along vessels leading to a combined traction/rhegmatogenous retinal detachment. Vitrectomy is required to repair a combined traction/ rhegmatogenous retinal detachment as soon as possible to minimize vision loss and limit progression of proliferative vitreoretinopathy.[9] The combined detachment often extends anteriorly and is usually associated with an attached posterior hyaloid.

VASCULAR OCCLUSIONS

Both branch and central retinal vein occlusions are associated with vitreous hemorrhage when then there is development of neovascularization.

In BRVO, when there is vitreous hemorrhage one should be particularly careful in the performing the preoperative ultrasound. It is important to assess the presence of fibrovascular proliferation as the adhesions are broad-based and unlike those as in proliferative diabetic retinopathty. Vitrectomy here too should be done from the periphery. Dissection of membranes here can be sometimes more difficult than in diabetics. Most commonly the membranes spread out to over the macula in which case all the traction has to be relieved.

In CRVO, the prognosis is usually very poor and one should check for rubeosis and the angles very carefully.[10] Vitrectomy should be taken up earlier in these cases since the eyes may go in for neovascular glaucoma very quickly. Extensive and aggressive laser should be done in these patients. Anterior retinal cryopexy can also be considered if necessary.

EALES' DISEASE

A large number of patients here are of the younger age group. Absence of PVD or presence of vitreoschisis is quite common. Staining of vitreous with TA is a very helpful step. If necessary restaining after the surgery has progressed to some extent can be done. Fibrovascular proliferations can extend to the far periphery. In some cases where dissection is incomplete or where a break has occurred perioperatively it may be necessary to put in an encirclage. It can defeat the purpose of doing 23 gauge surgery but anatomical stability of the retina should be the foremost criteria.

Those cases where there is extensive traction on the nasal side and the macular traction has been relieved completely it may be wiser to leave them alone.[11] Good laser photocoagulation staying about 2 disk diameters away should be done.

TRAUMA

Vitreous hemorrhage can be due to either penetrating or blunt trauma. In penetrating trauma where primary wound repair has been done it is best to wait for 10–14 days before taking up for resurgery. Even in case of blunt trauma an earlier surgery if there is no sign of heme clearing up should be contemplated. All trauma cases may have an associated anterior segment pathology like a cornea edema/wound or raised intraocular pressure or subluxated or cataractous lens. In the posterior segment along with the vitreous hemorrhage there may be a retinal pathology like a retinal tear or dialysis or a subretinal heme.[12] 23 gauge vitrectomy can easily be done in any of these cases. Manipulation is rather easier and the reduced surgical time gives better results.

SPECIAL CONSIDERATIONS IN MIVS FOR VITREOUS HEMORRHAGE

1. Dense vitreous hemorrhage may prevent the visualization of the cannula inside the vitreous cavity. Infusion must not be begun before seeing the tip of the cannula. Infusion cannula may be placed in the anterior chamber and anterior vitrectomy is done. Once the anterior vitreous is debulked, the cannula can be easily seen and the infusion cannula is placed in the cannula. Ohno et al proposed using longer 5.5 mm cannula instead of the regular 4 mm cannula for vitreous surgery for vitreous hemorrhage.[13] This longer cannula is more likely to be easily visualized within the vitreous cavity and prevent suprachoroidal placement of the cannula.
2. Minimally invasive 25, 27 and 30 gauge vitreous surgery is best suited for recurrent vitreous hemorrhage following vitrectomy, especially in diabetics. Vitreous lavage using 25 or 27 gauge allows the surgeon to identify areas of blood ooze and suitable cauterization. 30 gauge vitreous lavage was shown by Satyen et al to be useful for clearing the vitreous hemorrhage. However, this process does not allow cauterization or endolaser.

COMPLICATIONS SPECIFIC TO MIVS FOR VITREOUS HEMORRHAGE

1. Dense vitreous hemorrhage may clog the 25 gauge cutter during vitrectomy.[14] This problem is however less likely in the 23 gauge cutter due to the larger lumen. Hence, the vitreous surgeon may choose a suitable gauge depending upon the consistency of the vitreous hemorrhage.
2. Shinoda et al reported jamming of the 25 gauge cannula during instrument removal in vitrectomy for dense old vitreous hemorrhage.[15] The light pipe and cutter became locked and the cannula had to be removed with the instrument. Old vitreous hemorrhage was found to be present between the instrument and inner lumen of the cannula. This occurred in 3 of the 45 eyes that underwent 25 gauge vitrectomy for vitreous hemorrhage. Two of these eyes had formation of giant retinal breaks which were treated with encirclage and endotamponade. New cannulas were inserted in the original tract to allow completion of the surgery. Nam et al experienced a similar problem of jamming of the instrument with 23 gauge system in vitrectomy for severe vitreous hemorrhage in one patient of the 50 eyes operated.[16] They were however able to remove the instrument after stabilizing the collar of the cannula. No complications were noted by them.
3. Dark old vitreous hemorrhage may sometimes be seen subconjunctivally at the sclerotomy site after removal of cannulas. This must be cleared after conjuctival peritomy. Two methods that may prevent incarceration of the old vitreous hemorrhage in the sclerotomy are using valves and light pipe assisted removal of cannulas.

REFERENCES

1. Machemer R , Buettner H, Norton EWD, et al. Vitrectomy: A pars plana approach. Trans Am Acad Ophthalmol Otolaryngol. 1971;75:813.
2. Fujii G, de Juan E Jr, Humayun MS, et al. A new 25-gauge instrument system for transconjunctival sutureless vitrectomy surgery. Ophthamology. 2002;109:1807–12.
3. Fujii G, de Juan E Jr, Humayun MS, et al. Initial experience using the transconjunctival sutureless vitrectomy system for vitreoretinal surgery. Ophthalmology. 2002;109(10):1814–20.
4. Eckardt C. Transconjunctival sutureless 23-gauge vitrectomy. Retina. 2005;25:208–11.
5. Kunikata H, Nitta F, Meguro Y, et al. Difficulty in inserting 23 and 25-gauge trocar cannula during vitrectomy. Ophthalmologica. 2011;226:198–204.
6. Couch CM, Bakri SJ. Use of triamcinolone during vitrectomy surgery to visualize membranes and vitreous. Clin Ophthalmol. 2008;4:891–96.
7. Issa SA, Connor A, Habib M, et al. Comparison of retinal breaks observed during 23 gauge transconjunctival vitrectomy versus conventional 20 gauge surgery for proliferative diabetic retinopathy. Clin Ophthalmol. 2011;5:109–14.
8. Lakhanpal RR, Humayun MS, de Juan E, et al. Outcomes of 140 consecutive cases of 25-gauge transconjunctival surgery for posterior segment disease. Ophthalmology. 2005;112:817–24.

9. Ibara MS, Hermel M, Prenner JL, et al. Longer-term outcomes of transconjunctival sutureles 25-gauge vitrectomy. Am J Ophthalmol. 2005;139:831–6.
10. Chuang LH, Wang NK, Chen YP, et al. Vitrectomy and panretinal photocoagulation reduces the occurrence of neovascular glaucoma in central retinal vein occlusion with vireous haemorrhage. Retina. 2012 Oct 30.
11. Shukla D, Kanungo S, Prasad NM, et al. Surgical outcomes for vitrectomy in Eales' disease. Eye (Lond). 2008;22(7):900–4.
12. Ehlrich R, Polkinghorne P. Small gauge vitrectomy in traumatic retinal detachment. Clin Experimental Ophthalmol. 2011;39:429–33.
13. Hisato O, Kenji I. A Long Cannula for Microincision Vitrectomy. Retina. 2012;32(7):1435–7.
14. Natarajan S, Agarwal A. 25 guage suturless vitrectomy. Day Surg J India. 2006;2:23–7.
15. Shinoda H, Nakajima T, Shinoda K, Suzuki K, Ishida S, Inoue M. Jamming of 25-gauge instruments in the cannula during vitrectomy for vitreous haemorrhage. Acta Ophthalmol. 2008;86:160–4.
16. Nam DH, Ku M, Sohn HJ, Lee DY. Jamming of 23-gauge instruments in the micro-cannula during vitrectomy for severe vitreous haemorrhage. Acta Ophthalmologica. 2010;88(4):e134–5.

CHAPTER

13

MIVS for Retinal Detachment

Harsha Bhattacharya

INTRODUCTION

Rhegmatogenous retinal detachment is an important cause of painless diminution of vision with an annual incidence of 1 in 10,000. It complicates 0.4–1% of eyes undergoing phacoemulsification.[1] The two most common reattachment procedures are scleral buckling and pars plana vitrectomy.[2] The Scleral Buckling versus Primary Vitrectomy in Rhegmatogenous Retinal Detachment Study reflected a benefit of sclera buckling in phakic eyes with respect to best corrected visual acuity. Pars plana vitrectomy was recommended in pseudophakic eyes owing to no difference in best corrected visual acuity and better anatomic outcome compared to scleral buckling.[3] The current literature suggests that pars plana vitrectomy may represent a reasonable primary approach in selected cases.

The advent of microincisional vitrectomy surgery, wide-angle viewing systems, better endoillumination and perfluorocarbon liquids (PFCL) have increased the scope of pars plana vitrectomy in the management of rhegmatogenous retinal detachment.

HISTORICAL BACKGROUND

Microincision vitrectomy surgery (MIVS) is one of the most significant innovations in the field of vitreoretinal surgery since the development of modern vitrectomy by Machemer et al in early 1970. Machemer et al performed pars plana vitrectomy using a 17 gauge vitrector (1.5 mm diameter) through a 2.3 mm scleral incision.[4] O' Malley and Heintz introduced 20 gauge vitrector (0.9 mm diameter) in 1974.[5] This three port 20 gauge cannula entry system became the gold standard in vitreous surgery. This technique requires the conjunctival dissection and the creation of three 1.4 mm linear scleral incisions.

De Juan and Hickingbotham designed variety of 25 gauge vitreoretinal instruments (0.5 mm diameter) and the era of sutureless vitrectomy begins. 25 gauge transconjunctival vitrectomy system was introduced by Fujii et al in 2002.[6]

Eckardt introduced 23 gauge system (0.75 mm diameter) in 2005.[7] 27 gauge instruments have been used for macular surgeries. 27 gauge instruments (0.40 mm diameter) are being developed for complicated procedures.[8]

INSTRUMENTATION

The 23 gauge transconjunctival sutureless vitrectomy system consists of 23 gauge microcannular system and wide array of vitreoretinal instruments. 23 gauge microcannular system includes microcannulas, insertion trocars, an infusion cannula, plug forceps and cannula plugs.

The microcannula is a steel tube of 4 mm in length (without its head) with an external collar which can be grasped with the forceps. The internal diameter of the cannula is 0.65 mm and the external diameter is 0.75 mm. The external openings of two of three microcannulas are funnel shaped to facilitate insertion of instruments (Figure 13.1). Now-a-days a valved trocar-cannula system is available which prevents the reflux of fluid out of the ports following extraction of instruments out of the eye. Both the sharp and blunt insertion trocars are available for creating one step and two step scleral incisions respectively. The 23 gauge infusion cannula consists of a small steel tube that fits snugly into the microcannula.

A wide array of 23 gauge vitreoretinal instruments are available which includes pneumatic vitreous cutter, electromagnetic vitreous cutter, wide-angle endoillumination probe, flute needle with back flush handle, scissors, end-gripping forceps, endolaser probe, endodiathermy probe, Hem-stopper, radial optic neurotomy knife, retinal pick.

The three leading vitreoretinal surgery systems—Alcon's Accurus Surgical system, Alcon's Constellation Vision System, and Baush & Lomb's Millennium

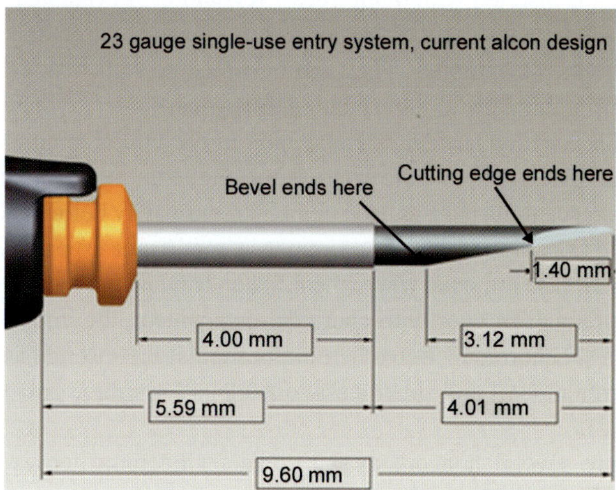

Fig. 13.1: Alcon 23 gauge trocar cannula

Transconjunctival Sutureless Vitrectomy System—are all the options for the 23 gauge vitreous surgery.

BASIC SURGICAL TECHNIQUE

Anesthesia

23 gauge surgery is usually performed under local anesthesia. General anesthesia is preferred in selected patients. 23 gauge surgery can be performed under topical anesthesia but duration and complexity of surgery should be evaluated before considering topical vitrectomy. A prospective study comparing 25 gauge and 23 gauge sutureless vitrectomy under topical 2% lignocaine gel to 25/23 gauge sutureless vitrectomy under peribulbar block showed no statistically difference in pain levels between the groups.[9]

Technique

The most essential step for the success of 23 gauge sutureless vitrectomy is the configuration of the sclerotomy to achieve self-sealing wound. This is achieved by misaligning the conjunctival and sclera entry sites and creating an oblique wound. Cotton tipped applicator can be used to displace conjunctiva slightly to induce misalignment between the conjunctival and scleral incision before insertion of microcannula into the eye. Two types of wound constructions have been described one step and two step incisions. One step incision involves the entry with the sharp trocar with overlying cannula. Two step incisions involves the initial entry through the conjunctiva, sclera and pars plana 3–4 mm from the corneoscleral limbus (depending on phakic status) with a 45° angled stiletto blade at an angle of 20° to 30° to sclera and then cannula is inserted with blunt trocar. Teixeira et al evaluated ultrasound biomicroscopy images of recent postoperative 23 gauge vitrectomy using one step and two step techniques. They demonstrated no statistical difference in sclerotomy site diameter at ultrasound biomicroscopy.[10]

After the insertion of first microcannula in the inferotemporal quadrant, infusion cannula is fitted into the external opening of the microcannula. The tip of the infusion cannula is visualized in the vitreous cavity before switching on the balanced salt solution. This is of immense importance especially in highly bullous retinal detachments, where the infusion cannula may inadvertently be placed sub-retinal. In eyes with choroidal detachment, the infusion cannula may remain subchoroidal. Two other microcannulas are inserted and plugged in the superotemporal and superonasal quadrants for a three port vitrectomy (Figure 13.2).

There are several noncontact and contact vitrectomy lenses with self-stabilizing system for intraoperative viewing.

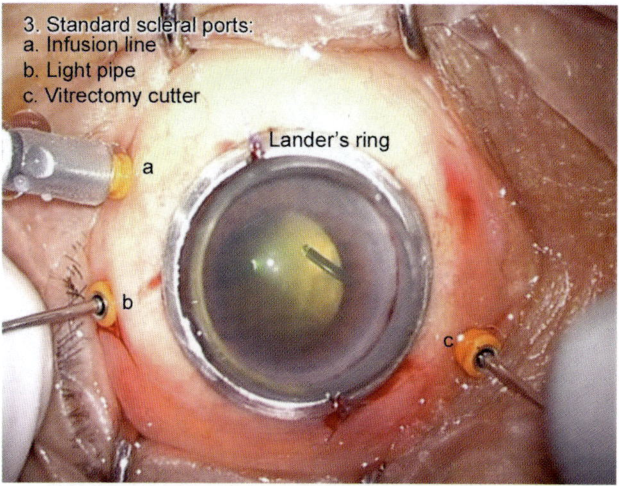

Fig. 13.2: 23 gauge three port vitrectomy

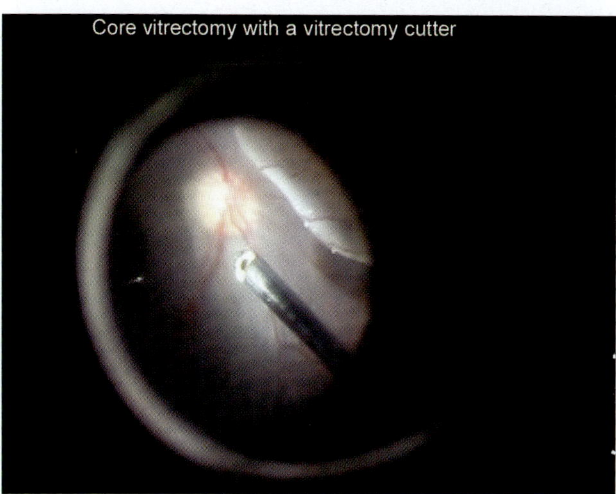

Fig. 13.3: Core vitrectomy (*Courtesy*: Dr Ronel Soibam)

It is necessary to utilize maximum cut settings and high aspiration power settings to achieve reasonable cutting and aspiration rates and avoid outflow occlusion with aspirated fragments of ocular tissue. The 23 gauge cutter port is 50% closer to the probe tip compared to 20 gauge cutter. This allows efficient vitreous shaving close to the retina without creating iatrogenic retinal breaks. Core vitrectomy (Figure 13.3) followed by separation and removal of posterior hyaloid membrane is performed. Peripheral vitrectomy is done with the help of scleral depression.

Air-fluid exchange (Figure 13.4) can be done using backflush needle through pre-existing retinal break or posterior retinotomy created with endodiathermy (Figure 13.5). Focal endolaser treatment is applied around

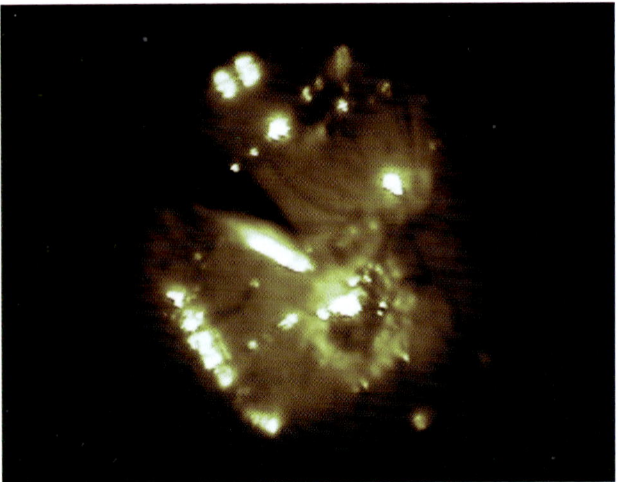

Fig. 13.4: Fluid-air exchange

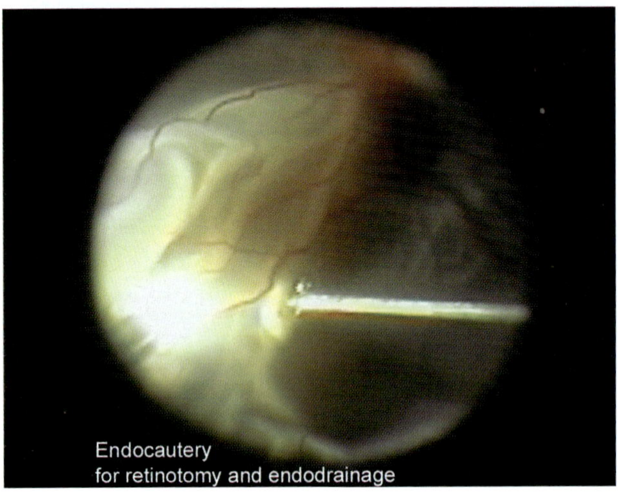

Fig.13.5: Endodiathermy (*Courtesy*: Dr Ronel Soibam)

the retinotomy site (Figure 13.6), retinal breaks and suspicious areas of peripheral retinal pathology. Parolini et al suggested placing two to three rows of laser burns posterior to vitreous base around the sclerotomy sites or bordering predisposing retinal lesions to lower the risk of iatrogenic retinal breaks because of traction and residual vitreous incarceration (Figure 13.7).[11] Air, gas or silicone oil can be used as a tamponading agent. The infusion line is held firmly with forceps to prevent the infusion line escape during silicone oil injection. Studies have revealed that silicone oil can be injected safely and effectively using 23 gauge transconjunctival sutureless vitrectomy system.[12,13]

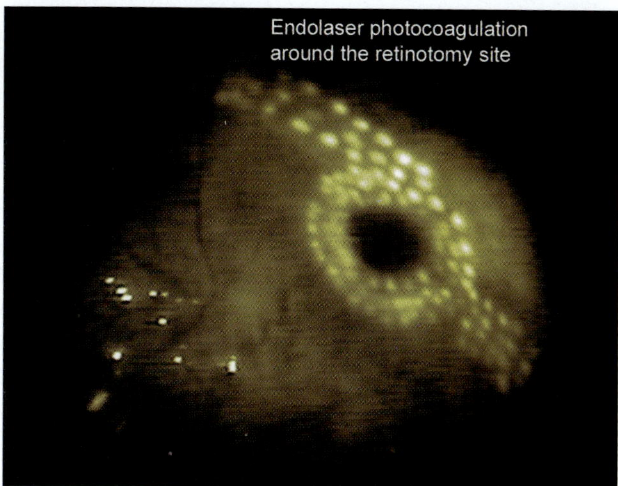

Fig. 13.6: Endolaser around the retinotomy site

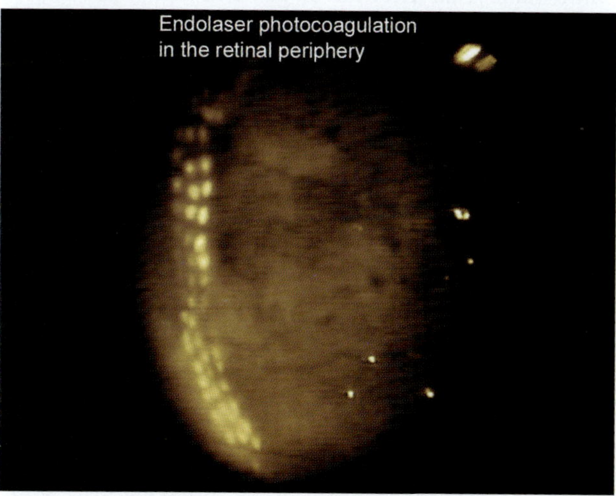

Fig. 13.7: Three rows of peripheral laser

Retinal periphery must be examined at the conclusion of the case with indirect ophthalmoscope or binocular indirect ophthalmomicroscope (BIOM) wide-angle viewing system incorporating scleral indentation.

Microcannula removal at the end of surgery is performed by grasping the external collar with the forceps and rolling over the conjunctival opening with a cotton tip to misalign the conjunctival and scleral openings. The superior microcannulas are removed first while the infusion is kept open to maintain chamber stability, optimize intraocular pressure and promote vitreous occlusion of the sclerotomies. The infusion tube with its attached cannula is then removed simultaneously.

COMPLICATIONS

23 gauge vitreous surgery involves the risks inherent to 20 gauge vitrectomy including inadvertent lens touch, cataract progression, iatrogenic retinal beaks, and ocular hypertension. There are some complications specifically related to the 23 gauge system.

Wound Leak and Hypotony

Open sclerotomies at the end of surgery can result in wound leak and hypotony which develops when the sclerotomy is not plugged internally by vitreous or externally with the conjunctiva. The hypotony resolves spontaneously within 1 week without any long-term complications. Occasionally wound leaks are significant and may necessitate suture. Some surgeons close the wound leak with a single 8-0 vicryl suture transconjunctivally. Others perform peritomy to close the wound, particularly if the wound leak cannot be visualized through the conjunctiva. It has been noted that suturing was more frequently required after fluid tamponade than after air or gas and was most frequent with the use of silicone oil. Intraocular gas improves wound closure by pushing the internal lips of the scleral tunnel against the external part of it. Batman et al has demonstrated that the tissue glue is efficacious in closing the sclerotomy ports when wound leakage is observed in transconjunctival sutureless vitreoretinal surgery.[14] Fine et al studied outcomes of 77 consecutive cases of 23 gauge vitreous surgery for posterior segment disease and found only 2.8% patient's had an intraocular pressure of $\leq$ 5 mm Hg on the first postoperative day.[15]

Endophthalmitis

Endophthalmitis in 23 gauge vitreous surgery may occur as a result of several mechanisms. Direct cannula insertion may inoculate the vitreous with conjunctival flora during trocar insertion, open sclerotomies and wound leaks may lead to increased influx of bacteria. Precautionary steps to curtail the risk includes sterilization of the surgical field with povidone iodine, conjunctival displacement prior to cannula insertion to misalign conjunctival and sclera openings, oblique cannula insertion and suture any wound leaks seen following cannula removal.

Parolini et al studied the incidence of endophthalmitis after 23 gauge vitrectomy and compared it with 20 gauge vitrectomy. Endophthalmitis developed in one of 3078 eyes after 20 gauge vitrectomy (0.03%) and in none of 943 eyes which underwent 23 gauge vitrectomy.[16]

Retinal Detachment

The incidence of retinal detachment after 20 gauge vitrectomy varies between 1.8–14%. Parolini et al studied postoperative complications and intraocular pressure in 943 cases of 23 gauge pars plana vitrectomy and they noted the incidence of retinal detachment was 0.2%. The explanation of low incidence was that they performed peripheral vitrectomy with careful cleaning of the vitreous at the sclerotomy sites to prevent vitreous incarceration and applied peripheral laser at the sclerotomy sites.[11]

Vitreous Hemorrhage

Parolini et al noted vitreous hemorrhage as the most common complication which resolved spontaneously in 1 week to 3 weeks. The bleeding from the sclerotomy sites was the causative factor.[11]

ADVANTAGES

The intraoperative time is reduced because there is no need for a conjunctival peritomy or closure of the sclerotomies.

The patient feels increased comfort because of less inflammation and avoidance of suture related problems such as foreign body sensation.

The conjunctival scarring is less which may be beneficial for the glaucoma patients who may require filtration surgery in future or patients who had undergone previous multiple surgeries.[17]

The fast visual recovery is attributed to elimination of astigmatism caused by sclera sutures as well as reduction in postoperative inflammation.

Advantages over 25 gauge vitrectomy include less flexible instrumentation, higher fluidics, long durability of instruments, brighter endoillumination and lesser learning curve.

23 GAUGE VITRECTOMY OUTCOMES

Shin et al studied 59 eyes which underwent primary vitrectomy for rhegmatogenous retinal detachment. They noted single operation anatomic success rate was 79.3% in 20 gauge group compared to 93.3% in 23 gauge group. The average operation time of the 23 gauge group was 80.2 minutes which was significantly shorter than the 94.8 minutes of the 20 gauge group. Transient ocular hypertension and progression of lens opacity were the most common complications in the both groups.[18]

Tsang et al reported the results of 23 gauge vitrectomy for the repair of rhegmatogenous retinal detachment. They found the anatomic success rate was 91.7%. Only one patient out of 24 had hypotony on postoperative day 1.[19] Several authors have shown that 23 gauge vitrectomy is safe and effective in the management of variety of vitreoretinal disorders including rhegmatogenous retinal detachment.[20-25]

CONCLUSION

Primary rhegmatogenous retinal detachment is an important cause of vision loss. The fundamental principles of retinal reattachment surgery are well defined. All the goals can be achieved by 23 gauge vitrectomy.

Recent advances in the field of vitreoretinal surgery have ushered in a new era of sutureless vitrectomy. This system allows for less invasive and more efficient surgery. Decreased surgical time, less trauma and inflammation and faster patient recovery has contributed to enhance patient care and satisfaction.

REFERENCES

1. Haddad WM, Monin C, Morel C, et al. Retinal detachment after phacoemulsification: A study of 114 cases. Am J Ophthalmol. 2002;133:630–8.
2. Schwartz SG, Flynn HW Jr. Pars plana vitrectomy for primary rhegmatogenous retinal detachment. Clinical Ophthalmol. 2008;2(1):57–63.
3. Heimann H, Bartz-Schmidt KU, Bornfeld N, et al. Scleral buckling versus primary vitrectomy in rhegmatogenous retinal detachment: A prospective randomized multicenter clinical study. Ophthamol. 2007;114(12): 2142–54.
4. Machemar R, Parel JM, Norton EW. Vitrectomy: A pars plana approach. Technical improvements and further results. Trans Am Acad Ophthalmol Otolaryngol. 1972;76:462–6.
5. O'Malley C, Heintz RM Sr. Vitrectomy with an alternate instrument system. Ann Ophthalmol. 1975;7;585–8;591–4.
6. Fujii GY, De Juan E Jr, Humayun MS, et al. A new 25 gauge instrument system for transconjunctival sutureless vitrectomy surgery. Ophthalmol. 2002;109:1807–12.
7. Eckardt C. Transconjunctival sutureless 23 gauge vitrectomy. Retina. 2005;25:208–11.
8. Sakaguchi H, Oshima Y, Tano Y. 27 gauge transconjunctival nonvitrectomizing vitreous surgery for epiretinal membrane removal. Retina. 2007;27(9):1302–4.
9. Theocharis IP, Alexandridou A, Tomic Z. A two year prospective study comparing lidocaine 2% jelly verus peribulber anaesthesia for 25 gauge and 23 gauge sutureless vitrectomy. Graefes Arch Clin Exp Ophthalmol. 2007;245:1253–8.
10. Teixeira A, Allemann N, Yamada AC, et al. Ultrasound biomicroscopy in recently postoperative 23 gauge transconjunctival vitrectomy sutureless self-sealing sclerotomy. Retina. 2009;29(9):1305–9.
11. Parolini B, Prigione G, Romanelli, et al. Postoperative complications and intraocular pressure in 943 consecutive cases of 23 gauge transconjunctival pars plana vitrectomy with 1 year follow-up. Retina. 2010;30:107–11.
12. Oliveira LB, Reis PA. Silicone oil tamponade in 23 gauge transconjunctival sutureless vitrectomy. Retina. 2007;27:1054–8.
13. Siqueira RC, Gil AD, Jorge R. Retinal detachment surgery with silicone oil injection in transconjunctival sutureless 23 gauge vitrectomy. Arq Bras Oftalmol. 2007;70:905–9.
14. Batman C, Ozdamar Y, Aslan O, et al. Tissue glue in sutureless vitreoretinal surgery for the treatment of wound leakage. Ophthalmic Surg Lasers Imaging. 2008;39(2):102–6.
15. Fine HF, Iranmanesh R, Iturralde D, et al. Outcomes of 77 consecutive cases of 23 gauge transconjunctival vitrectomy surgery for posterior segment disease. Ophthalmol. 2007;114:1197–1200.
16. Parolini B, Romanelli F, Prigione G. Incidence of endophthalmitis in a large series of 23 gauge and 20 gauge transconjunctival pars plana vitrectomy. Graefes Arch Clin Exp Ophthalmol. 2009;247:895–8.
17. Spirn MJ. Comparison of 25, 23 and 20 gauge vitrectomy. Curr Opin Ophthalmol. 2009;20:195–9.

18. Shin MK, Lee JE, Oum BS. Comparison between 20 gauge and 23 gauge vitrectomy system in primary vitrectomy for rhegmatogenous retinal detachment. J Korean Ophthalmol Soc. 2009;50(3):405-11.
19. Tsang CW, Cheung BT, Lam RF, et al. Primary 23 gauge transconjunctival sutureless vitrectomy for rhegmatogenous retinal detachment. Retina. 2008;28:1075-81.
20. Kim MJ, Park KH, Hwang JM, et al. The safety and efficacy of transconjunctival sutureless 23 gauge vitrectomy. Korean Journal of Ophthalmol. 2007;21(4):201-7.
21. Schweitzer C, Delyfer MN, Colin J, Korobelnik JF. 23 gauge transconjunctival sutureless pars plana vitrectomy: Results of a prospective study. Eye (Lond) 2009;23(12):2206–14.
22. El-Batamy AM. Transconjunctival 23 gauge vitrectomy for vitreoretinal diseases: Outcome of 30 consecutive cases. Middle East Afr J Ophthalmol. 2008;15:99–105.
23. Tewari A, Shah GK, Fang A. Visual outcomes with 23 gauge transconjunctival sutureless vitrectomy. Retina. 2008;28:258–62.
24. Lott MN, Manning MH, Singh J, et al. 23 gauge vitrectomy in 100 eyes: Short-term visual outcomes and complications. Retina. 2008;28(9):1193–200.
25. Gupta OP, Ho AC, Kaiser PK, et al. Short-term outcomes of 23 gauge pars plana vitrectomy. Am J Ophthalmol. 2008;146(2):193–7.

CHAPTER

14

MIVS in Macular Edema

Atul Kumar, Subijay Sinha, Varun Gogia

Pars plana vitrectomy as a technique has revolutionized retinal surgery since its advent and initial report by Machemer et al.[1] It allowed the removal of traction by an internal method, essential in retinal detachment procedures, as well as provided an active management modality for vitreous hemorrhage and opened the door for surgical intervention in a myriad.

Since that time, the evolution of vitrectomy surgery has seen experimentation and implementation of smaller surgical instruments aimed at greater functionality and minimalization of ocular trauma. The basis of a sutureless pars plana sclerotomy was to stabilize intraocular pressure (IOP) during surgery[2] with a truly closed system, as well as reduce surgical time by removing the need for sutured wound closure. Wound and suture related complications such as leakage, irritation, and scleral pigmentary changes could also be avoided. Concerns regarding wound competence in a sutureless procedure have seen the modification of the conventional straight incision to such techniques as angled, beveled and oblique scleral tunnel incisions.

In 1996, Chen[3] described a technique for creating a self-sealing, pars plana sclerotomy. This involved an initial scleral incision based 6 mm posterior to the limbus, creating a scleral flap that was theoretically self-sealing. De Juan and Hickingbotham[4] devised and introduced a range of 25 gauge instruments in 1990 for use through conventional sclerotomies. However, it was only in 2002, with the advent of the microcannulae array, that the 25 gauge transconjunctival sutureless vitrectomy (TSV) system was introduced by Fujii et al. This was followed by the introduction of a 23 gauge system by Eckardt in 2005.[5] Initially, both 23 and 25 gauge systems were available with a limited gamut of intraocular instruments. However, as the techniques rapidly became widely utilized, almost all intraocular instruments have been developed and made available for sutureless vitrectomy.

The benefits of sutureless vitrectomy, regardless of the instrument gauge, are similar to those experienced with sutureless cataract phacoemulsification. A decrease in intraoperative time, patient discomfort (suture and nonsuture related), and postoperative inflammation has been reported.[6-8] There have also been reports of less surgery induced astigmatism and more rapid visual recovery.[9,10] Damage to the conjunctiva is also minimalized with a transconjunctival, sutureless approach. This will be of clinical significance in those patients requiring glaucoma filtration surgery in the future. This benefit is also relevant to those few patients undergoing multiple vitreoretinal procedures. Comparison of 25 gauge TSV wounds to conventional 20 gauge wounds in the same patient revealed a much faster healing rate of 15 days as opposed to 6–8 weeks, using UBM to assess the wound.[11] As with standard pars plana vitrectomy, sutureless vitrectomy has inherent complications. These include iatrogenic retinal breaks and detachment, lens touch, cataract progression, and endophthalmitis. The fact that the sclerotomies are not sutured at the end of the procedure has led to an incidence of wound leak and subsequent ocular hypotony. Concerns have been made regarding the possibility of an increase in endophthalmitis incidence related to sutureless procedures, including vitrectomy. Other complications reported with sutureless vitrectomy include decompression retinopathy, postoperative retinal detachment, retinal breaks, and intraoperative instrument breakage.[12,13] Increased instrument flexibility, a result of their smaller gauge, as well as increased time for an oil fill have been highlighted as limiting factors in certain posterior segment procedures by many vitreoretinal surgeons.

MACULAR EDEMA IN VASCULAR OCCLUSIONS

Together with central retinal vein occlusion and hemicentral retinal vein occlusion, BRVO is the second most common cause of retinal vascular disease, exceeded only by diabetic retinopathy.[14] In all but a few rare cases, the BRVO occurs at crossing sites where the artery is passing anteriorly (superficially) to the vein.[15] The upper temporal vascular arcade is more often involved than the lower temporal vascular arcade.[15-18] Most BRVOs involve the area inside the temporal vascular arcades (macular BRVO), whereas peripheral BRVOs are more rarely seen partly because they tend to be asymptomatic.

Branch retinal vein occlusion (BRVO) is a common retinal vascular disease that often causes macular edema, which is the main reason for visual impairment in these patients.[19,20] The macula is important for detailed vision, especially the fovea that consists entirely of cones.[21] In humans, histological studies have shown that macular edema is associated with swelling of the Müller cells, especially in the outer plexiform layer of the neurosensory retina.[22-24]

Accordingly, macular edema may affect retinal function and lead to visual impairment in BRVO patients. Various factors might be involved in the pathogenesis of macular edema associated with BRVO. Recently, it has been reported that the vitreous level of vascular endothelial growth factor (VEGF) is elevated in BRVO patients with macular edema, and that vitreous VEGF levels are correlated with the nonperfused area of the retina and with the severity of macular edema[25,26] VEGF directly increases vascular permeability and VEGF expression by retinal glial cells is up regulated due to hypoxia.[27,28]

The edema associated with BRVO may cause a reduction in visual acuity if it reaches the fovea, notably if cystoid edema develops.[22,24] The smaller the sector of the perifoveal arcades that is involved, the better the prognosis. If the perifoveal collaterals are not involved, visual acuity often will remain normal (Figures 14.1A and B), but foveal vision may be affected by edema and hard exudate leaking from collaterals at a distance of several hundred micrometers.

Thus, VEGF may contribute to the occurrence of macular edema in patients with BRVO, and a decrease of VEGF production may be related to the improvement of macular edema in BRVO patients who undergo pars plana vitrectomy (PPV). Recently, PPV combined with posterior vitreous detachment has been reported to effectively reduce macular edema and improve visual acuity in BRVO patients.[29,30] Various studies by Fujimoto, Figueroa, Charbonnel, and Becquet also support the premise that vitrectomy improves macular edema and visual acuity, whether or not arteriovenous sheathotomy is performed.[31-34]

Natural history data from the Central Vein Occlusion Study (CVOS) showed that patients with poor visual acuity at the first visit (<20/200) had an 80% chance of having a visual acuity less than 20/200 at final visit, whether perfused or nonperfused initially.[35] It is hypothesized that vitrectomy with removal of the ILM would allow the congested, hemorrhagic retina to decompress by facilitating the release of extracellular fluid and blood into the vitreous, which would, in turn, restore normal retinal thickness, reduce opacities within the retina that might interfere with light transmission to photoreceptors, and allow vision to improve.

Macular edema associated with a central retinal vein occlusion was improved by vitrectomy and internal limiting membrane removal in studies by Mandelcorn and Radetzky.[36,37] The mechanism for improvement is uncertain, but is it possible that removal of the posterior hyaloid by vitrectomy may improve oxygenation of the retina, as was suggested by Steffanson.[38] Alternatively, vitrectomy may improve diffusion of harmful cytokines that promote increased vascular permeability, such as vascular endothelial growth.

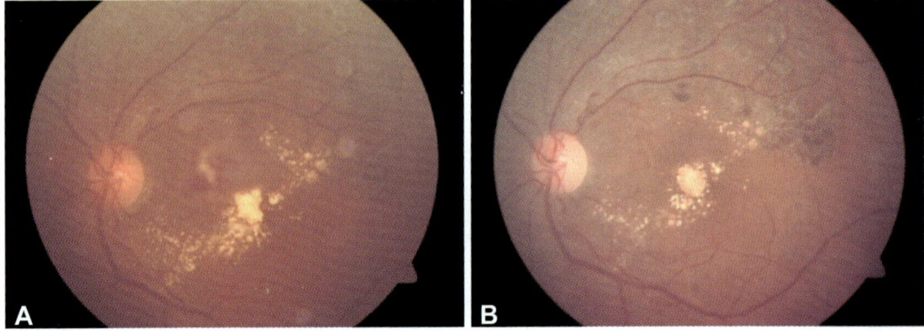

Figs 14.1A and B: (A) Preoperative BRVO with extensive macular edema and VA:3/60; (B) Postoperative 8 weeks, after PPV and ILM peel shows, resolution of intraretinal edema and VA:6/24

VITRECTOMY IN DIABETIC MACULAR EDEMA

The vitreous has been implicated as a cause of macular edema in people with diabetes via several mechanical and physiologic mechanisms, all of which are postulated to lead to increased vascular permeability.[39-41] Suggested mechanisms include, destabilization of the vitreous by abnormal glycation and cross-linking of vitreal collagen, leading to traction on the macula; accumulation and concentration of factors causing vasopermeability in the premacular vitreous gel, and accumulation of chemo attractant factors in the vitreous, leading to cellular migration to the posterior hyaloid, contraction, and macular traction.

Edema Arises due to Disruption of the Balance between Capillary Hydrostatic Forces and Plasma Osmotic Pressure Gradients

The observation that release of mechanical traction on the macula with subsequent reduction in DME, either by spontaneous posterior vitreous detachment or with vitrectomy, lends support to this line of reasoning.[41]

In a recent prospective study, published by DRCR net writing committee, 87 eyes undergoing vitrectomy for DME associated with at least moderate visual loss and investigator-determined vitreomacular traction, the median

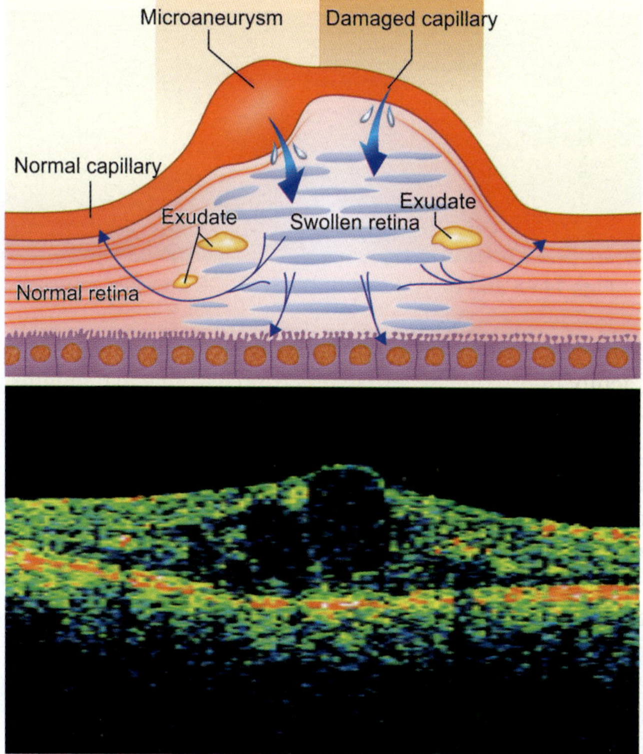

Fig. 14.2: Pathophysiology of DME

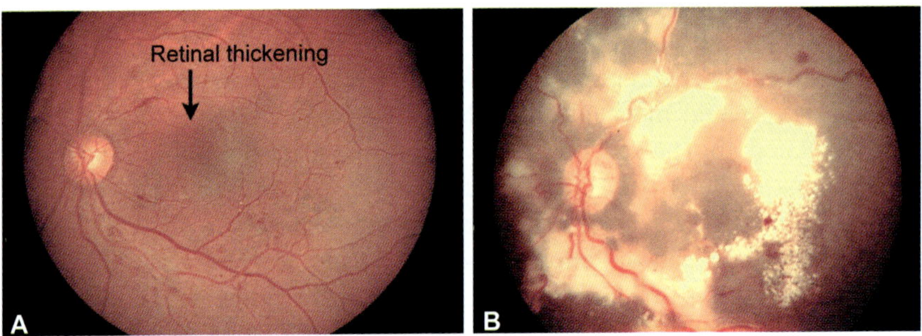

Figs 14.3A and B: (A) Focal macular edema; (B) Diffuse macular edema

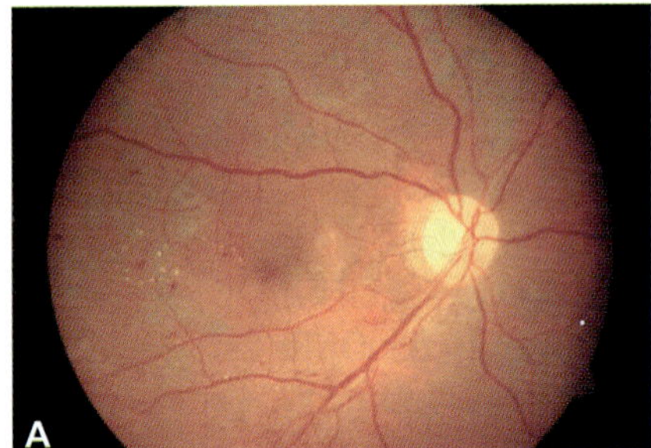

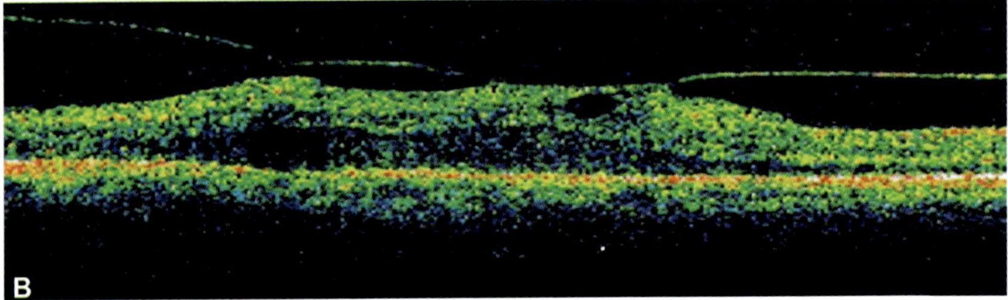

Figs 14.4A and B: (A) Focal CSDME; (B) OCT reveals associated VMT

change in visual acuity at 6 months was an improvement of 3 letters, with visual acuity improving by ≥10 letters from baseline to 6 months in 38% (95% CI, 28%–49%) and worsening by ≥10 letters in 22% (95% CI, 13%–31%). Reduction in OCT central subfield thickness to <250 microns occurred in almost half, and most eyes had a reduction of thickening of ≥50%.[56]

Another randomized, prospective study from our center compared the outcomes of vitrectomy with ILM peel and grid laser in 24 eyes of 24 patients with metabolically stable diabetes and with diffuse diabetic macular edema. The result showed no clinically significant difference of visual acuity between the two groups at the end of 6 months. However, foveal thickness and macular volume decreased significantly more in the ILM group compared to the laser group.[42]

Other studies have also suggested benefits of vitrectomy for diabetic macular edema and various mechanisms by which the vitreous may contribute

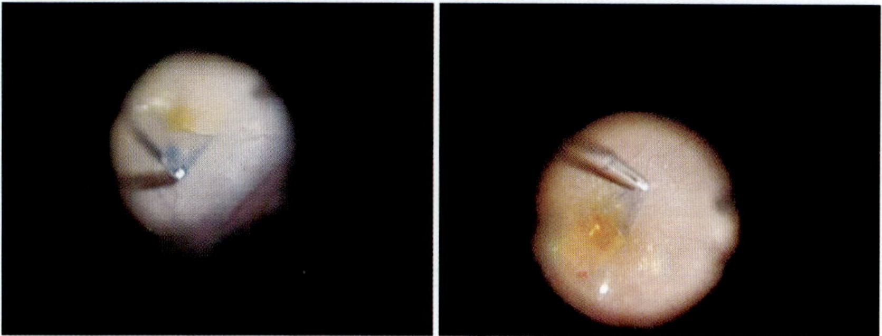

Fig. 14.5: Shows Brilliant blue G stained ILM peel in an eye with tractional diabetic macular edema (DME)

to the formation of DMO have been postulated. These include vitreomacular traction, which may range from the taut thickened hyaloid described by Lewis et al through partial vitreomacular separation to microtraction resulting from an abnormal PVD resulting in posterior vitreoschisis and a persistent premacular vitreous adhesion.[43-46] Relief of traction is not the only postulated mechanism for improved structure and function after vitrectomy; Stefansson has long advocated that improved transvitreal oxygenation of the retina may be the causative mechanism.[47,48] Others have suggested that removal of a growth factor reservoir in the premacular hyaloid is important.[49] It is known that the diabetic vitreous is abnormal with enzyme-mediated vitreous collagen cross linking and nonenzymatic glycation; with reduced permeability potentially increasing the concentration of a premacular growth factor.

Now-a-days, pars plana vitrectomy is being combined with peeling of ILM as the modified treatment for this type of diabetic macular edema. Gandorfer et al first reported rapid improvement in visual acuity soon after surgery with ILM peeling and early absorption of edema.[50] Subsequently a number of authors have evaluated the effects of ILM peeling in resolution of diabetic macular edema, most of whom have reported fairly promising results in resolution of the macular edema and improvement in visual acuity following the surgery.

Surgical ILM peeling for diffuse diabetic macular edema can be a useful alternative to laser photocoagulation as it provides rapid resolution of fluid in outer retinal layers, increased oxygenation of the macula and most importantly removes all tangential and anteroposterior traction over the edematous macula, which causes the incompetent capillaries to leak. Studies by Kuhn, Rosenblatt, Avci, and Dillinger demonstrated improved diabetic macular edema following internal limiting membrane removal in the absence of a taut posterior hyaloid.[51-54]

The mechanism by which ILM peeling improves in resolution of DME has been recently hypothesized that in diabetic patients the ILM thickness and amount of heparin sulphate, proteoglycan, fibronectin, Type-I, III, IV, and

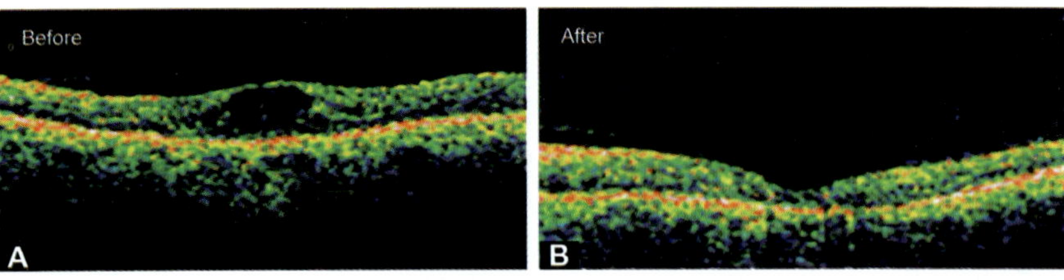

Figs 14.6A and B: (A) Preoperative OCT of nontractional DME not responding to laser and anti-VEGF; (B) Postoperative OCT of same undergone 23 gauge MIVS and ILM peel reveals resolution of macular edema

V collagen increases. It is speculated that ILM thickening contributes to the structural and functional disturbance of water movement between the vitreous and retina resulting in diabetic maculopathy.[55] Egress of intraretinal fluid post-ILM peel also contributes in decreasing the edema. Also the removal of the ILM guarantees complete separation of the posterior hyaloid from the macular surface. Egress of fluid from the outer retinal layers (outer plexiform layer, outer nuclear layer) post-ILM peel also contributes in decreasing the edema.

ACKNOWLEDGMENT

Sh. Mahender Singh (AIIMS)—Data layout and script preparation.

REFERENCES

1. Machemer R, Buettner H, Norton EW, Parel JM. Vitrectomy: A pars plana approach. Trans Am Acad Ophthalmol Otolaryngol. 1971;75:813–20.
2. Kwok AK, Tham CC, Lam DS, Li M, Chen JC. Modified sutureless sclerotomies in pars plana vitrectomy. Am J Ophthalmol. 1999;127:731–3.
3. Chen JC. Sutureless pars plana vitrectomy through self-sealing sclerotomies. Arch Ophthalmol. 1996;114:1273–5.
4. De Juan E, Jr, Hickingbotham D. Refinements in microinstrumentation for vitreous surgery. Am J Ophthalmol. 1990;109:218–20.
5. Eckardt C. Transconjunctival sutureless 23 gauge vitrectomy. Retina. 2005;25:208–11.
6. Chen E. 25 gauge transconjunctival sutureless vitrectomy. Curr Opin Ophthalmol. 2007;18:188–93.
7. Lakhanpal RR, Humayun MS, de Juan E, Jr, Lim JI, Chong LP, Chang TS, et al. Outcomes of 140 consecutive cases of 25 gauge transconjunctival surgery for posterior segment disease. Ophthalmol. 2005;112:817–24.
8. Rizzo S, Genovesi-Ebert F, Murri S, Belting C, Vento A, Cresti F, et al. 25 gauge, sutureless vitrectomy and standard 20 gauge pars plana vitrectomy in idiopathic epiretinal membrane surgery: A comparative pilot study. Graefes Arch Clin Exp Ophthalmol. 2006;244:472–9.
9. Tewari A, Shah GK, Fang A. Visual outcomes with 23 gauge transconjunctival sutureless vitrectomy. Retina. 2008;28:258–62.
10. Yanyali A, Celik E, Horozoglu F, Nohutcu AF. Corneal topographic changes after transconjunctival (25 gauge) sutureless vitrectomy. Am J Ophthalmol. 2005;140:939–41.

11. Keshavamurthy R, Venkatesh P, Garg S. Ultrasound biomicroscopy findings of 25 gauge Transconjuctival Sutureless (TSV) and conventional (20 gauge) pars plana sclerotomy in the same patient. BMC Ophthalmol. 2006;6:7.
12. Rezende FA, Regis LG, Kickinger M, Alcantara S. Decompression retinopathy after 25 gauge transconjunctival sutureless vitrectomy: Report of 2 cases. Arch Ophthalmol. 2007;125:699–700.
13. Inoue M, Noda K, Ishida S, Nagai N, Imamura Y, Oguchi Y. Intraoperative breakage of a 25 gauge vitreous cutter. Am J Ophthalmol. 2004;138:867–9.
14. Orth DH, Patz A. Retinal branch vein occlusion. Surv Ophthalmol. 1978;22:357–76.
15. Weinberg D, Dodwell DG, Fern SA. Anatomy of arteriovenous crossings inbranch retinal vein occlusion. Am J Ophthalmol. 1990;109:298–302.
16. Becker B, Post LT Jr. Retinal vein occlusion. Clinical and experimental observations. Am J Ophthalmol. 1951;34:677–86.
17. Blankenship GW, Okun E. Retinal tributary vein occlusion. History and management by photocoagulation. Arch Ophthalmol. 1973;89:363–8.
18. Gutman FA, Zegarra H. The natural course of temporal retinal branch vein occlusion. Trans Am Acad Ophthalmol Otolaryngol. 1974;78:178–92.
19. Michels RG, Gass JD. The natural course of retinal branch vein obstruction. Trans Am Acad Ophthalmol Otolaryngol. 1974;78:166–77.
20. Gutman FA, Zegarra H. The natural course of temporal retinal branch vein occlusion. Trans Am Acad Ophthalmol Otolaryngol. 1974;78:178–92.
21. Hogan MJ, Alvarado JA, Weddell JE. Histology of the Human Eye: An Atlas and Textbook. Philadelphia, Saunders; 1971;492-7.
22. Fine BS, Brucker AJ. Macular edema and cystoid macular edema. Am J Ophthalmol. 1981;92:466–81.
23. Tso MO. Pathology of cystoid macular edema. Ophthalmol. 1982; 89:902–15.
24. Yanoff M, Fine BS, Brucker AJ, Eagle RC Jr. Pathology of human cystoid macular edema. Surv Ophthalmol. 1984;28:505–11.
25. Noma H, Minamoto A, Funatsu H, Tsukamoto H, Nakano K, Yamashita H. Intravitreal levels of vascular endothelial growth factor and interleukin 6 are correlated with macular edema in branch retinal vein occlusion. Graefes Arch Clin Exp Ophthalmol. 2006;244:309–15.
26. Noma H, Funatsu H, Yamasaki M, Tsukamoto H, Mimura T, Sone T. Aqueous humour levels of cytokines are correlated to vitreous levels and severity of macular oedema in branch retinal vein occlusion. Eye. 2008;22:42–8.
27. Senger DR, Galli SJ, Dvorak AM, Perruzzi CA, Harvey VS, Dvorak HF. Tumor cells secrete a vascular permeability factor that promotes accumulation of ascites fluid. Science. 1983;219:983–5.
28. Behzadian MA, Wang XL, Shabrawey M, Caldwell RB. Effects of hypoxia on glial cell expression of angiogenesis-regulating factors VEGF and TGF-β. Glia. 1998;24:216–25.
29. Tachi N, Hashimoto Y, Ogino N. Vitrectomy for macular edema combined with retinal vein occlusion. Doc Ophthalmol. 1999;97:465–9.
30. Saika S, Tanaka T, Miyamoto T, Ohnishi Y. Surgical posterior vitreous detachment combined with gas/air tamponade for treating macular edema associated with branch retinal vein occlusion: Retinal tomography and visual outcome. Graefes Arch Clin Exp Ophthalmol. 2001;239:729–32.
31. Fujimoto R, Ogino N, Kumagai K, Demizu S, Furukawa M. The efficacy of arteriovenous sheathotomy for macular edema in branch retinal vein occlusion. Nippon Ganka Gakkai Zasshi. 2004;108:144–9.

32. Figueroa MS, Torres R, Alvarez MT. Comparative study of vitrectomy with and without vein decompression for branch retinal vein occlusion: A pilot study. Eur J Ophthalmol. 2004;14:40–7.
33. Charbonnel J, Glacet-Bernard A, Korobelnik JF, et al. Management of branch retinal vein occlusion with vitrectomy and arteriovenous adventitial sheathotomy, the possible role of surgical posterior vitreous detachment. Graefes Arch Clin Exp Ophthalmol. 2004;242:223–8.
34. Becquet F, Le Fouic JF, Zanlonghi X, et al. Efficiency of surgical treatment for chronic macular edema due to branch retinal vein occlusion. J Fr Ophtalmol. 2003;26:570–6.
35. The Central Vein Occlusion Study Group. Natural history and clinical management of central retinal vein occlusion. Arch Ophthalmol. 1997;115:486–91.
36. Mandelcorn MS, Nrusimhadevara RK. Internal limiting membrane peeling for decompression of macular edema in retinal vein occlusion: A report of 14 cases. Retina. 2004;24:348–55.
37. Radetzky S, Walter P, Fauser S, et al. Visual outcome of patients with macular edema after pars plana vitrectomy and indocyanine green-assisted peeling of the internal limiting membrane. Graefes Arch Clin Exp Ophthalmol. 2004;242:273–8.
38. Stefansson E, Novack RL, Hatchell DL. Vitrectomy prevents retinal hypoxia in branch retinal vein occlusion. Invest Ophthalmol Vis Sci. 1990;31:284–9.
39. Dillinger P, Mester U. Vitrectomy with removal of the internal limiting membrane in chronic diabetic macular oedema. Graefes Arch Clin Exp Ophthalmol. 2004;242:630–7.
40. Figueroa MS, Contreras I, Noval S. Surgical and anatomical outcomes of pars plana vitrectomy of diffuse nontractional diabetic macular edema. Retina. 2008;28:420–6.
41. Foos RY, Kreiger AE, Forsythe AB, Zakka KA. Posterior vitreous detachment in diabetic subjects. Ophthalmol. 1980;87:122–8.
42. Kumar A, Sinha S, Azad R, Sharma YR, Vohra R. Comparative evaluation of vitrectomy and dye-enhanced ILM peel with grid laser in diffuse diabetic macular edema. Graefes Arch Clin Exp Ophthalmol. 2007;245:360–8.
43. Lewis H. The role of vitrectomy in the treatment of diabetic macular edema. Am J Ophthalmol. 2001;131:123–5.
44. Massin P, Duguid G, Erginay A, Haouchine B, Gaudric A. Optical coherence tomography for evaluating diabetic macular edema before and after vitrectomy. Am J Ophthalmol. 2003;135:169–77.
45. Shah SP, Patel M, Thomas D, Aldington S, Laidlaw DA. Factors predicting outcome of vitrectomy for diabetic macular edema: Results of a prospective study. Br J Ophthalmol. 2006;90:33–6.
46. Kishi S, Demaria C, Shimizu K. Vitreous cortex remnants at the fovea after spontaneous vitreous detachment. Int Ophthalmol. 1986;9:253–60.
47. Stefansson E. Ocular oxygenation and the treatment of diabetic retinopathy. Surv Ophthalmol. 2006;51:364–80.
48. Stefansson E. The therapeutic effects of retinal laser treatment and vitrectomy. A theory based on oxygen and vascular physiology. Acta Ophthalmologica Scandinavica. 2001;79:435–40.
49. Stolba U, Binder S, Gruber D, Krebs I, Aggermann T, Neumaier B. Vitrectomy for persistent diffuse diabetic macular edema. Am J Ophthalmol. 2005;140:295–301.
50. Gandorfer A, Messmer EM, Ulbig MW, Kamplik A. Resolution of diabetic macular edema after surgical removal of the posterior hyaloid. Ophthalmol. 2000;103:1796–1806.

51. Kuhn F, Kiss G, Mester V, Szijarto Z, Kovacs B. Vitrectomy with internal limiting membrane removal for clinically significant macular edema. Graefes Arch Clin Exp Ophthalmol. 2004;242:402–08.
52. Rosenblatt BJ, Shah GK, Sharma S, Bakal J. Pars plana vitrectomy with internal limiting membranectomy for refractory diabetic macular edema without a taut posterior hyaloid. Graefes Arch Clin Exp Ophthalmol. 2005;243:20–5.
53. Avci R, Kaderli B, Avci B, et al. Pars plana vitrectomy and removal of the internal limiting membrane in the treatment of chronic macular edema. Graefes Arch Clin Exp Ophthalmol. 2004;242:845–52.
54. Dillinger P, Mester U. Vitrectomy with removal of the internal limiting membrane in chronic diabetic macular edema. Graefes Arch Clin Exp Ophthalmol. 2004; 242:630–7.
55. Matsunaga N, Ozeki H, Hirabayashi Y, Shimada S, Ogura Y. Histopathologic evaluation of the internal limiting membrane surgically excised from eyes with diabetic maculopathy. Retina. 2005;25:311–6.
56. Diabetic Retinopathy Clinical Research Network Committee. Vitrectomy outcomes in eyes with diabetic macular edema and vitreomacular traction. Ophthalmol. 2010;117;1087–93.

CHAPTER

15

Silicone Oil in MIVS

Shalabh Sinha

Silicone oil (polydimethylsiloxane) has been used for providing long-term tamponade to the retina in various conditions including rhegmatogenous retinal detachment complicated with proliferative vitreoretinopathy or chorio-retinal coloboma, tractional retinal detachment, endophthalmitis, uveitis, posterior segment trauma, infectious retinal and chorioretinal pathologies, etc. Though the silicone oil study report 11 did not find much difference between silicone oil and long acting gas for retinal detachment with PVR, closer analysis did favor the use of silicone oil. Gas filled eyes had higher rates of re-retinal detachment in the early postoperative period, and a greater incidence of hypotony and worse visual outcome in comparison to oil removed eyes in the long-term.[1]

Various grades of viscosity of silicone oil are currently available, such as 1000 cst, 1300 cst and 5000 cst. The higher the viscosity, the lesser is the likelihood of emulsification. However, there are no fixed guidelines as to which grade of silicone oil should be used for a particular condition. Generally, it is choice of the treating surgeon to decide which silicone oil must be used for a given pathology. In certain countries, 5000 cst is the preferred grade while in India 1000 cst is primarily used.

There are a number of reports of the use of silicone oil in MIVS. Shah et al reported that 25 gauge MIVS with silicone oil was safe in complicated retinal detachments and was an alternative to 20 gauge.[2] Altan et al used 1000 cst silicone oil in tractional retinal detachment with 25 gauge.[3] Erakgun reported 23 gauge instrumentation to be feasible, effective and safe for vitrectomy with silicone oil injection in diabetic tractional retinal detachments and proliferative vitreoretinopathy.[4]

INJECTION OF SILICONE OIL

Conventional means of injecting silicone oil is by 19/20 gauge needle either manually or by an automated silicone oil pump. While it is easier to inject 1000 cst or 1300 cst silicone oil manually using a large 20 mL syringe, 5000 cst silicone oil requires an automated pump. Manual injection of 5000 cst though possible takes a great deal of effort and time.

With the arrival of MIVS, the 25 gauge cannula was too thin to allow injection of silicone oil. Reimann et al devised a new system for injecting silicone oil using a 24 gauge angiocatheter.[5] This needle was exchanged with the 25 gauge cannula, and then silicone oil 1000 cst or 5000 cst could be infused. For 23 gauge, either a similar needle could be directly inserted through the cannula or a separate infusion line was connected to the cannula to allow injection of silicone oil.[6] A specially designed cannula (Figures 15.1 and 15.2) can be used for injection of silicone oil. The wall is very thin and silicone oil can be easily injected or aspirated using this cannula.

Caution needs to be exercised while injecting silicone oil when used in combination with 'valved' cannula system. Removal of the valve as in the DORC system or the use of a vent as in the Alcon system, is necessary to allow escape of air and prevent increase in intraocular pressure while injecting the silicone oil (Figures 15.3A to C).

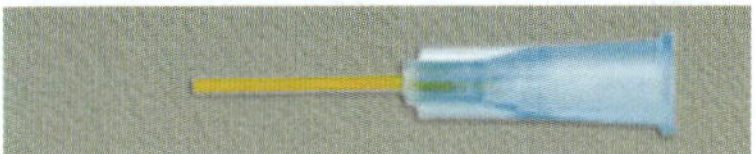

Fig. 15.1: Long 7 mm silicone oil injection/removal cannula DORC

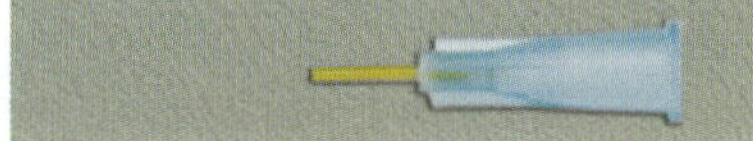

Fig. 15.2: Short 4 mm silicone oil injection cannula DORC

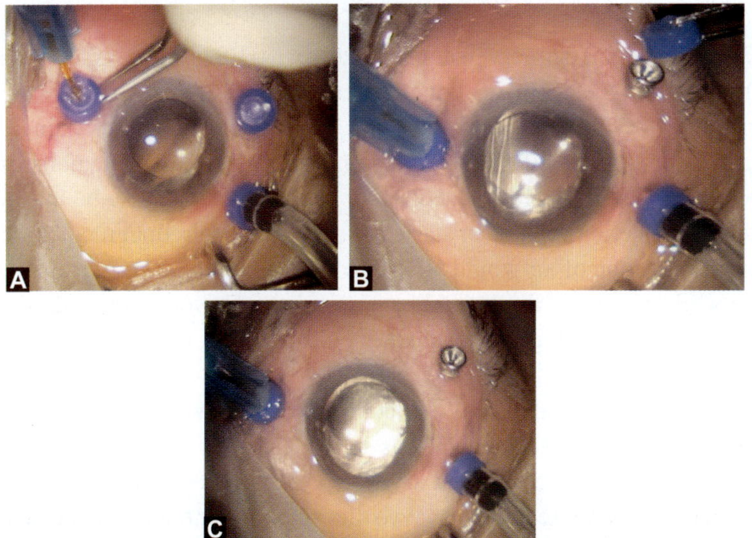

Figs 15.3A to C: (A) Silicone oil cannula inserted; (B) Valve removed before injection; (C) 23 gauge silicone oil injection. Note valve has been removed to allow egress of air

In retinal detachments with giant retinal tears, while perflurocarbon liquids have a special role in flattening the retina during surgery,[7] silicone oil may be required for long-term endotamponade. A direct perflurocarbon liquid (PFCL) silicone oil exchange is possible. Care must be taken to first dry the edges of the retinal detachment and where fluid collects in the slope of the PFCL meniscus before beginning to passively/actively remove the PFCL bubble. This maneuver prevents slipping of the GRT more commonly seen if a fluid-air exchange is performed. In pseudophakic eyes with an open posterior capsule, no fogging of the IOL is encountered (Figures 15.3D and E).

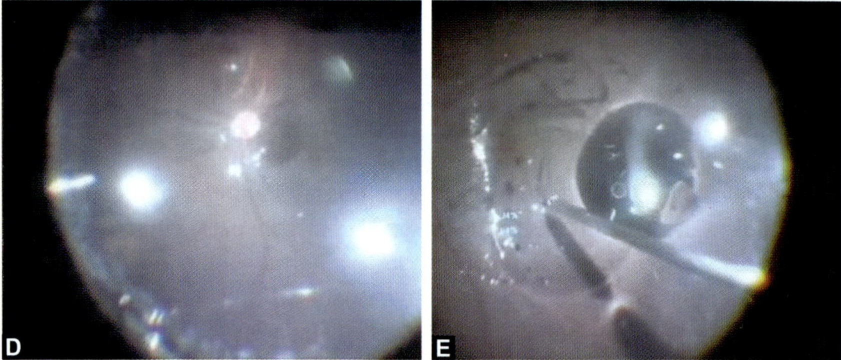

Figs 15.3D and E: (D) Edges of GRT are dried; (E) Direct PFCL silicone oil exchange (*Courtesy:* Dr Manish Nagpal)

Subsilicone oil surgery using 25 gauge MIVS system is of value in recurrent retinal detachments complicated with PVR. Also termed 'interface vitrectomy'[8] by Steve Charles, this saves a great deal of time. Using small gauge system, egress of silicone oil is minimal. Epiretinal membranes can be removed, and retina reattached. A bubble of PFCL can also be injected to flatten the posterior pole, open starfolds and expose epiretinal membranes for removal. Injection of air would allow the silicone oil to be pushed against the retina while subretinal fluid could be passively or actively aspirated. Silicone oil top-up using a 25 gauge cannula would ensure a complete fill (Figures 15.3F to I).

Continuous infusion of heavy silicone oil while undertaking repeat surgery for inferior retinal redetachment has been shown to be possible using the 23 gauge system by Natarajan et al. Here a relaxing retinectomy is done and subretinal fluid aspirated while heavy silicone oil is continuously infused. The heavy silicone oil effectively tamponades the inferior retina.[9] No meniscus was observed between the regular and heavy silicone oil in such eyes.

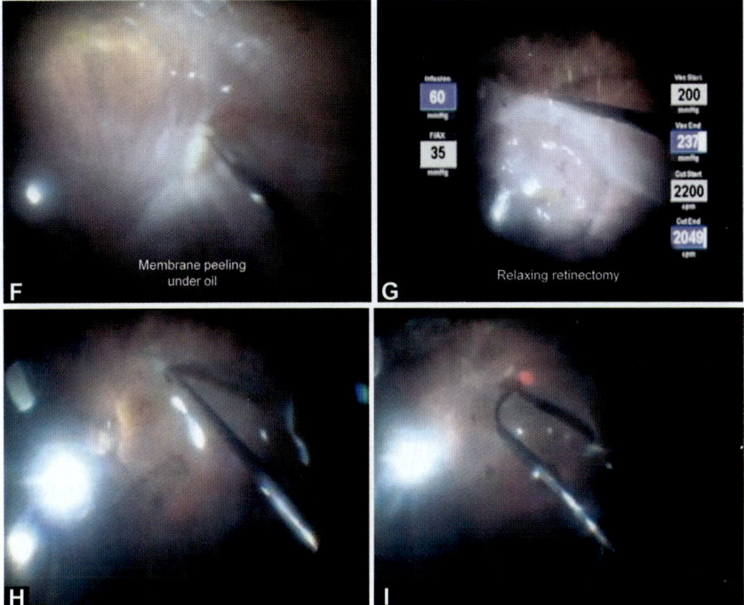

Figs 15.3F to I: (F) Membrane peeling under silicone oil; (G) Relaxing retinectomy under silicone oil. Note PFCL stabilizes posterior pole; (H) SRF drainage under silicone oil; (I) Endolaser under silicone oil (*Courtesy*: Dr Manish Nagpal)

TO SUTURE OR NOT TO SUTURE THE SCLEROTOMIES WHILE USING SILICONE OIL?

This decision must be made on table by the operating surgeon. If the sclerotomy leaks silicone oil, it must be sutured. In patients with thin sclera or low scleral rigidity as in a high myope or in children, the sclerotomy should be sutured. In patients undergoing a repeat surgery, the sclerotomies ideally must be sutured. Two methods of suturing include either a transconjunctival approach, where the sclerotomy is visible or by performing a localized peritomy, and then suturing the sclerotomy. The conjunctiva may either be sutured or approximated using bipolar cautery.

REMOVAL OF SILICONE OIL

The timing of silicone oil removal remains controversial. In the silicone oil study, early removal of silicone oil was advocated. It is however unlikely to advocate this modality in all clinical conditions. The major criteria for silicone oil removal must be the achievement of "complete" retinal reattachment, closure of "all" retinal breaks and the absence of proliferative membranes over or under the retina. The final decision must be individualized to each patient, the presence or absence of complications and the status of the fellow eye.

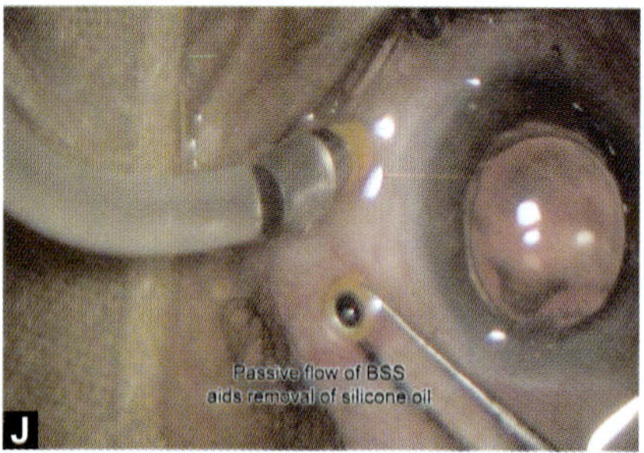

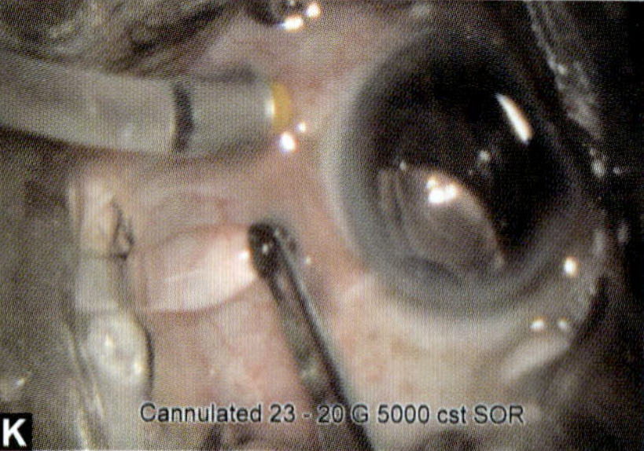

Figs 15.3J and K: (J) 23 Gauge passive silicone oil removal; (K) 23–20 gauge 5000 cst passive silicone oil removal

Conventional means of silicone oil removal is by a 19 gauge needle ideally attached to a vacuum pump. Active removal of 1000 cst silicone oil by 25 gauge TSV was first reported by Kapran et al without the need to close the sclerotomies with sutures.[10] They later reported passive removal of 1000 cst silicone by the 25 gauge system.[11] Passive removal of silicone oil by 23 gauge cannula system was first shown by Naresh et al [12] (Figure 15.3J). Patwardhan et al compared the safety and efficacy of 1000 cst silicone oil removal with 23 gauge and conventional sutured 20 gauge, wherein fluid-air exchange and 360° endolaser was done in all the eyes.[13] They reported hastening of recovery and similar efficacy as 20 gauge. Cekic et al have reported 23 gauge instrumentation for passive removal of 5000 cst silicone oil.[14] 5000 cst silicone oil is more easily removed passively using a single nonvalved 20 gauge cannula combined with 2 ports of 23 gauge (Figure 15.3K). Silicone oil can be actively aspirated using polyamide needle passed through the cannula. Alternatively an aspiration line is directly attached to the cannula and connected to an automated pump with a vacuum of 400–600 mm Hg. Removal of heavy silicone oil is possible only actively since this does not float up by the injected BSS. This is possible with 23 gauge transconjunctival system as was reported by Romano et al.[15]

COMBINED SURGERY WITH SILICONE OIL

The advent of MIVS has shifted the treatment paradigm for co-existing lenticular opacities with posterior segment pathologies. Combining phacoemulsification and intraocular lens implantation with vitreous surgery is preferred for its relatively atraumatic nature coupled with the advantage of lesser number of surgeries. While some retinal surgeons would prefer to tackle the posterior segment pathology first, it may be difficult to undertake the vitreous surgery in the presence of significant cataract. It is hence advisable in certain situations to first replace the cataract with an intraocular lens and wait for at least a week before undertaking the second posterior segment surgery. This would prevent most of the complications of posterior synechiae, fibrin deposition, closure of peripheral iridectomy and migration of silicone oil into the anterior chamber.

Combining phacoemulsification with silicone oil removal is another alternative wherein the lenticular opacification was not significant enough during the primary surgery, or developed in time following the vitrectomy. Some anterior segment surgeons have shown silicone oil removal to be possible via a posterior capsulotomy following cataract removal. But this is insufficient in removing all the tiny bubbles of silicone oil. MIVS can play a special role in this combined procedure allowing complete removal of the silicone oil.

COMPLICATIONS OF SILICONE OIL IN MIVS

Subconjunctival or sub-Tenon's silicone oil has been seen more often where MIVS was performed without suturing the sclerotomies.[16] This collects as multiple small bubbles which are difficult to drain or remove and may cause repeated episodes of inflammation postoperatively. Nearly one third of patients could have subconjunctival blebs corresponding to silicone oil, and nearly 90% have an inflammatory response.

Suprachoroidal infusion of silicone oil can occur if the cannula gets pulled or displaced during vitrectomy and it goes unrecognized. Hence, it is imperative that the cannula is visualized in the vitreous cavity before beginning silicone oil infusion, or a relatively longer infusion cannula (Figure 15.1) be used. The flow of silicone oil into the vitreous cavity can also be ascertained before removing the light pipe from the cannula.

Retinal redetachment has been reported after removal of silicone oil. The main cause is failure to identify and close peripheral breaks, whether iatrogenic or missed, by cryopexy or by laser photocoagulation. This can happen both in the primary surgery and secondary surgery to remove the silicone oil. Indirect ophthalmoscopy with scleral depression at the end of the procedure before fluid-air exchange should be done. With increasing use of wide-angle viewing system, the ability to visualize the peripheral retina under high magnification helps to rule out the presence of retinal breaks. 360° laser photocoagulation performed either a month before removing the silicone oil or during the surgery[17] itself has been found to reduce the rate of retinal detachments. Incomplete removal of the vitreous base in the primary surgery may leave behind residual traction leading to retinal redetachment following silicone oil removal.[18]

Hypotony following silicone oil removal can occur. Kim et al studied various factors including age, number of previous pars plana vitrectomies, number of intraoperative endolaser applications, extent of remaining posterior proliferative vitreoretinopathy and the degree of proliferative vitreoretinopathy removal, number of preoperative antiglaucoma ophthalmic solutions, duration of postoperative anterior chamber inflammation, axial length, preoperative intraocular pressure, and duration of oil tamponade, showed that only axial length was significantly associated with the development of postoperative transient hypotony. Most cases recovered within a week.[19]

Other complications of the use of silicone oil such as glaucoma, keratopathy, silicone oil emulsification, subretinal migration of silicone oil, cataract, etc. can also occur in MIVS procedure.

Heavy Silicone Oil

Heavy silicone oil, a mixture of polydimethylsiloxane with perfluorohexyloctane (Densiron) is a new addition. This silicone oil is heavier than water and provides better tamponade inferiorly. This is converse to the regular silicone oil that is lighter than water and does not provide good tamponade inferiorly. Its use is advocated in complex inferior retinal detachments either primarily or in previously failed retinal detachments with regular silicone oil. Auriol et al studied the use of heavy silicone oil in complicated retinal detachment involving a large inferior retinectomy.[20] While the heavy silicone oil provided efficient endotamponade inferiorly, it was complicated with inflammatory reaction in almost half the patients. Joussen et al compared standard silicone oil versus heavy silicone oil in inferior PVR but could not demonstrate any difference in efficacy.[21] Romano et al compared 23 gauge vitrectomy with Densiron and 20 gauge vitreous surgery with scleral buckle and SF6 in retinal detachment with inferior breaks.[22] They reported no difference in outcome of both the procedures. Sandner et al reported a poor anatomical success of 33.3% with Densiron in primary surgery that went up to 75% following reoperation.[23] Wong et al reported a better success rate of 81% with one operation and 93% after reoperations using heavy silicone oil.[24]

Heavy silicone oil must be removed after a period of 2 to 3 months. Longer use is likely to cause a pressure necrosis of the retina.

REFERENCES

1. Abrams GW, Azen SP, McCuen BW, Flynn HW, Lai MY, Ryan SJ. Vitrectomy With Silicone Oil or Long-Acting Gas in Eyes With Severe Proliferative Vitreoretinopathy: Results of Additional and Long-term Follow-up: Silicone Study Report 11 Arch Ophthalmol. 1997;115(3):335–44.
2. Shah CP, Ho AC, Regillo CD, Fineman MS, Vander JF, Brown GC. Short-term outcomes of 25 gauge vitrectomy with silicone oil for repair of complicated retinal detachment. Retina. 2008;28(5):723–8.
3. Altan T, Acar N, Kapran Z, Unver YB, Ozdogan S. Transconjunctival 25 gauge sutureless vitrectomy and silicone oil injection in diabetic tractional retinal detachment. Retina. 2008;28(9):1201–6.
4. Erakgun T, Egrilmez S. Surgical outcomes of transconjunctival sutureless 23 gauge vitrectomy with silicone oil injection. Indian J Ophthalmol. 2009;57(2):105–9.
5. Riemann CD, Miller DM, Foster RE, Petersen MR. Outcomes of transconjunctival sutureless 25 gauge vitrectomy with silicone oil infusion. Retina. 2007;27(3):296–303.
6. Rubens Camargo Siqueira, Aline Degasperi Cote Gil, Rodrigo Jorge. Retinal detachment surgery with silicone oil injection in transconjunctival sutureless 23 gauge vitrectomy. Arq Bras Oftalmol. 2007;70(6):905–9.

7. Chang S , Lincoff H, Zimmerman NJ, et al. Giant retinal tears. Surgical techniques and results using perfluorocarbon liquid. Arch Ophthalmol. 1989;107:761–6.
8. Steve Charles. The Interface Vitrectomy Technique. Retina Today February 2010.
9. Natarajan S. Densiron Infusion Sandwich Technique; Presented at the 16th Afro Asian Congress of Ophthalmology, Istanbul, Turkey June 2012.
10. Kapran Z, Acar N. Removal of silicone oil with 25 gauge transconjunctival sutureless vitrectomy system. Retina. 2007;27(8):1059–64.
11. Kapran Z, Acar N, Unver YB, Altan T, Ocak B. Passive removal of silicone oil with a 25 gauge sutureless system. Jpn J Ophthalmol. 2008;52(1):63–6.
12. Naresh B, Ramchandani B, Dhawan A, Shukla D, Kim R. 23G Transconjunctival sutureless silicone oil removal. Presented at the Vitreo Retina Society India Annual Conference 2008.
13. Patwardhan SD, Azad R, Shah V, Sharma Y. The safety and efficacy of passive removal of silicone oil with 23 gauge transconjunctival sutureless system. Retina. 2010;30(8):1237–41.
14. Cekiç O, Cakir M, Yilmaz OF. Passive silicone oil removal in 23 gauge transconjunctival vitrectomy. Ophthalmic Surg Lasers Imaging. 2011;42(6):514–5.
15. Romano MR, Groenwald C, Das R, Stappler T, Wong D, Heimann H. Removal of Densiron-68 with a 23 gauge transconjunctival vitrectomy system. Eye (Lond). 2009;23(3):715–7.
16. Cunha LP, Primiano Júnior HP, Nakashima A, Trein Júnior JA, Ghanem RC, Santo RM, et al. Subconjunctival deposit of silicone oil after vitreoretinal surgery. Arq Bras Oftalmol. 2007;70(4):589–92.
17. Falkner-Radler CI, Smretschnig E, Graf A, Binder S. Outcome after silicone oil removal and simultaneous 360° endolaser treatment. Acta Ophthalmol. 2011 Feb;89(1):e46–51.
18. Unlü N, Kocaoğlan H, Acar MA, Sargin M, Aslan BS, Duman S. Outcome of complex retinal detachment surgery after silicone oil removal. Int Ophthalmol. 2004;25(1):33-6.
19. Kim SW, Oh J, Yang KS, Kim MJ, Rhim JW, Huh K. Risk factors for the development of transient hypotony after silicone oil removal. Retina. 2010;30(8):1228–36.
20. Sylvain Auriol, Vẹronique Pagot-Mathis, Laurence Mahieu, Claudia Lemoine, André Mathis. Efficacy and safety of heavy silicone oil Densiron 68® in the treatment of complicated retinal detachment with large inferior retinectomy. Graefe's Archive for Clinical and Experimental Ophthalmology. 2008;246(10):1383–9.
21. Joussen AM, Rizzo S, Kirchhof B, Schrage N, Li X, Lente C, et al. HSO-Study Group Heavy silicone oil versus standard silicone oil in as vitreous tamponade in inferior PVR (HSO Study): Interim analysis. Acta Ophthalmol. 2011;89(6):e483–9.
22. Romano Mario R; Angi Martina; Valldeperas Xavier; Costagliola Ciro; Vinciguerra Paolo. Twenty-three–gauge pars plana vitrectomy, Densiron-68, and 360° endolaser versus combined 20 gauge pars plana vitrectomy, scleral buckle, and Sf6 for pseudophakic retinal detachment with inferior retinal breaks. Retina. 2011;31(4):686–91.
23. Sandner D, Herbrig E, Engelmann K. High-density silicone oil (Densiron) as a primary intraocular tamponade: 12-month follow up. Graefes Arch Clin Exp Ophthalmol. 2007;245(8):1097–105.
24. Wong D, van Meurs JC, Stappler T, Groenewold C, Pearce IA, McGalliard JN, et al. A pilot study on the use of a perfluorohexyloctane/silicone oil solution as a heavier than water internal tamponade agent. Br J Ophthalmol. 2005;89:662–5.

CHAPTER

16

Combined Cataract and Vitreoretinal Surgery

Shobhit Chawla

Cataract exists as comorbidity in fair number of patients with posterior segment disorders, especially diabetes.[1] Vitrectomy itself contributes to cataractogenesis.[2,4,5] With the evolution of technology combined cataract extraction and vitrectomy have become safe and effective.[13] Combined cataract and vitreoretinal surgery gives us an opportunity to address both the cataract and posterior segment pathology as a single step approach.[11] Elderly patients with pre-existing nuclear sclerosis are suitable candidates for combined surgical procedure. Rapid visual rehabilitation is one of the main advantages of this procedure.

Cataract removal during surgery aids in better visualization of the posterior segment. It allows maximum access to the anterior vitreoretinal structures. Combined surgery is thus recommended in patients having significant cataract that limits the ability to perform finer marginal maneuvers like membrane dissection, both at the posterior fundus and also when tractional membranes exist anteriorly.[10]

At the time when modern vitreoretinal technique were under evolution cataract surgery in eyes with posterior segment pathology especially proliferative diabetic retinopathy was linked to the development of neovascular glaucoma but modern surgical techniques used for cataract like phacoemulsification have decreased the incidence of these complications.[7]

In patients who undergo macular hole surgery there is a high rate of nuclear cataract progression of up to 81.1% in 2 years and at least 25% patients will require postoperative cataract surgery.[3] Thus, patients who undergo combined macular hole and cataract surgery can enjoy a faster postoperative rehabilitation with improvement in visual acuity.[9]

In one series 47% have shown progression or appearance of nuclear sclerosis for after vitrectomy idiopathic epiretinal membrane while virtually no changes in anterior subcapsular cataract and posterior subcapsular cataract.[3,4,6]

Indications

1. **In Diabetic Retinopathy**[12]
   In conjunction with almost any complication of diabetic retinopathy; Taut posterior hyaloid membrane, epiretinal membranes in diabetic retinopathy, vitreous hemorrhage, tractional retinal detachments requiring vitreous surgery with unimanual or bimanual dissection and during reoperations like vitreous lavage for recurrent vitreous hemorrhage and silicone oil removal.
2. **Macular Hole Surgery**: Combined Surgery in macular hole as a single step approach if grade II nuclear sclerosis coexists.[9]
3. **Epiretinal Membrane Surgery**: Epiretinal membrane surgery if cataract of grade I + or so exists.[3]
4. **Rhegmatogenous Retinal Detachments**: Vitrectomy for Rhegmatogenous retinal detachment when cataract coexists and in some cases to achieve meticulous vitreous base excision.[10]
5. **Vitreous Hemorrhage with Coexistant Cataract of Unknown Etiology**:[13] Many times the diagnosis of such patients is established intraoperatively.
6. Ocular trauma cases with lens injury or where lens has to be removed to facilitate other maneuvers (Figures 16.1A to C).

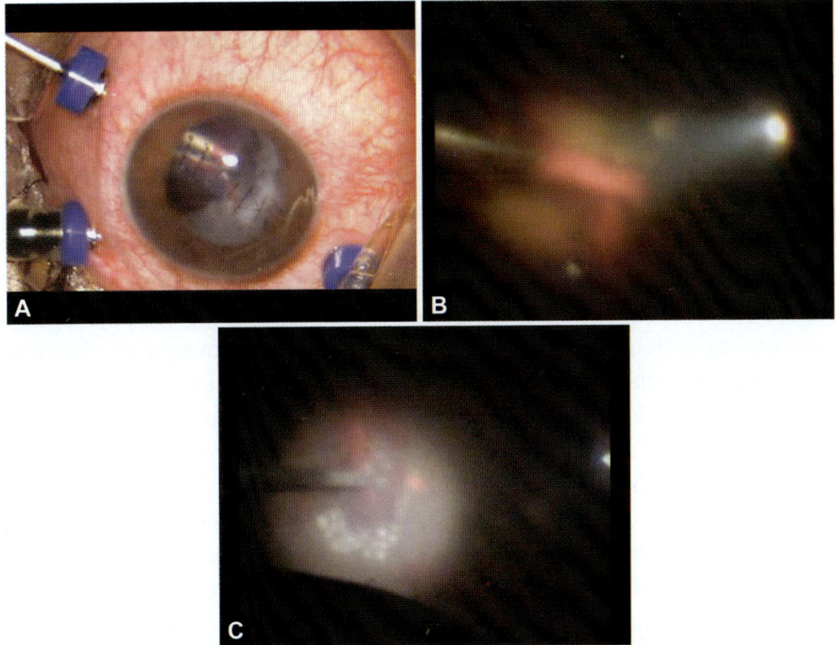

Figs 16.1A to C: (A) Lensectomy and anterior vitrectomy being done using 23 gauge valved cannulas. *Note* Corneal sutures; (B) Vitrectomy for postpenetrating injury vitreous hemorrhage; (C) Endolaser being done surrounding area of retinochoroidal penetrating injury site

Technique

With the evolution of technology the technique of combined surgery has made a paradigm shift. At present the preferred technique in our hands is a coaxial microincision phacoemulsification and 23 gauge vitrectomy.[13] The reason for preference of coaxial microincision phacoemulsification is that the 2.2 mm wound is very stable and the 2 mm intracorneal course provides excellent stability to bear the strains of a 23 gauge vitreous surgery procedure on the globe (Figure 16.2A). The procedure can start with the preplacement of pars plana infusion. This is mandatory if a 20 gauge surgery is being planned; but can be deferred till after the phacoemulsification if a 23 or 25 gauge procedure is being done. Postplacement of suture on the cataract wound depends on the wound stability and the technique of phacoemulsification adopted.[8] IOL implantation, in most cases Acrylic foldable implants whether hydrophobic or hydrophilic, as per choice of the surgeon is done at conclusion of the phacoemulsification prior to starting vitrectomy (Figure 16.2B). The vitreous surgery is accomplished mostly with either 23 gauge (Figure 16.2C) or 25 gauge procedure transconjunctivally unless the conjunctiva has been opened for buckling or a 20 gauge approach is deemed necessary. We personally prefer the single step 9° approach with the trocar cannula system for both 23 gauge and 25 gauge sclerotomies as it seals better. The main advantage intraoperatively is observed in cases of proliferative diabetic retinopathy, where using wide-angle viewing anterior vitreous gel or hemorrhage can be removed and the peripheral retina can be well ablated by photocoagulation in this psuedophakic situation, in contrast to phakic situation. Similar advantage is observed when excising the vitreous base in eyes with rhegmatogenous retinal detachments with and without PVR. Of course the clear view in the center aids in dissection in cases of tractional retinal detachments of the posterior pole, ILM peeling in macular holes (Figure 16.2D) and epiretinal membrane removal. Here the contact lens viewing systems offer excellent view for these fine maneuvers, but one can also use the macula lens of noncontact wide-angle viewing systems. At conclusion of the three port vitrectomy procedure a routine fluid air exchange can be done using about 30 to 40 mm Hg air pressure using active or passive fluid extrusion technique (Figure 16.2E). This ensures proper sealing of the sclerotomies. Later on, nonexpansile gas mixture or silicone oil can be used if warranted in the particular situation. We like to use an extrusion needle placed in midvitreous cavity during infusion of nonexpansile gas as this ensures a complete replacement of air with the gas mixture. If any leak is noticed on removal of the cannulae, sclerotomies can be sutured transconjunctivally with a single 6-0 vicryl suture.

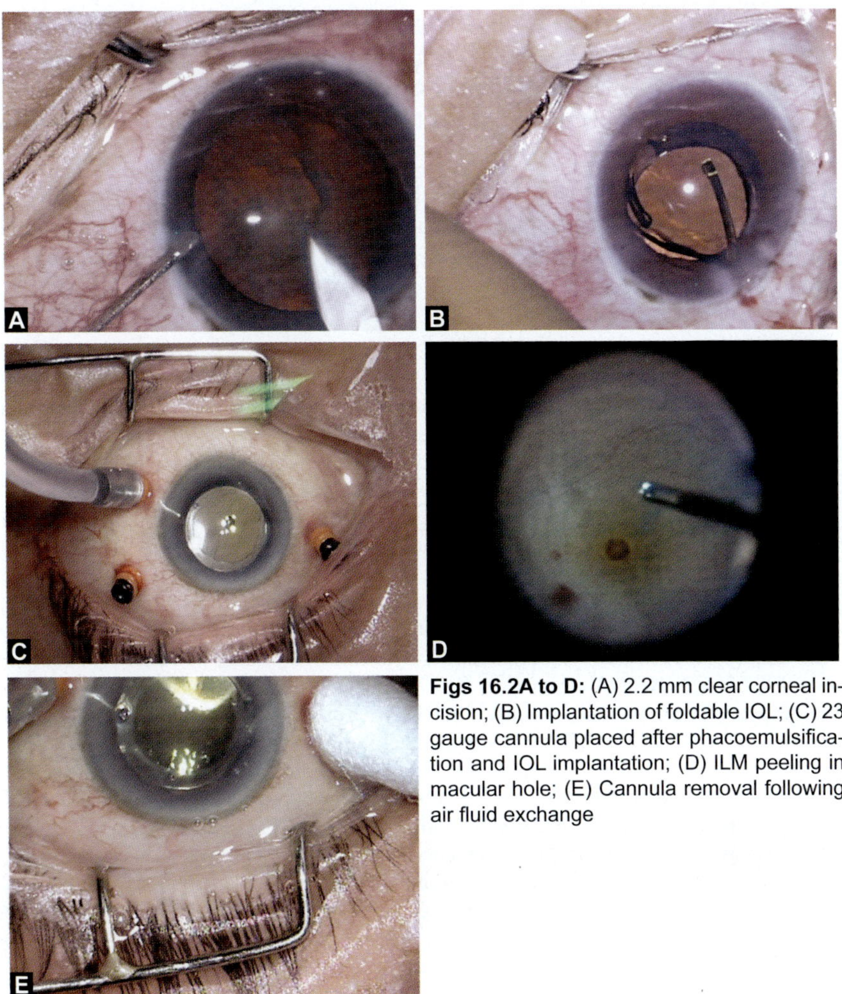

Figs 16.2A to D: (A) 2.2 mm clear corneal incision; (B) Implantation of foldable IOL; (C) 23 gauge cannula placed after phacoemulsification and IOL implantation; (D) ILM peeling in macular hole; (E) Cannula removal following air fluid exchange

SOME PEARLS

Many patients especially diabetics undergoing combined surgery should ideally have a cornea friendly surgery with use of viscoelastic to ensure a clear cornea for the posterior segment procedure. As most of us use clear corneal phacoemulsification, hydration of corneal ports should not be done prior to the vitreoretinal procedure; but instead the viscoelastic should be retained after IOL implantation to maintain a stable anterior chamber. The anterior chamber should not be over deepened so as to avoid injury to the zonular apparatus while inserting the trocar and cannulae.

Special Considerations of Combined Surgery in Uveitic Eyes

Patients with complicated cataract needing vitrectomy for posterior or intermediate uveitis should be put on intensive steroid therapy starting at least a week before surgery and continuing postoperatively for another few months.

Posterior synechiolysis helps in dilating the pupil thereby providing proper view of the posterior segment.

Cyclitic membranes tends to restrict the proper entry of the infusion port. Cataract removal helps to visualize the infusion sleeve before the surgeon starts the infusion.

Cataract removal helps in proper visualization of the vitreous base thereby assisting in cyclitic membrane peeling. Postoperative hypotony is a real complication in cases with extensive cyclitic membranes. Silicone oil should be injected whenever in doubt.

REFERENCES

1. Klein BE, Klein R, Moss SE. Incidence of cataract surgery in the Wisconsin epidemiologic study of diabetic retinopathy. Am J Ophthalmol. 1995;119(3):295–300.
2. Petermeier K, Szurman P, Bartz-Schmidt UK, Gekeler F. Pathophysiology of cataract formation after vitrectomy, KlinMonblAugenheilkd. 2010;227(3):175–80.
3. Thompson JT. The role of patient age and intraocular gas use in cataract progression after vitrectomy for macular holes and epiretinal membranes. Am J Ophthalmol. 2004;137(2):250–7.
4. Chung CP, Hsu SY, Wu WC. Cataract formation after pars plana vitrectomy, Kaohsiung J Med Sci. 2001;17(2):84–9.
5. Blodi BA, Paluska SA. Cataract after vitrectomy in young patients, Ophthalmol. 1997;104(7):1092–5.
6. Hsuan JD, Brown NA, Bron AJ, Patel CK, Rosen PH. Posterior subcapsular and nuclear cataract after vitrectomy. J Cataract Refract Surg. 2001;27(3):437–44.
7. Wensheng L, Wu R, Wang X, Xu M, Sun G, Sun C. Clinical complications of combined phacoemulsification and vitrectomy for eyes with coexisting cataract and vitreoretinal diseases. Eur J Ophthalmol. 2009;19(1):37–45.
8. Demetriades AM, Gottsch JD, Thomsen R, Azab A, Stark WJ, Campochiaro PA, et al. Combined phacoemulsification, intraocular lens implantation, and vitrectomy for eyes with coexisting cataract and vitreoretinalpathology. Am J Ophthalmol. 2003;135(3):291–6.
9. Lahey JM, Francis RR, Fong DS, Kearney JJ, Tanaka S. Combining phacoemulsification with vitrectomy for treatment of macular holes. Br J Ophthalmol. 2002;86(8):876–8.
10. Ogino N, Kumagai K. Advantage of combined procedure in vitreous surgery, Semi Ophthalmol. 2001;16(3):137–8. Review.
11. Mochizuki Y, Kubota T, Hata Y, Miyazaki M, Suyama Y, Enaida H, et al. Surgical results of combined pars plana vitrectomy, phacoemulsification, and intraocular lens implantation. Eur J Ophthalmol. 2006;16(2):279–86.
12. Diolaiuti S, Senn P, Schmid MK, Job O, Maloca P, Schipper I. Combined pars planavitrectomy and phacoemulsification with intraocular lens implantation in severe proliferative diabetic retinopathy. Ophthalmic Surg Lasers Imaging. 2006;37(6):468–74.
13. Yazici AT, Kara N, Bozkurt E, Cakir M, Goker H, Demirok A, et al. Combined 23 gauge transconjunctival sutureless vitrectomy and cataract surgery in cases with cataract and posterior segment diseases. Middle East Afr J Ophthalmol. 2010;17(4):359–64.

CHAPTER

17

Hybrid Vitrectomy

Manish Nagpal

INTRODUCTION

Pars plana vitrectomy as a technique has revolutionized retinal surgery since its advent and initial report by Machemer et al.[1] It allowed the removal of traction by an internal method, essential in retinal detachment procedures, as well as provided an active management modality for vitreous hemorrhage and opened the door for surgical intervention in a myriad of retinal pathologies.

The last decade has seen a general trend toward efficient, minimal invasive interventions in several areas of medicine.[2-5] Cataract surgery was revolutionized by the introduction of phacoemulsification and foldable IOLs. This technology enabled a reduction in the size of the incision and avoided the necessity of using sutures. This transition shortened surgical time, reduced complications, and increased the satisfaction and comfort of the patient. The same transition is occurring in vitreous surgery. Ever since the introduction of pars plana vitrectomy over 30 years ago, the instrumentarium of posterior segment surgery, too, has been subject to incessant change. In this, two objectives have been in the foreground: One is reducing surgical time, and the other is speeding the recovery of the eye. The primary means of reaching these targets lies in instruments that are smaller and thus induce less surgical trauma and at the same time are more efficient, while affording improved visualization and illumination of the operating field.

Traditional 20 gauge pars plana vitrectomy requires a conjunctival peritomy prior to making the sclerotomies. It requires sutures to close the sclerotomy and conjunctiva. Sutures can warp the surface of the eye, leading to temporary postoperative astigmatism. In addition, suture-induced granulomatous reaction can rarely occur. Finally, extra time in the operating room is required to close up the sclerotomies and conjunctiva.

In 2002, Eugene de Juan, MD, introduced 25 gauge transconjunctival sutureless vitrectomy (TSV).[6] This system permits 3 port pars plana vitrectomy using microcannulas, trocars, and 25 gauge instrumentation, without requiring sutures to close the sclerotomies. Subsequently, Claus Eckardt, MD, developed a similar technique, but with 23 gauge instrumentation.[7] While the

20 gauge vitrectomy system still is considered the 'gold standard' of pars plana vitrectomy, the last 5 years, in particular, have seen fast paced innovation in the field of the posterior segment instrumentarium toward smaller, more efficient 25 and 23 gauge vitrectomy systems, which now-a-days are routinely used.

The advent of smaller gauge instrumentation allows for minimally invasive vitreoretinal surgery (MIVS) as compared to conventional pars plana vitrectomy. To perform minimally invasive surgery has many advantages for both the surgeon and the patient. Small gauge sutureless vitrectomy technique is becoming increasingly popular because of the minimal surgical trauma, less exchange of intraocular fluids and better stabilization of the detached retina while the vitreous is removed, faster wound healing, decreased convalescence period, improved postoperative comfort and reduced post-operative astigmatism associated with this technique.[8-10] Because small surgical incisions do not require sutures, the operation times for vitrectomy and the postoperative inflammation are reduced, and patient recuperation is more rapid.

Nonetheless, the original MIVS procedure did pose some unique difficulties. The major issue arose from the excessive flexibility of the first generation 25 gauge instruments, making it difficult for surgeons to adequately shave the vitreous base and to rotate the eye. As a result, procedures that put stress on the instruments at the sclerotomy sites, such as removal of anterior fibrovascular proliferation, were more difficult to perform. The smaller diameter of its light probes also created a problem with inadequate illumination. Postoperative leakage of gas or silicone oil from the sclerotomies into the subconjunctival space was another concern with this new procedure. Furthermore, an incomplete repertoire of 25 gauge instruments severely limited the types of procedures performed by MIVS. For instance, the lack of a 25 gauge curved laser probe made peripheral photocoagulation difficult. In addition, since MPC scissors and illuminated instruments were not available in 25 gauge, MIVS was not used in cases of severe PVR or tractional retinal detachment. Other procedures, such as removal of silicone oil or dense vitreous hemorrhage, were not performed with MIVS due to the low flow rate caused by the smaller inner lumen diameter.

After Eckardt introduced 23 gauge MIVS in 2005,[7] this addressed the major concerns present in the first generation 25 gauge vitrectomy system. The stiffer shaft of the 23 gauge instrumentation feels much like that of a 20 gauge instrument, improving both vitreous gel removal and vitreous base shaving relative to 25 gauge instruments; in addition, the larger diameter of the 23 gauge provides improved illumination and higher flow rate, increasing the ease with which silicone oil and other dense materials can be removed. Furthermore, it retained all of the advantages of 25 gauge vitrectomy over the 20 gauge procedure.

HOW RECENT ADVANCES HAVE ADDRESSED EARLY SMALL GAUGE CONCERNS

- **Instrument Rigidity**: Rigidity of instruments is a problem with 25 gauge, as instruments are more pliable and can bend and break, and moving the globe around can be cumbersome. This is not a problem with 23 gauge, as rigidity is similar to that of 20 gauge. In addition, several companies have made new 25 gauge instruments more rigid and/or reducing the length to achieve the same purpose.
- **Instrumentation Availability**: Although initially instrumentation was limited to forceps in small gauge, at present a full armamentarium of instruments is available in small gauges, including extrusion cannulas for silicone oil injection and removal, scissors, dual-bore cannulas for perfluorocarbon injection, diathermy, multidirectional laser probes, chandeliers, and 40 gauge cannulas for subretinal injections. In essence, at present the same range of instruments used in 20 gauge is available in 23 and 25 gauge, with the exception of a fragmatome. Nevertheless, several companies are working on developing a 23 gauge fragmatome to address dislocated nuclei.
- **Illumination**: Since the number of light fibers is reduced, particularly in 25 gauge procedures, brighter light sources are needed such as the Photon (Synergetics Inc, O'Fallon, MO) and Xenon (Alcon Labs, Fort Worth, TX). Alcon's new Constellation system has a light that is much brighter than the actual Xenon, and Baush & Lomb (Rochester, NY) uses the Photon, so light is not an issue any longer.
- **Cutting Efficiency**: Slow vitreous removal is a problem with 25 gauge at present but this challenge is addressed in the new Constellation machine. The new 25 gauge probe has a bigger opening and a longer duty cycle (amount of time the port is open). This allows for increased aspiration rate while having high-speed cutting rates. The 23 gauge system will benefit from the same duty cycle improvement. Plus the probe is different, and it does not have a spring mechanism to open it so it can stay open longer during each cut, allowing greater aspiration. Thus, the rapidity of vitreous removal with 23 and 25 gauge will be markedly improved. Cutting rates of up to 5000 cpm are available with Constellation, allowing for shaving of the vitreous base and safer vitrectomy even in detached retinas.
- **Wound Architecture**: Achieving proper wound architecture is the most important aspect of small gauge surgery, as complications of endophthalmitis and retinal breaks are associated with the wounds. Initially, wounds were made in 25 gauge procedures by direct entry, which is potentially a cause of hypotony and other potential problems, including increased endophthalmitis rates. Displacement of the conjunctiva and 2 plane wounds with fluid-air exchange at the end of the procedure allow for reduced wound leaks and less risk of endophthalmitis and hypotony. The DORC (Zuidland, The Netherlands) 23 gauge and the new Alcon 23 gauge

TSV systems have a flat-blade trocar system that produce a slit wound, which closes better than the actual chevron wound made by the round trocar blade system. Wound construction in our view is the most important aspect of this surgery and the most important aspect of the learning curve, but if in doubt, just suture. Our threshold to suture a sclerotomy tends to be lower in complicated cases where silicone oil needs to be used.

- **Surgical Outcomes**: Outcomes are excellent. Benefits include astigmatic neutral surgery, important in this age of refractive surgery, shortened time, and less inflammation and patient discomfort. We truly believe that the increased incidence of endophthalmitis is technique-dependent. With adequate preoperative povidone preparation, good wound construction in 2 steps with a partial or total fluid-air exchange at the end of the procedure, and subconjunctival antibiotics, the complications of hypotony and endophthalmitis can be kept to a minimum.
- **Learning Curve**: The learning curve for wound construction and for 25 gauge at present is due to lack of rigidity. The TSV 23 gauge system has less of a learning curve, as instruments feel just like 20 gauge.

In a nutshell, 23 gauge has been more user-friendly due to the light (comparable to 20 gauge), rigidity, and increased flow through the instruments (aspiration rates like 20 gauge). With the new improvements of the 25 gauge system, at least with the Constellation system, 25 gauge surgery will feel more like 23 gauge as rigidity, aspiration, and light will be increased significantly. These improvements have led to a wider acceptance of MIVS.

There are also some drawbacks to performing 25 and 23 gauge vitrectomy. To date certain instrumentation is still limited compared to 20 gauge vitrectomy. In cases, where fragmentation, MPC scissors, or bimanual surgery is preferred, 20 gauge may offer certain advantages. Silicone oil infusion as well as removal can be cumbersome and time consuming with small gauge vitrectomy.

In spite of its considerably widened range of applications, 25 gauge vitrectomy to date continues to be associated with certain disadvantages: the high flexibility, slower gel removal time and delicate nature of 25 gauge instruments that require specific prior training on the part of the surgeon, while rendering some surgical manipulation altogether impossible. For these reasons, and also in view of its reduced flow rate, 25 gauge vitrectomy is still not an option for all applications and is not an all purpose vitrectomy system.

The 23 gauge system provides faster speed of vitrectomy and the instruments have stiffer shafts, but it requires a larger incision.

Therefore, 25 gauge is suitable in macular surgery and for less complex cases, while 23 gauge allows the performance of complex retinal detachment. Patients suffering from more severe pathologies with poor visual recovery are still managed with 20 gauge technology.

To overcome these limitations of small gauge vitrectomy and to expand the existing indications for surgery, use of combined systems, using a single

20 gauge superior vitrector port and two small gauge ports, namely one superior port for endoillumination and one inferotemporal infusion port have been advocated.

Indications

1. *Dropped lens matter*: Fragmatomes are not yet available in a small gauge version. Generally, posteriorly dislocated lens or dropped nucleus are contraindications for this sutureless technique.[11] One sclerotomy can be enlarged for phacofragmenter use for lensectomy or removal of dislocated lens material.
2. *Intraocular foreign body*: Use of the forceps (Machemer-Parel diamond-coated, Wilson's forcep) for intraocular foreign body removal also necessitates enlarging one port. Utilizing one 20 gauge sclerotomy with two 25 gauge sclerotomies to address the mechanical properties of the dropped nucleus and the physical size of the intraocular foreign body was found to be safe and effective.
3. *Silicone oil removal*: This type of hybrid arrangement is also ideal for silicone oil removal. Because only one port needs to be larger—the one used to remove the silicone oil—the infusion port and the illumination port can remain 25 or 23 gauge. This retains most of the advantages attributed to the small gauge procedure, while eliminating the disadvantage of slow and cumbersome silicone oil removal.
4. *Complex cases requiring silicone oil infusion*: Because MIVS preserves ocular structures and minimizes scarring of the conjunctiva, sclera, and tenon's layer, it is an excellent choice for patients who have had multiple previous ocular surgeries or may require surgery in the future (i.e. a glaucoma patient with an existing, or a likelihood of a future, trabeculectomy). MIVS, however, may not always be optimal in certain circumstances; nonetheless, small gauge instrumentation need not be abandoned, even in complicated cases. For instance, in the rare case where MIVS is unsuccessful at repairing a retinal detachment, one of the ports can be enlarged to 20 gauge and the procedure can be completed. One port can be enlarged in cases requiring silicone oil injection. This enables easy and quick infusion of silicone oil and suturing the port decreases any chances of oil leak postoperatively. While now-a-days silicone oil may be infused through a 25 gauge sclerotomy, this process clearly prolongs surgery times.
5. *Bimanual surgery with multipurpose instruments*: The 20/25 technique can also be used for 20 gauge conformal forceps, end gaugeripping diamond-coated forceps, the Chang end-aspirating laser probe, the disposable bipolar endoilluminator, or certain illuminated instruments for so-called bimanual surgery. For example, during a complex tractional retinal detachment repair, the surgeon may use a forceps in one hand and an illuminated pick in the other to facilitate delamination of membranes.

These techniques allow the advantages of small gauge to be combined with the advantages of one special purpose 20 gauge sclerotomy.

Instrumentation

Transconjunctival sutureless vitrectomy consists of a 23 gauge or 25 gauge microcannula system and a wide array of vitreoretinal instruments specifically designed for this operating system. The microcannula consists of a thin-walled tube 4 mm in length. A collar is present at the extraocular portion and can be grasped with a forceps to manipulate the microcannula. The insertion trocar has a sharp tip that forms a continuous bevel with the microcannula, allowing ease to entry through the conjunctiva into the eye. A wide array of vitreoretinal microsurgical instruments complying with the 23/25 gauge standards has been designed. These include vitreous cutters, illumination probes, intraocular forceps, microvitreoretinal blades, tissue manipulator, aspirating picks, aspirators, soft-tip cannulas, curved scissors, extendable curved picks, intraocular laser probes, and diathermy probes.

TROCAR-CANNULA SYSTEM

The newer noncoring trocars require less insertion force when compared with competitive hypodermic based coring type design. The cannula fits over the trocar, which allows a 23 or 25 gauge sclerotomy and simultaneous insertion of a cannula. The cannula maintains the alignment between the conjunctival and scleral openings and facilitates instrument insertion, thus, preventing the breaks at the vitreous base due to repeated insertion of instrumentation. The earlier generation cannulas were metallic and the incisions made by the older blade were chevron-shaped and patulous, thus increasing the chances of wound leak. The newer EdgePlus MVR blades (Alcon Laboratories, Inc.) have a hump perpendicular to the horizontal plane of the blade, which stretches the tissue in the direction perpendicular to the horizontal plane of the blade and thus ensures a slit-like incision (Figures 17.1A and B). The slit-like incision is always better as it is not patulous and is stable.

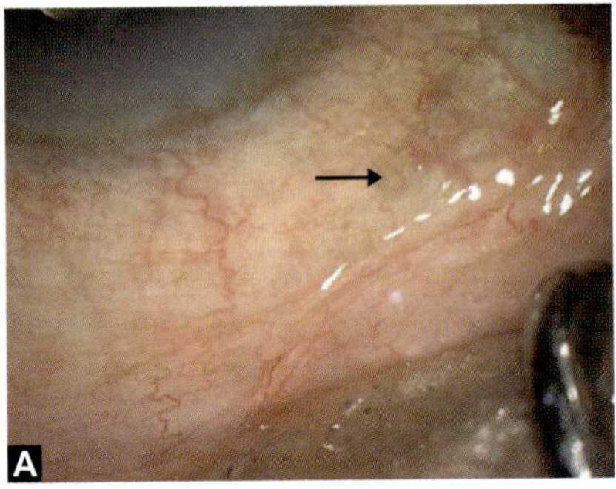

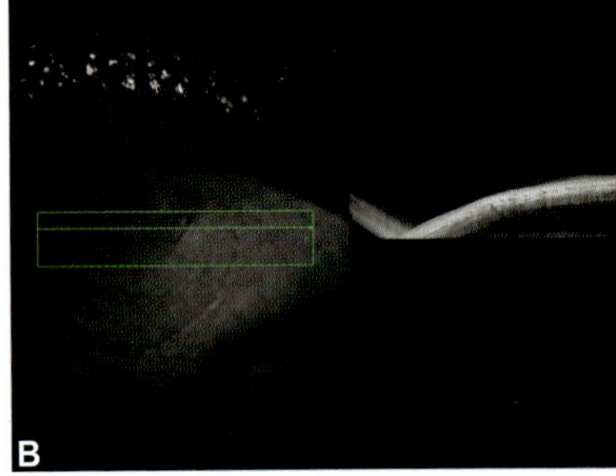

Figs 17.1A and B: (A) Linear incision; (B) Anterior segment OCT showing the well closed linear incision

DIFFERENT TYPES OF INCISIONS

Stab incision: For 25 gauge vitrectomy, direct entry is made with small gauge trocars after conjunctival displacement at the pars plana at the required distance from the limbus depending on the phakic status of the patient. The disadvantage to this incision is that leakage of intraocular fluid can occur, increasing the risk of endophthalmitis.

Oblique incision: The entry is made in an oblique fashion with the trocar 30º to the sclera. The length of the incision should be adequate. The disadvantage to the oblique incision is that the inner tissues are often disrupted, resulting in an insecure postoperative wound.[12]

Biplanar incision: The incision is two-stepped: Initially, the blade is inserted at a 30º angle and then entry is made perpendicular to the sclera.[13] The advantages of this incision is that it prevents hypotony and the wound is more secure.

Surgical Technique

A small gauge (23/25) two port setup for infusion and illumination was used along with a 20 gauge vitrectomy through a third port. Small gauge vitrectomy is usually performed with the patient under local anesthesia. General anesthesia is only used in selected cases. Intravenous sedation may also be helpful in selected cases. After appropriate anesthesia, the operative field is prepared using antiseptic solutions. Preoperatively, the eyelash margins are scrubbed with povidone-iodine solution. The microcannulas are inserted through the conjunctiva into the eye by means of a trocar. Insertion is accomplished by first displacing the conjunctiva laterally by approximately 2 mm, blocking direct access into the eye and thus reducing the risk of infection. The pressure plate forceps have an incorporated caliper to measure distance from the limbus apart and have serrations on the undersurfaces, allowing a good hold on the conjunctiva for misalignment over the proposed scleral entry. Initially, the blade is inserted obliquely into the sclera at an angle of about 30º to 45º up to the cannula mark. Then, the direction of the blade is adjusted perpendicular to the sclera as it is inserted into the vitreous cavity. The biplanar incision not only holds the cannula in place but also prevents egress of fluid in the postoperative period. We use the biplanar incision for both 23 and 25 gauge procedures. The biplanar incision has the added advantage of reducing the chance of inadvertent slipping of the cannula during instrument withdrawal. Initially a small gauge port is made for infusion inferotemporally. The pressure plate forceps allow a stable fixed globe while making the biplanar incision. The pressure plate forceps' inner margins slide into the groove of the cannula, allowing an easy trocar withdrawal without disturbing the integrity of the cannula. Another similar port is made for the illumination probe. The third port included a localized peritomy and sclerotomy with a 20 gauge microvitreoretinal blade. The vitrectomy probe or fragmatome was introduced

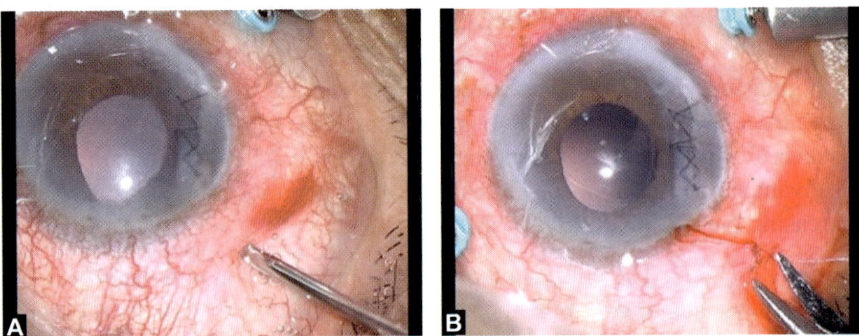

Figs 17.2A and B: (A) 20 gauge port for phacoframentor; (B) Port is sutured at end of surgery

through the 20 gauge port and the surgery is completed. Infusion pressure may be raised to combat hypotony (Figures 17.2A and B).

Cannula Removal and Closure

After the vitrectomy, we plug the cannulae to prevent egress of fluid. We remove the cannulae by holding them with plain forceps and we decrease the infusion pressure to 15 mm Hg. The lower infusion pressure prevents egress of intraocular fluid during removal. We then massage the wound area with a blunt tip applicator for 10 to 15 seconds to encourage the stretched scleral fibers to regain their elastic memory (Figure 17.3). This technique allows a better sealing of the scleral fibers and prevents any inadvertent vitreous incarceration. The site inspected for any wound leak which was sutured with a single stitch, only if found leaking. The displaced conjunctiva was repositioned with a cotton swab or smooth forceps while the single 20 gauge opening was sutured with 8-0 vicryl. Care was taken to examine for sclerotomy leakage at physiological pressure. A 8-0 vicryl conjunctival suture used at the inflection point of an L-shaped miniconjunctival flap. A drop of povidone-iodine is then instilled. At the end of the procedure, we administer a subconjunctival antibiotic injection in the inferonasal quadrant. We avoid all other quadrants to prevent accidental entry of antibitotics into the vitreous cavity, which may lead to retinal toxicity. Postoperative day 1, we examine the incision sites for leakage.

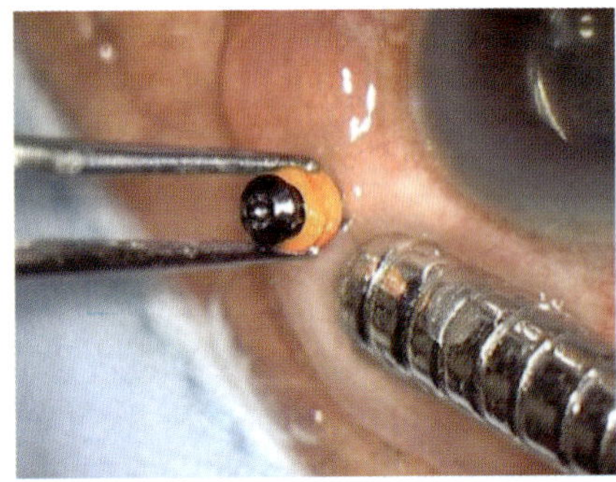

Fig. 17.3: Blunt tipped instrument to gently massage port area after removal of cannula

Advantages of one over the Other

Sutureless self-sealing pars plana vitrectomy was first described by Chen in 1996.[14] Combined vitrectomy, however, allows more thorough peripheral and more complex vitreoretinal maneuvers like near-complete vitreous base dissection, use of complex instruments in diabetic eyes for relieving traction, proliferative vitreoretinopathy (PVR) cases and eyes with intraocular foreign body (IOFB), eyes with dislocated lens and for silicon oil removal. The presence of two sutureless ports allows for low postoperative inflammation, good patient comfort, decreased conjunctival scarring and limited astigmatism. Furthermore, the single-suture 20 gauge sclerotomy in this technique may help shorten the surgical opening and closing times.

Advantages of combination vitrectomy over a small gauge vitrectomy are faster gel removal and enhanced ability to manipulate with a wide array of 20 gauge instruments.Thus, with combined 20 gauge with small gauge vitrectomy, the indications for vitrectomy can be vastly expanded besides making it economically viable for the surgeon as he need not duplicate all 20 gauge instruments to small gauge. Hence, it can be used as an alternative combination modality to the existing vitrectomy systems.

Even in complex cases where we need a variety of scissors and forceps and/or injection of silicone oil, 25 gauge or 23 gauge sclerotomies can be used for the infusion and illumination probe, and a 20 gauge sclerotomy can be performed for instruments and the injection or removal of silicone oil at the end of surgery. This enables the surgeon to use 20 gauge instruments and reduce the costs of replacing all 20 gauge instruments.

EXTENDED HYBRID TECHNIQUES

The ability to combine an encircling band or buckle in combination with MIVS system brings the best out of both the procedures. Some indications for vitreous surgery that may necessitate the placement of an encirclage (Figure 17.4A) or buckle (Figure 17.4B) include inferior breaks in rhegmatogenous retinal detachment, rhegmatogenous retinal detachment complicated by PVR or giant retinal tears, foreign body removal (Figure 17.4C), etc. Using the MIVS system allows the surgeon to bring the benefits of the use of the valved cannula system for these complicated cases. A special modification while making the incision is to have a longer scleral tunnel. This will prevent the cannula from coming out during instrument removal or exchange.

Difficulties encountered during hybrid vitrectomy: Intraoperative hypotony can occur because of fluid leakage through the 20 gauge opening. To prevent this, infusion pressure can be increased or alternatively suction settings can be decreased. Another problem with this technique (during the vitrectomy or lensectomy) is the difficulty in interchanging hands if the second superior port needs to be enlarged. However, for all subjects, conversion of the second port to 20 gauge sclerotomy is not required.

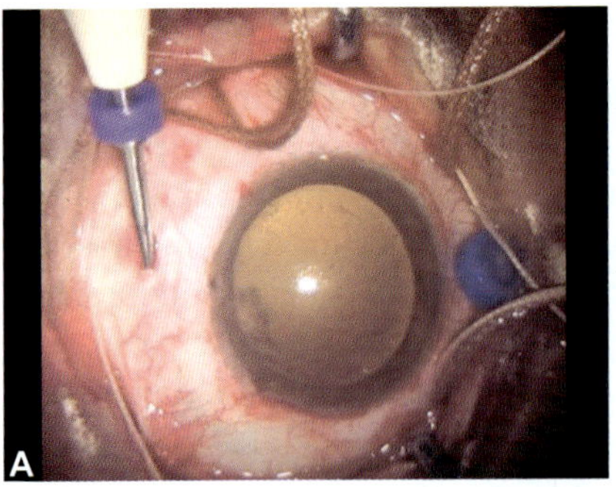

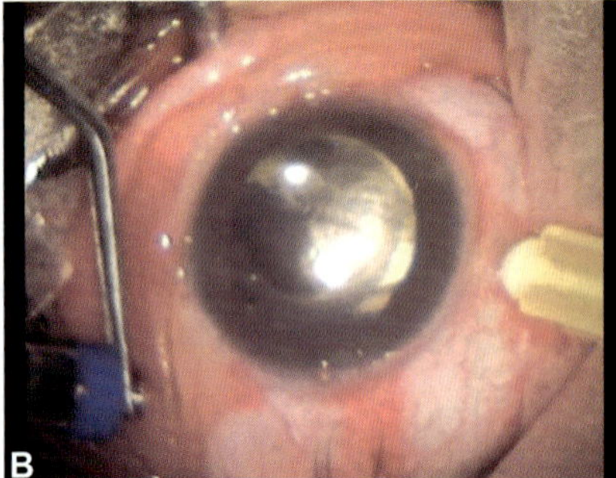

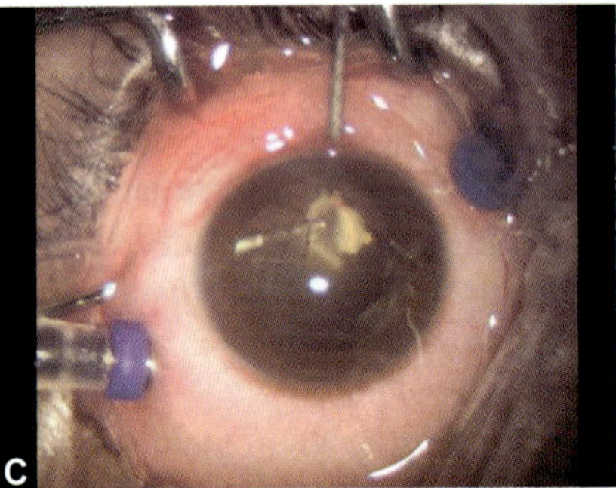

Figs 17.4A to C: (A) Encircling band in combination with 23 gauge valved cannula system; (B) Segmental buckle with 23 gauge valved cannula system. Gas being injected at completion with 30 gauge needle before cannula removal; (C) IOFB removal through corneal tunnel incision. Note one of the 23 gauge valved cannula has been removed, and sclerotomy is enlarged to allow use of 20 gauge forceps

Complications: Small gauge ports, however, are not without their challenges.

Hypotony: An increased risk of transient hypotony has been reported with both 25 gauge[15-17] and 23 gauge vitrectomies.[18,19] However, some recent reports[20,21] have not supported these findings, and others[17,22] have demonstrated that the now-standard oblique incision reduces the incidence of hypotony relative to the original perpendicular incision.

Endophthalmitis: There have been reports of increased incidence of endophthalmitis associated with MIVS. This increased risk may be due to entry of organisms from ocular surface into the eye due to wound gape during blinking. The early hypotony may provide a suction force to draw surface organisms further into the posterior chamber; the incarcerated vitreous at the wound may also act as a wick for bacteria to gain entry into the posterior chamber.[23] The association between 25 gauge vitrectomy and an elevated incidence of endophthalmitis is controversial, however, with two large (N≥4400) retrospective studies reporting an increased risk[24,25] and three similar studies (N≥3500) reporting no difference in endophthalmitis rates between 20 gauge and 25 gauge vitrectomies.[26-28] Interestingly similar apprehensions have been expressed in connection with clear cornea incisions in cataract surgery, but despite some case reports[29,30] again no increased rate of endophthalmitis could be confirmed. This variance may be due to the type of incision used with the 25 gauge surgeries. Both of the studies showing no difference in endophthalmitis rates reported using primarily oblique incisions, whereas at least one of the two studies demonstrating increased endophthalmitis rates with 25 gauge vitrectomy used primarily perpendicular incisions.

Silicone oil leak: Silicone oil, a long-acting tamponade frequently used in surgery for proliferative or diabetic vitreoretinopathy, can escape through unsutured sclerotomies during the postoperative course. Subconjunctival silicone deposits are frequently found in eyes that have undergone sutureless vitrectomy. Patients may experience chronic conjunctival swelling and redness combined with foreign body sensation. Ptosis and muscle disturbances may occur as a result of large silicone deposits.

We have observed this complication in eyes with a transient rise in intraocular pressure (IOP) after vitrectomy and in eyes with recurrent retinal detachment. An increase in IOP may cause silicone to prolapse through the unsutured wound. In the case of recurrent retinal detachment, the silicone is pushed more anteriorly, which can also facilitate transscleral escape. Because silicone is embedded in tissue in hard droplets that must be opened one by one, removal can be time-consuming. Therefore, we believe that silicone oil use should also include tight wound closure. Small-incision instrumentation can still be used. The patient may experience discomfort in the first postoperative week due to the sutures; however, he or she is not likely to experience chronic irritation and redness from subconjunctival silicone deposits.

REFERENCES

1. Machemer R, Buettner H, Norton EW, et al. Vitrectomy: A pars plana approach. Trans Am Acad Ophthalmol Otolaryngol. 1971;75:813–20.
2. Godstein DJ, Oz MC. Current statuss and future directions of minimally invasive cardiac surgery. Curr Opin Cardiol. 1999;14:419–25.
3. Harell AG, Heniford BT. Minimally invasive abdominal surgery: Lux et veritas past present and future. Am J Surg. 2005;190:239–43.
4. Koh CH, Janik GM. Laparoscopic microsurgery: Current and future status. Curr Opin Obstet Gynecol. 1999;11:401–7.
5. Lundell L. Anti reflux surgery in laparoscopic era. Baillieres Best Prac Res Clin Gastroenterol. 2000;18:272–7.
6. Fujii GY, De Juan E Jr, Humayun MS, et al. Initial experience using the transconjunctival sutureless vitrectomy system for vitreoretinal surgery.Ophthalmol. 2002;109(10):1814–20.
7. Eckardt C. Transconjunctival sutureless 23 gauge vitrectomy. Retina. 2005;25(2): 208–11.
8. Kadonosono K, Yamakawa T, Uchio E, Yanagi Y, Tamaki Y, Araie M. Comparison of visual function after epiretinal membrane removal by 20 gauge and 25 gauge vitrectomy. Am J Ophthalmol. 2006;142(3):513–5.
9. Rizzo S, Genovesi-Ebert F, Murri S, et al. 25 gauge, sutureless vitrectomy and standard 20 gauge pars plana vitrectomy in idiopathic epiretinal membrane surgery: A comparative pilot study. Graefes Arch Clin Exp Ophthalmol. 2006;244(4):472–9.
10. Yanyali A, Celik E, Horozoglu F, Nohutcu AF. Corneal topographic changes after transconjunctival (25 gauge) sutureless vitrectomy. Am J Ophthalmol. 2005;140(5):939-41.

11. Fine HF, Bhatnagar P, Spaide R. 23 gauge vitrectomy. In: Bhavsar AR, editor. Surgical techniques in ophthalmology: Retina and vitreous surgery. China: Saunders Elsevier, China; 2009:51–8.
12. Singh A, Stewart JM. 25 gauge sutureless vitrectomy: Variations in incision architecture. Retina. 2009;29(4):451–5.
13. Singh RP, Bando H, Brasil OF, Williams DR, Kaiser PK. Evaluation of wound closure using different incision techniques with 23 gauge and 25 gauge microincision vitrectomy systems. Retina. 2008;28(2):242–8.
14. Chen JC. Sutureless pars plana vitrectomy through self-sealing sclerotomies. Arch Ophthalmol. 1996;114:1273–5.
15. Acar N, Kapran Z, Unver YB, Altan T, Ozdogan S. Early postoperative hypotony after 25 gauge sutureless vitrectomy with straight incisions. Retina. 2008;28(4):545–52.
16. Byeon SH, Lew YJ, Kim M, Kwon OW. Wound leakage and hypotony after 25 gauge sutureless vitrectomy: Factors affecting postoperative intraocular pressure. Ophthalmic Surg Lasers Imaging. 2008;39(2):94–9.
17. Inoue M, Shinoda K, Shinoda H, Kawamura R, Suzuki K, Ishida S. Two-step oblique incision during 25 gauge vitrectomy reduces incidence of postoperative hypotony. Clin Experiment Ophthalmol. 2007;35(8):693–6.
18. Misra A, Ho-Yen G, Burton RL. 23 gauge sutureless vitrectomy and 20 gauge vitrectomy: A case series comparison. Eye. 2009;23(5):1187–91.
19. Woo SJ, Park KH, Hwang JM, Kim JH, Yu YS, Chung H. Risk factors associated with sclerotomy leakage and postoperative hypotony after 23 gauge transconjunctival sutureless vitrectomy. Retina. 2009;29(4):456–63.
20. Lai MM, Ruby AJ, Sarrafizadeh R, et al. Repair of primary rhegmatogenous retinal detachment using 25 gauge transconjunctival sutureless vitrectomy. Retina. 2008;28(5):729–34.
21. Nagpal M, Wartikar S, Nagpal K. Comparison of clinical outcomes and wound dynamics of sclerotomy ports of 20, 25, and 23 gauge vitrectomy. Retina. 2009;29(2): 225–31.
22. Hsu J, Chen E, Gupta O, Fineman MS, Garg SJ, Regillo CD. Hypotony after 25 gauge vitrectomy using oblique versus direct cannula insertions in fluid-filled eyes. Retina. 2008;28(7):937–40.
23. C Scott IU, Flynn HW Jr, Dev S, et al. Endophthalmitis after 25 gauge and 20 gauge pars plana vitrectomy: Incidence and outcomes. Retina. 2008;28(1):138–42.
24. Kunimoto DY, Kaiser RS. Incidence of endophthalmitis after 20 and 25 gauge vitrectomy. Ophthalmol. 2007;114(12):2133–7.
25. Scott IU, Flynn HW Jr, Dev S, et al. Endophthalmitis after 25 gauge and 20 gauge pars plana vitrectomy: Incidence and outcomes. Retina. 2008;28(1):138–42.
26. Mason JO, III, Yunker JJ, Vail RS, et al. Incidence of endophthalmitis following 20 gauge and 25 gauge vitrectomy. Retina. 2008;28(9):1352–4.
27. Shimada H, Nakashizuka H, Hattori T, Mori R, Mizutani Y, Yuzawa M. Incidence of endophthalmitis after 20 and 25 gauge vitrectomy causes and prevention. Ophthalmol. 2008;115(12):2215–20.
28. Hu AYH, Bourges JL, Shah SP, et al. Endophthalmitis after pars plana vitrectomy: A 20 and 25 gauge comparison. Presented at: American Society of Retina Specialists (ASRS) annual meeting, Maui, Hawaii; October 14, 2008.
29. Miller KM, Glasgow BJ. Bacterial endophthalmitis following sutureless cataract surgery. Arch Ophthalmol. 1993;111:377–9.
30. Stonecipher KG, Parmley VC, Jensen H, Rowsey JJ. Infectious endophthalmitis following sutureless cataract surgery. Arch Ophthalmol. 1991;109:1562–3.

CHAPTER

18

20 Gauge Sutureless Vitrectomy

C Claes, AP Lafetá

INTRODUCTION

Sutureless pars plana vitrectomy was first proposed Chen[1] and it was based on 20 gauge self-sealing scleral tunnels. Many complications were reported and other authors have described modifications for this technique trying to avoid problems such as wound leakage, dehiscence, hemorrhage, incarceration of vitreous and/or retina, retinal tears and dialyses.[2-7]

The use of trocars for sutureless vitrectomy was first described by Fugii et al.[8,9] A scleral perpendicular 25 gauge incision was used and they suggested that the holes would be closed because they were small and the conjunctiva would also cover it, serving as a protection. But in the concept of minimal surgery, the closure of the sclerotomies is essentially made by the peripheral vitreous, what might increase the risk of incarceration and secondary retinal detachment. If this peripheral vitreous were removed leakage would happen.

Strauma and hasten postoperative recovery, some problems such as flexibility and fragility[10] of the instruments, low infusion and aspiration rates[8] and, of course, higher costs, have limited its use. Since then, many attempts have been done to improve sutureless vitreoretinal surgery.

Eckardt[11] presented, as an alternative to the 25 gauge, a new method using a 23 gauge system. He has used a 30° to 40° tunnel incision made with a stiletto and inserted the cannulas using a blunt inserter. This system offers the advantages of a sutureless surgery but it also requires a complete different set of instruments, also flexible which would still keep surgery costs high and its indications still limited.

To avoid the leakage mentioned before in the 25 gauge surgeries, Lópes-Guajardo[12] proposed that the sclerotomies should be made in the same way Eckardt described for his 23 gauge ones, creating scleral tunnels with displacement of the conjunctiva.

We introduced, in 2007,[13] the 20 gauge transconjunctival trocar system (DORC, Zuidland, Holland) that allows the use of the conventional

20 gauge vitrectomy in sutureless surgeries. It is analogous to the 23 gauge one, a tangential tunnel is also made with a bend stiletto and the trocars are introduced with a blunt inserter in a two step technique.

INSTRUMENTATION AND TECHNIQUE

The first generation trocars were designed in 2004 but the intense leakage of infusion fluids through those gaping 20 gauge ports caused severe conditions of hypotony at various moments during the surgery. To solve these problem silicone disposable valves (Figure 18.1) were developed. The valves keep the eye sealed after retraction of the instruments reducing the consumption of infusion fluids and allowing the surgeon to have complete control of the intra-ocular pressure. They fit the distal trocar tip and are easily removable (Figures 18.2 and 18.3). A set (Figure 18.4) includes: one blunt infusion inserter, that measures 11.5 mm, one infusion trocar measuring 8.5 mm with a 4.0 mm intraocular extension; two blunt trocar-inserters, measuring 10.0 mm to place the 6.5 mm trocars, also with a 4.0 mm intraocular extension. The external diameter for the infusion and trocars is of 1.0 mm and the internal one is of 0.9 mm. The trocars protect the entry sites from erosion and plugs are not needed when using this system. In the second generation of trocars the basic difference is the tip of the infusion line that fits in any one of the trocars.

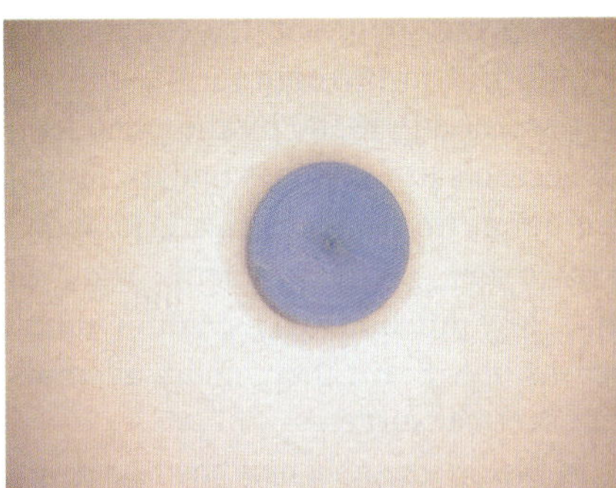

Fig. 18.1: Valve

Fig. 18.2: Trocars in place with valves

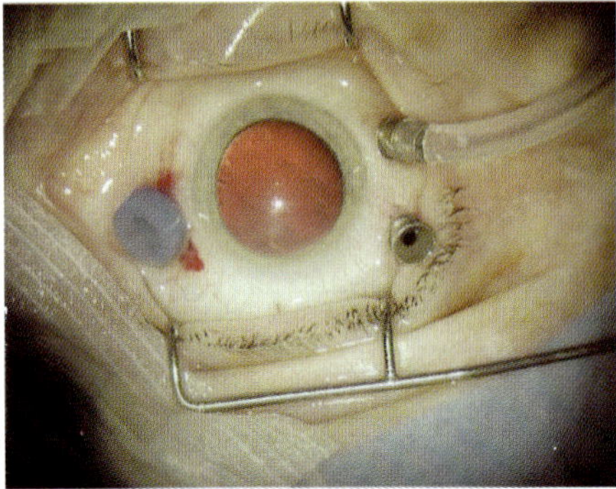

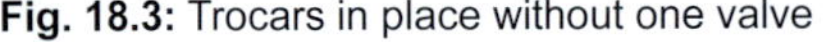

Fig. 18.3: Trocars in place without one valve

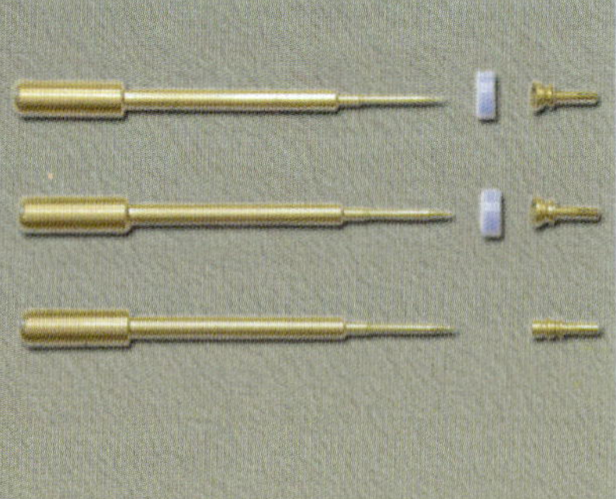

Fig. 18.4: A complete set

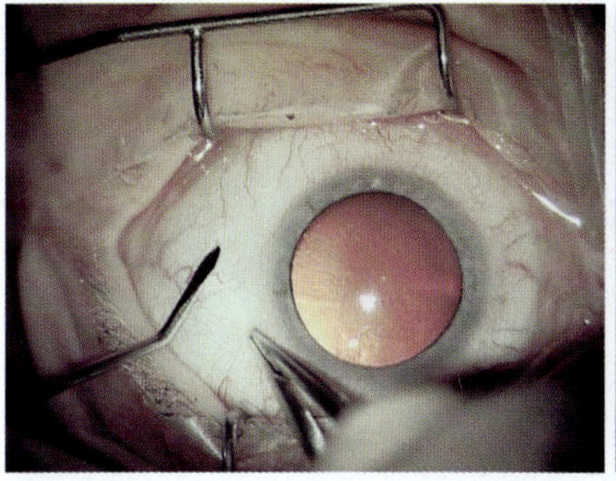

Fig. 18.5: Incision made with 20 gauge stiletto at a 10° angle through the conjunctiva

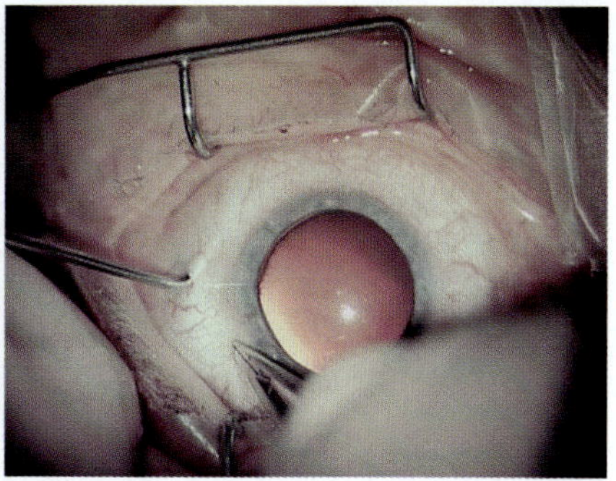

Fig. 18.6: Scleral tunnel limbus-parallel made with stiletto

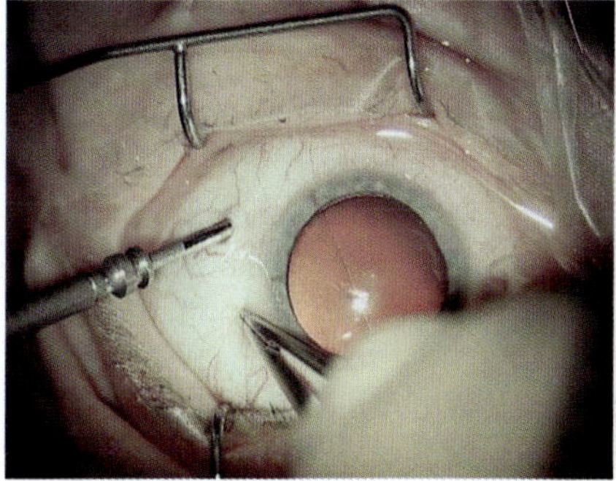

Fig. 18.7: Placement of the infusion trocar

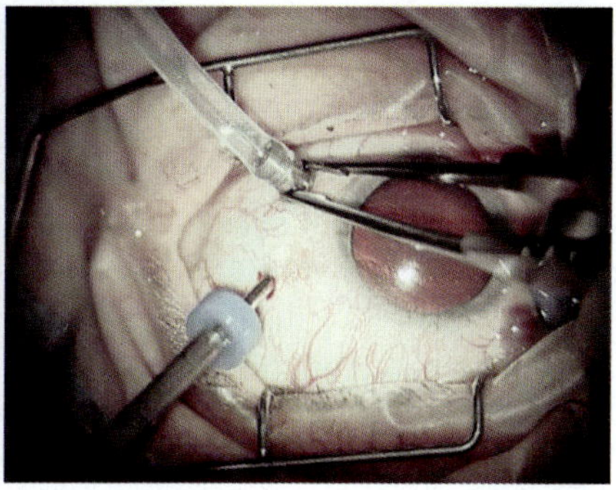

Fig. 18.8: Placement of the valved trocar

The procedure is initiated using a 20 gauge bend stiletto (45° angle; 0.9 mm; Blumenthal; BD Visitec) that is inserted at a 10° angle through the conjunctiva, without displacement (Figure 18.5), to create a 3.5 mm scleral tunnel. Incisions are radially made at 3 mm from the limbus and tunnels are made limbus-parallel (Figure 18.6). The infusion trocar is first placed into the inferotemporal tunnel (Figure 18.7) and then trocars are placed at the superior quadrants (Figure 18.8). With the second generation of trocars you can easily change your infusion to the superior ports and also exchange it for a silicone oil infusion.

By being less traumatic a two-step procedure is preferred creating first the tunnels with the stiletto knife and placing the trocars after. This creates better sclerotomies with slit configurations as you can see in this intraoperative picture where the trocar was removed (Figure 18.9), and is considered decisive for good wound closure.

At the end, the eye is pressurized at 20 mm Hg and the infusion is closed and before removing the two trocars from the superior quadrants. Then, the infusion is reopened, increasing the eye pressure for a few seconds with simultaneous cotton tip massage at the entry-ports in order to close the tunnels (Figure 18.10). The massaging is continued until the absence of leakage.

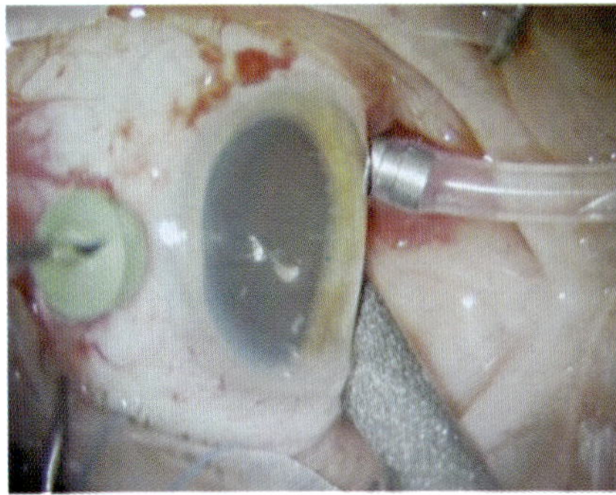

Fig. 18.9: Inside vision from incision

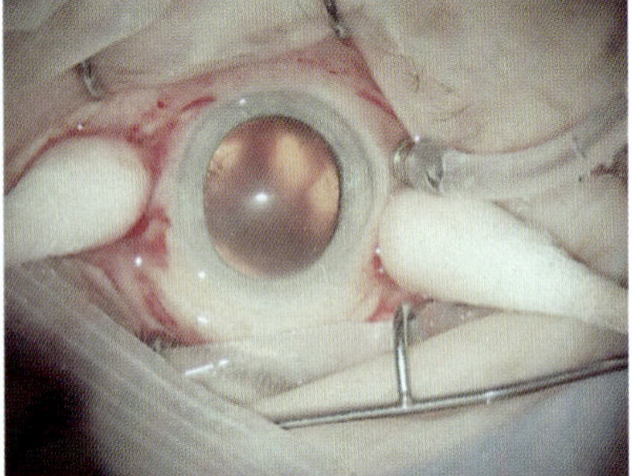

Fig. 18.10: Massage at entry ports

Since a complete vitrectomy with careful shaving of the vitreous base is our routine in all patients, after the removal of the first two trocars, the closure of the tunnels is obtained by the apposition of its walls when the infusion pressure is raised. So, using 10° incisions, we create longer tunnels, which close easier. The last one, the infusion trocar, is removed after closing the infusion with simultaneously massages at its entry port. In case of hypotony, after the trocars removal, air is injected through the pars plana using a 3 cc syringe and a 30 gauge needle. Additional diathermy can be applied to close conjunctival buttonholes.

The surgery is performed using the regular straight or adapted curved 20 gauge instruments. Many curved instruments can easily pass through the trocars. The illuminated spatula (Figure 18.11) is our preferred instrument to dissect membranes in difficult PVR and diabetic cases. The illuminated fork (Figure 18.12) is very useful in preventing retinal breaks when pulling membranes. As the 20 gauge lumen is big enough, by inserting a 27 gauge optic fiber through the infusion and placing another one through the sclera, bimanual surgery can be performed under excellent illumination conditions. Indentation can be executed without difficulty and the periphery is easily accessible. Also, the 20 gauge system is the only one that has a special coated facofragmentation probe to use with the trocars (Figure 18.13).

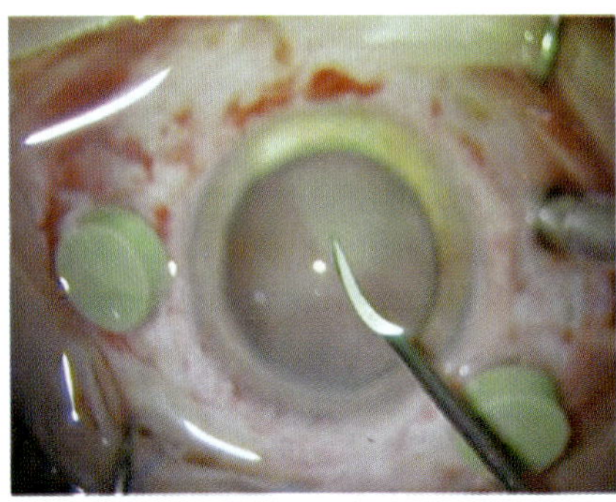

Fig. 18.11: Illuminated spatula

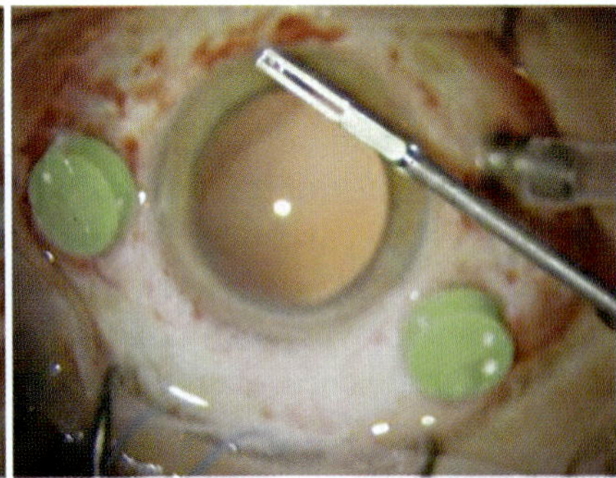

Fig. 18.12: Illuminated fork

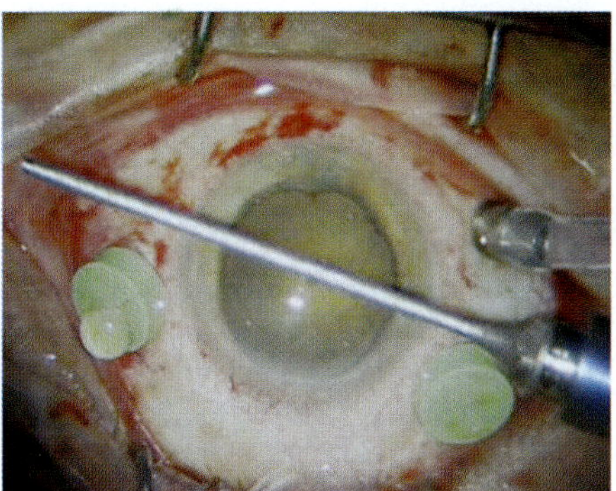

Fig. 18.13: Coated facofragmentor probe

DISCUSSION

The 20 gauge system presents advantages over the 25/23 gauges without their inconveniences. It shortens the procedure for being transconjunctival and sutureless. It also provides faster healing and less postoperative inflammation given a superior postoperative comfort to the patient, as well as others existing trocar systems. Small conjunctival hemorrhages caused by the grasping forceps used to hold the eye during the insertion of the trocars do not cause any discomfort to the patients.

The 20 gauge trocars, together with the high speed cutters an the IOP control in combination with valves, allow, by using high infusion/aspiration rates, faster vitreous removal with easier clearance of organized vitreous. This combination also reduces iatrogenic traction and hypotony periods giving more control to the surgeon. It is easier and faster to work with silicone oil than the smaller gauge systems, even with 5000 centistokes (Cs).

The learning curve is short. At first you feel a reduced freedom in moving the instruments inside the eye. However, by getting used to the system, this minor discomfort completely disappears and is replaced by more control and safety. The instruments used are basically the same as in 20 gauge conventional vitrectomy, probes, scissors, forceps and many others. Some new curved instruments that could pass trough the trocars have been developed. Starting with straightforward cases, after experiencing the absence of major complications, the system can now be used in almost all vitreoretinal surgeries. It provides easy access to the entire periphery with nonflexible instrumentation. Also the coated facofragmentation probe allows aspiration of the hardest cataracts from the posterior pole. The 20 gauge trocar system can be used with air, gas, BSS and silicone oil tamponade.

Summarizing, in this era of sutureless surgeries, this 20 gauge trocar system with valves is a safe, comfortable and less expensive alternative to conventional, 25 and 23 gauge vitrectomy.

Furthermore, it offers a complete set of instrumentation as the conventional 20 gauge vitrectomy, allowing the surgeon to deal with all kinds of pathologies, from dropped nucleus to macular translocation.

REFERENCES

1. Chen JC. Sutureless pars plana vitrectomy through self-sealing sclerotomies. Arch Ophthalmol. 1996;114:1273–5.
2. Milibak T, Suveges I. Complications of sutureless pars plana vitrectomy through self-sealing sclerotomies [letter]. Arch Ophthmol. 1998;116:119.
3. Kwok AK, Tham CC, Lam DS, et al. Modified sutureless sclerotomies in pars plana vitrectomy. Am J Ophthalmol. 1999;127:731–33.
4. Schmidt J, Nietgen GW, Briedan S. Selbstverchliessende, nahtlose SKlerotomie zur Pars-plana-Vitrektomie. Klin Monatsbl Augenheilkd. 1999;215:247–51.
5. Jackson T. Modified sutureless scleroromies in pars plana vitrectomy [letter]. Am J Ophthalmol. 2000;129:116–7.
6. Assi AC, Scott RAH, Charteris DG. Reversed self-sealing pars plana sclerotomies. Retina. 2000;689–92.
7. Rahman R, Rosen PH, Riddell C, Towler H. Self-sealing sclerotomies for sutureless pars plana vitrectomy. Ophthalmic Surg Lasers. 2000;31:462–6.
8. Fugii GY, de Juan E Jr, Humayun MS, et al. A new 25 gauge instrument system for transconjunctival sutureless vitrectomy surgery. Ophthalmology. 2002;109:1807–12.
9. Fugii GY, de Juan E Jr, Humayun MS, et al. Initial experience using the transconjunctival sutureless vitrectomy system for vitreoretinal surgery. Ophthalmology. 2002;109:1814–20.
10. Inoue M, Noda K, Ishida S, Nagai N, et al. Intra-operative breakage of a 25 gauge vitreous cutter. Am J Ophthalmol. 2004;138(5)/867–9.
11. Eckardt C. Transconjunctival sutureless 23 gauge vitrectomy. Retina. 2005;25:208–11.
12. Lópes-Guajardo L, Pareja-Esteban, Jésus, Teus-Guezala M. Oblique sclerotomy for prevention of incompetent wound closure in transconjunctival 25 gauge vitrectomy. Am J Ophthalmol. 2006;141:1154–6.
13. Lafetá AP, Claes C. Twenty gauge tansconjunctival suturelees vitrectomy trocar system. Retina. 2007;27:1136–41.

CHAPTER

19

Complications of MIVS

Priyank Garg, Arindam Chakravarti, Sundaram Natarajan

With technological advancements and increased experience, our understanding of the complications associated with pars plana vitrectomy has grown. Traditional pars plana vitrectomy has been associated with a myriad of complications. These same risks are associated with MIVS. Due to the nature of this surgical technique, additional concerns have risen regarding potential hypotony, wound healing, and those associated with incomplete removal of vitreous gel.

INTRAOPERATIVE COMPLICATIONS[1]

While performing MIVS, concerns often arise regarding the insertion and use of small incision trocars. The original Entry Alignment System (EAS) for use with the Transconjunctival Sutureless Vitrectomy system (TSV-25) available from Bausch & Lomb Surgical (St. Louis, MO, USA) featured hollow-bore trocars that occasionally required excessive force for introduction of the cannulas.[37] The globe could potentially be pushed deep into the orbit in patients with abundant periorbital tissue, causing distortion of the normal anatomy and potential injury to intraocular contents such as the crystalline lens. The potential risk of scleral tissue coring with the use of hollow trocars has not proven to be valid. The cannula insertion trocars used with the Accurus 25 gauge vitrectomy system from Alcon Surgical (Ft. Worth, TX, USA) were designed with solid, sharper trocars that allow for easier placement of the cannulas. The second-generation EAS has been redesigned to allow easier, smoother cannula placement compared to the predecessor. After the cannulas are inserted, they most often will stay in position throughout the surgery. Occasionally, the cannulas may become displaced as the instruments are removed from the eye, resulting in chemosis or subconjunctival entrapment of fluid/air, depending on what is currently being infused. Cannula replacement with the trocar makes it possible to continue with the surgery; however, the surgeon must take care to modify his surgical technique accordingly to avoid further conjunctival trauma. Certain cannulas with valves that fit on top of the cannula (DORC) may also pose the problem of valve displacement. One important modification is that instruments should go into and out of the eye in the same direction as while inserting the trocar-cannula. This would minimize the chances of cannula or valve displacement.

In eyes with choroidal edema such as rhegmatogenous retinal detachment or endophthalmitis, the cannula may inadvertently be placed subchoroidally. If infusion fliud is started without seeing the tip of the cannula in the vitreous cavity, choroidal detachment will result. An extremely oblique entry may place the cannula below the retina in a patient with a high retinal detachment. Hence, the infusion cannula must be clearly visualized before the infusion is switched on. Intraoperative manipulations may sometimes pull on the infusion cannula resulting in subretinal or subchoroidal infusion of balanced salt solution. Use of wide-angle viewing system would allow early recognition of such an event and corrective steps would be taken (Figures 19.1A and B).

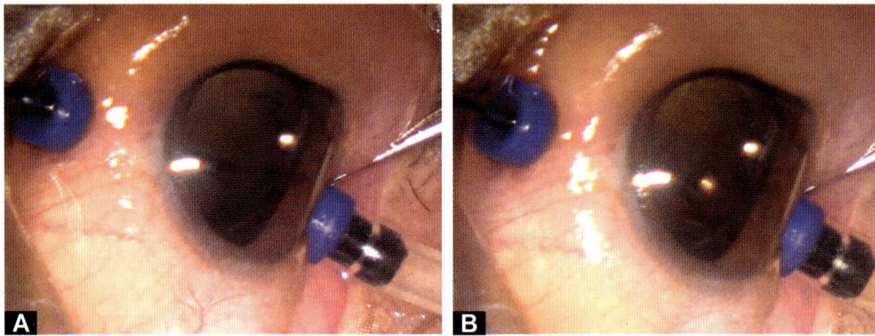

Figs 19.1A and B: (A) Subchoroidal cannula; (B) Choroid is gently teased off the cannula with blunt tipped instrument

Intraoperative fluid leaks through the nonvalved cannula can result in bleeding, vitreous prolapse with secondary vitreoretinal traction, miosis due to hypotony, or even retinal prolapse. Due to the free flow of fluid through the nonvalved cannulas, every time an instrument is removed, the loss of balanced salt solution can cause fluctuations in intraocular pressure. This may lead to hemorrhagic choroidal detachment. Hisato et al have reported unexplained postoperative retinal hemorrhages in patients undergoing 23 gauge MIVS and have speculated that fluctuating intraocular pressure may be one of the factors responsible.[31] The valved cannula protects against such fluctuations in intraocular pressure and resists loss of fluid, thus maintaining a uniform intraocular pressure.

Nam et al have reported two patients with presumed sclerotomy site hemorrhage into the anterior chamber with pseudophakic retinal detachment and gas tamponade.[19] The bleeding occurred 10–20 seconds after removal of the 23 gauge cannula. The hemorrhage cleared in 7–14 days. Microbleeds have been documented by intraocular endoscope in minimally invasive surgery.[20] These bleeds stop spontaneously. Cannulas made of polyamide material are delicate and may break either at the junction of the tip and collar or in between. Chen et al have reported a suprachoridal hemorrhage due to breakage of the tip of a 25 gauge cannula.[23] Hence, it is important to inspect the cannula after removal and attempt to remove the tip if it is found to be broken.

The instruments used in conjunction with MIVS are obviously finer than those used in 20 gauge surgery. During the initial learning period, it is not uncommon for the surgeon to attempt to torque the eye rather than rotating the instruments about the cannulas. This may result in unintentionally bending or breaking the instruments. The illuminating light pipes and laser probes are particularly fragile, and must be handled in a fashion unique to the MIVS. There have even been reports of breakage of the tip of the vitreous cutter during surgery.[2]

POSTOPERATIVE COMPLICATIONS[3]

After removal of the cannulas, the incisions are designed to be self-sealing. The open nature of the sclerotomies has led to concerns of hypotony, wound leakage, and vitreous incarceration. In addition, late complications of vitrectomy including retinal tears, retinal dialysis, and vitreous hemorrhage have also been associated with the creation of self-sealing sclerotomies.[4]

WOUND LEAK/HYPOTONY

Postoperative wound leaks have been a concern since MIVS was introduced. Wound leaks may lead to hypotony, defined as intraocular pressure lower than 5 mm Hg, resulting in choroidal detachments, bleeding, vitreous volume enhancement, or reoperations to suture the wounds. The incidence of open sclerotomies is directly proportional to the presence of ciliochoroidal detachment and hypotony.[28] Fluid air exchange at completion of the surgery should aid in closing the sclerotomy. The surface tension effect of an air bubble can reduce or eliminate wound leaks and prevent vitreous wicks until fibrin seals the wound, just as gas bubbles are used to "seal" retinal breaks and macular holes. Also the misalignment between conjunctival and scleral wounds helps in reducing incidence of hypotony.[5] Wound leaks can cause conjunctival ballooning especially with conjunctival displacement, with either air, gas or silicone oil.

WOUND HEALING

Sclerotomy wound healing is a concern with incisions that are purportedly self-sealing. In order to evaluate the timing of wound closure, integrity of overlying conjunctiva, and presence of vitreous incarceration, ultrasound biomicroscopy (UBM) was used to evaluate sclerotomies of patients undergoing vitrectomy with the TSV-25 system. UBM scans were obtained on postoperative day 1, week 1, and month 1. Postoperative day 1 UBM evaluation of sclerotomies uniformly showed open sclerotomies with intact overlying conjunctiva.

By postoperative week 1, all sclerotomies were closed, with variable amounts of vitreous gel incarcerated in all wounds. Postoperative month 1 UBM evaluation did not appreciably differ from postoperative week 1 scans.[6,7] Subclinical choroidal detachment and scleral gap at the sclerotomy sites was seen using AS-OCT at day 1 in a majority of eyes undergoing 23 gauge transconjunctival surgery. These features predispose eyes to hypotony in the immediate postoperative period, though these resolve without any intervention in the next few days.[21]

CATARACT

Cataract progression is a known complication of 20 gauge standard pars plana vitrectomy.[8,9] Decreased ocular manipulation and surgical time with 25 gauge transconjunctival vitrectomy may theoretically lead to a decreased rate of cataract formation. In a series of consecutive phakic patients with no previous intraocular surgery undergoing 25 gauge vitrectomy, the severity of nuclear, cortical, and posterior subcapsular lens opacities was graded on slit-lamp examination during preoperative and follow-up examinations.[10] After a mean follow-up of over 1 year, 28% of eyes had cataract progression. Two thirds of these eyes had gas tamponade.

Comparison of surgical techniques in this patient population is difficult due to the heterogeneous patient group; however, the rate of cataract progression following 25 gauge transconjunctival pars plana vitrectomy may be lower than 20 gauge standard pars plana vitrectomy. Decreased posterior segment manipulation, lower intraoperative infusion volumes, and case selection with 25 gauge transconjunctival vitrectomy may contribute to a lower rate of postoperative cataract progression.

Lens trauma may occur due to globe rotation and improper placement of trocars. This may complicate the procedure, and may even necessitate removal of the lens.[33] Preoperative biometry should be done in all cases even in the absence of cataract so as to have an accurate intraocular lens power, should lens removal and IOL implantation be required.

ENDOPHTHALMITIS

Acute onset postoperative endophthalmitis is uncommon but remains one of the most serious complications associated with devastating visual loss or blindness, despite appropriate treatment.[11-13] The reported incidence of infectious endophthalmitis after conventional 20 gauge vitrectomy has decreased to 0.03% to 0.05% during the past decades because of improved surgical techniques and recognition of the importance of perioperative antiseptic preparations.[14-16] There is a growing concern that microincision vitrectomy surgery may increase the risk of postoperative endophthalmitis compared with conventional 20 gauge vitrectomy because of the transconjunctival approach and sutureless nature of the procedure.[17] Unsutured 25 gauge incisions even with conjunctival displacement showed India ink in the incisions in a lab setting. This points towards the potential risk of ocular surface contaminants to enter the eye.[24] Oblique 25 gauge incisions would allow good wound apposition and prevent chances of endophthalmitis. Incomplete vitrectomy in the early 25 gauge vitrectomy series instead of near total vitrectomy as in 20 gauge vitrectomy, coupled with decreased fluid irrigation may also have been a contributory factor in increasing the incidence of endophthalmitis. Çekiç et al have reported endophthalmitis following 23 gauge vitrectomy wherein the peripheral vitreous was not removed.[27] Near total vitrectomy in MIVS, complete air fluid exchange, and the use of light pipe assisted cannula removal may decrease the chances of vitreous prolapse in the incisions, thus decreasing the likelihood of endophthalmitis. Use of preoperative antibiotics, 10% povidone iodine instillation in the conjunctival cul-de-sac in the preoperative period would decrease the conjunctival bacterial load.

Single or small samples of reports of endophthalmitis following MIVS had sounded alarm bells for the procedure. But large scale studies have failed to demonstrate an increased incidence for endophthalmitis. A large series comparison of 23 gauge versus 20 gauge vitrectomy over a period of 5 years did not show an increase in the incidence of endophthalmitis with the MIVS procedure.[25] Another large series comparing 25 gauge versus 20 gauge vitrectomy too provided no difference in the incidence of endophthalmitis. A careful perioperative anti-infective regimen was however advised.[26] In a recent multicenter study by Japan Microincision Vitrectomy Group,[18] the endophthalmitis rates were 0.034% from 20 gauge Vitrectomy and 0.054% after MIVS with no significant difference between groups. Although the incidence in 25 gauge cases (0.073%) was greater than in 23 gauge cases (0.030%). Another large scale multicenter study comparing 20, 23 and 25 gauge vitrectomy over a 5 year period failed to demonstrate an increase in postvitrectomy endophthalmitis for small gauge.[29]

VITREOUS HEMORRHAGE

In some reports, vitreous hemorrhage, which spontaneously cleared within 3 weeks, was the most common complication. The bleeding responsible was likely to be derived from the sclerotomy sites.[34,35]

VITREOUS INCARCERATION AND RETINAL DETACHMENT

The vitreous plug inducing wound closure in 23 and 25 gauge vitrectomy systems is thought to result in peripheral vitreous and retinal traction causing peripheral retinal breaks and subsequent retinal detachment. The incidence of retinal detachment varies from 1.8% to 14% in different studies.[36] The rate is significantly less in 25 than 23 gauge systems which is about 2%.[14,17] The vitrectomy procedure should be aimed to shave as much as vitreous base to prevent incarceration of any vitreous strands, attached to the retina, into the sclerotomy. With the recent 23 gauge system the larger less flexible instruments allow more peripheral vitreous skirt removal, reducing the incidence of vitreous incarceration at sclerotomy site thereby reducing the risk of subsequent retinal detachment.

OTHERS

1. Macular infarction was reported following 23 gauge vitrectomy and subconjunctival gentamicin for a macular pucker.[32] The author reported that the injection was given adjacent to the sclerotomy and the flow of injection was visible on retroillumination. This is likely to happen in the presence of an leaky/open sclerotomy. Hypotony in the postoperative period with a fluid filled eye would also predispose eyes to such complications. Subconjunctival injections of antibiotics should be given in the inferonasal quadrant far away from the sclerotomy. Gentamicin should be replaced with amikacin or ceftazidime which are less likely to cause macular toxicity. Fluid air exchange and face down positioning for a few hours postoperatively would prevent the antibiotics from reaching the vitreous cavity through an open incision.
2. Conjunctival pigmentation may occur in the region of the sclerotomy following small gauge surgery. This may be due to the prolapse of uveal pigments underneath the conjunctiva during removal of the cannula. Cha et al have reported sympathetic ophthalmia following 23 gauge vitrectomy in which dense conjunctival pigmentation had developed following two interventions.[30] Conjunctival pigmentation may be a preceeding sign for sympathetic ophthalmia.

CONCLUSION

MIVS represent a major leap forward in our ability to provide less invasive solutions to complicated ocular problems. The creation of self-sealing wounds has not been shown to be disadvantageous to the patient in the short or long-term. 25 gauge transconjunctival vitrectomy complication rates are comparable to and may be lower than standard 20 gauge pars plana vitrectomy.[38] Direct comparison to historical controls is limited for a number of reasons, including variable baseline characteristics and open entry criteria. Immediate recognition and appropriate treatment of any complication is important for optimal anatomic and functional outcomes.

REFERENCES

1. Chen C, Gupta A, Savar L, et al. 25 gauge transconjunctival vitrectomy: Intraoperative safety. Invest Ophthalmol Vis Sci (ARVO Abstracts). 2005;46:5455.
2. Inoue M, Noda K, Ishida S, Nagai N, Imamura Y, Oguchi Y. Intraoperative breakage of a 25 gauge vitreous cutter. Am J Ophthalmol. 2004;138:867–9.
3. Mango C, Gupta A, Chen C, et al. 25 gauge transconjunctival vitrectomy: Postoperative complications, Invest Ophthalmol Vis Sci (ARVO Abstracts). 2005;46:5459.

4. Chen JC. Sutureless pars plana vitrectomy through self-sealing sclerotomies. Arch Ophthalmol. 1996;114:1273–5.
5. Gupta A, Gonzales C, Lee S, et al. Transient postoperative hypotony following transconjunctival 25 gauge vitrectomy, Association for Research in Vision and Ophthalmol (ARVO) Annual Meeting, Fort Lauderdale, FL 2003.
6. Gonzales CR, Gupta A, Lee SY, et al. Ultrasound Biomicroscopic Evaluation of Sclerotomies Created by Transconjunctival 25 gauge Vitrectomy. Invest Ophthalmol Vis Sci. 2003;44.
7. Teixeira A, Allemann N, Yamada, Ana CN, et al. Ultrasound biomicroscopy in recently postoperative 23 gauge transconjunctival vitrectomy sutureless self-sealing sclerotomy. Retina. 29(9):1213–380.
8. Ghartey KN, Tolentino FI, Freeman HM, McMeel JW, Schepens CL, Aiello LM. Closed vitreous surgery. XVII. Results and complications of pars plana vitrectomy. Arch Ophthalmol. 1980;98:1248–52.
9. Melberg NS, Thomas MA. Nuclear sclerotic cataract after vitrectomy in patients younger than 50 years of age. Ophthalmol. 1995;102:1466–71.
10. Gupta A, Chen C, Savar L, et al. 25 gauge transconjunctival vitrectomy: Cataract progression. Invest Ophthalmol Vis Sci (ARVO Abstracts). 2005;46:5458.
11. May DR, Peyman GA. Endophthalmitis after vitrectomy. Am J Ophthalmol. 1976;81(4):520–1.
12. Blankenship GW. Endophthalmitis after pars plana vitrectomy. Am J Ophthalmol. 1977;84(6):815–7.
13. Ho PC, Tolentino FI. Bacterial endophthalmitis after closed vitrectomy. Arch Ophthalmol. 1984;102(2):207–10.
14. Cohen SM, Flynn HW Jr, Murray TG, Smiddy WE. Endophthalmitis after pars plana vitrectomy. The Postvitrectomy Endophthalmitis Study Group. Ophthalmol. 1995;102(2):705–12.
15. Aaberg TM Jr, Flynn HW Jr, Schiffman J, Newton J. Nosocomial acute-onset postoperative endophthalmitis survey. A 10 year review of incidence and outcomes. Ophthalmol. 1998;105(6):1004–10.
16. Eifrig CW, Scott IU, Flynn HW Jr, Smiddy WE, Newton J. Endophthalmitis after pars plana vitrectomy: Incidence, causative organisms, and visual acuity outcomes. Am J Ophthalmol. 2004;138(5):799–802.
17. Lewis H. Sutureless microincision vitrectomy surgery: Unclear benefit, uncertain safety. Am J Ophthalmol 2007;144(4):613–5.
18. Oshima Y, Kadonosono K, Yamaji H, et al. Multicenter survey with a systemic overview of acute-onset endophthalmitis after Transconjunctival microincision vitrectomy surgery. Am J Ophthalmol. 2010;150:716–25.
19. Nam DH, Yoon SC, Lee DY, Sohn HJ. Presumed sclerotomy site bleeding inflowing into the anterior chamber after the removal of a 23 gauge microcannula in 23 gauge sutureless vitrectomy. Indian J Ophthalmol. 2010;58:543–5.
20. Koch FH, Luloh KP, Singh P, Scholtz S, Koss M. 'Mini gauge' pars plana vitrectomy: 'Inside-out view' with the GRIN solid rod endoscope. Ophthalmologica. 2007;221:356–62.
21. Guthoff R, Riederle H, Meinhardt B, Goebel W. Subclinical Choroidal Detachment at Sclerotomy Sites after 23 gauge Vitrectomy: Analysis by Anterior Segment Optical Coherence Tomography. Ophthalmologica. 2010;23:224(5):301–7.
22. Ooto S, Kimura D, Itoi K, Mukuno H, Kusuhara S, Miyamoto N, et al. Suprachoroidal fluid as a complication of 23 gauge vitreous surgery. Br J Ophthalmol. 2008;92:1433–4.

23. Chen CJ, Satofuka S, Inoue M, Ishida S, Shinoda K, Tsubota K. Suprachoroidal hemorrhage caused by breakage of a 25 gauge cannula. Ophthalmic Surg Lasers Imaging. 2008;39(4):323–4.
24. Singh A, Chen JA, Stewart JM. Ocular surface fluid contamination of sutureless 25 gauge vitrectomy incisions. Retina. 2008;28(4):553–7.
25. Barbara Parolini, Federica Romanelli, Guido Prigione, Grazia Pertile. Incidence of endophthalmitis in a large series of 23 gauge and 20 gauge transconjunctival pars plana vitrectomy Graefe's Archive for Clinical and Experimental Ophthalmol.2009;247 (7):895-8.
26. Hu AY, Bourges JL, Shah SP, Gupta A, Gonzales CR, Oliver SC, et al. Endophthalmitis after pars plana vitrectomy a 20 and 25 gauge comparison. Ophthalmol. 2009;116(7):1360–5.
27. Osman Çekiç, Mehmet Çakir, Serpil Yazgan, Ö Faruk Yilmaz. Acute endophthalmitis following 23 gauge sutureless transconjunctival vitrectomy. Indian J Ophthalmol. 2011;59(2):160–2.
28. Yamane S, Inoue M, Arakawa A, Kadonosono K. Early postoperative hypotony and ciliochoroidal detachment after microincision vitrectomy surgery. Am J Ophthalmol. 2012;32(3):613–6.
29. Kuo HK, Lee JJ. Macular infarction after 23 gauge transconjunctival sutureless vitrectomy and subconjunctival gentamicin for macular pucker: A case report. Can J Ophthalmol. 2009;44(6):720–1.
30. Cha DM, Woo SJ, Ahn J, Park KH. A case of sympathetic ophthalmia presenting with extraocular symptoms and conjunctival pigmentation after repeated 23 gauge vitrectomy. Ocul Immunol Inflamm. 2010;18(4):265–7.
31. Hisato Ohno, Kenji Inoue. Unexplained postoperative retinal hemorrhage after 23 gauge sutureless vitrectomy. Clin Ophthalmol. 2011;5:1027–9.
32. Kuo HK, Lee JJ. Macular infarction after 23 gauge transconjunctival sutureless vitrectomy and subconjunctival gentamicin for macular pucker: A case report. Can J Ophthalmol. 2009;44(6):720–1.
33. Susanne Binder. Rare complications of vitrectomy with small gauge instrumentation can significantly affect vision. RETINA PEARLS: Incision-related Complications of Sutureless Vitrectomy 2010.
34. Eckardt C. Transconjunctival sutureless 23 gauge vitrectomy. Retina. 2005;25:208–11.
35. Barbara, P, Guido P, Federicka R, et al. Postoperative complications and intraocular pressure in 943 consecutive cases of 23 gauge transconjunctival pars plana vitrectomy with one year follow-up. Retina. 2010;30:107–11.
36. Wimpissinger B, Binder S. Entry-site–related retinal detachment after pars plana vitrectomy. Acta Ophthalmol Scand, 2007;85:782–5.
37. Fujii GY, De Juan E Jr, Humayun MS, et al. Initial experience using the transconjunctival sutureless vitrectomy system for vitreoretinal surgery. Ophthalmol. 2002;109:1814–20.
38. Ibarra MS, Hermel M, Prenner JL, Hassan TS. Longer-term outcomes of transconjunctival sutureless 25 gauge vitrectomy. Am J Ophthalmol. 2005;139:831–6.

CHAPTER

20

Improved Visualization for Microincision Vitreous Surgery

Meena Chakrabarti, Sonia Rani John, Arup Chakrabarti

INTRODUCTION

Visualization is crucial in surgery, and ophthalmol is no exception. However, vitrectomy surgery poses a number of unique challenges. Many of the tissues involved are nearly transparent, the globe is relatively small in size, and hence special optical systems are necessary before a view is possible.[1] Even then, some structures are optically inaccessible without special manipulation, and just a few drops of blood in the surgical field can completely obscure the view.

Improved visualization during vitrectomy, therefore, remains an ongoing quest for vitreoretinal surgeons. Several innovations have been introduced. Wide-angle viewing systems and the use of endoscopy during vitrectomy provides an unfettered view to areas that were previously inaccessible—namely the peripheral retina and vitreous base, wherein a vast amount of vitreoretinal pathology is present. The advent of small gauge, sutureless vitrectomy has also prompted the need for improved endoillumination through smaller instruments or from an additional fourth sclerotomy site. Tissue dyes have also been used to improve visualization and accurately remove thin and transparent tissues, such as staining of the internal limiting membrane (ILM) during macular hole repair and epiretinal membrane removal.

Intraoperative hemorrhage is a major concern as it obscures the view during vitrectomy. Various pharmaceutical agents and instruments are used to decrease hemorrhage and improve visualization. For example, preoperative bevacizumab (Avastin, Genentech) is used to decrease intraoperative hemorrhage during tractional retinal detachment repair in proliferative diabetic retinopathy. Intraoperative thrombin and use of an end-aspirating endoilluminator (Alcon Laboratories, Fort Worth, Texas) also decrease bleeding.

WIDE-ANGLE VITRECTOMY LENS SYSTEMS

Lens systems for vitrectomy initially employed plano concave or biconcave lenses, which afforded only a 20° to 35° view.[1] The retinal periphery was difficult to visualize, as even prism lenses could not provide visualization much past 60°.[2] Wide-angle viewing systems were introduced and took advantage of the same principle on which the indirect ophthalmoscope is based: The astronomical telescope. In this system, the cornea and lens act together as the objective and the high-plus condensing lens as the eyepiece. This produces a real inverted aerial image of the retina and vitreous. However, performing bimanual surgery in an inverted fashion is counterintuitive for humans. Stereoscopic image inversion systems solve this problem typically with the use of 2 adjoining but orthogonally oriented prisms that can be moved into or out of the viewing path of the microscope[3] in either a manual or mechanized manner.

Two types of wide-angle viewing systems for vitrectomy surgery exist: Noncontact systems and contact systems. Each type has advantages and disadvantages.

Contact Systems

Contact systems typically provide a wider field of view with fewer aberrations and reflections. This is because the lens is directly coupled to the cornea via a viscous agent such as viscoelastic, e.g. Healon, or hydroxypropyl methylcellulose. However, either a lens ring must be sewn on or a skilled assistant will be required to maintain the image quality. Contact lens systems include those produced by: Advanced Visual Instruments, Inc. (New York); Volk Optical, Inc. (Mentor, Ohio); and Ocular Instruments, Inc. (Bellevue, Wash). Yasuo Tano, MD,[4] developed a sutureless ring system to hold a contact lens on the cornea by yoking it to the ocular speculum; this device is especially useful for MIVS. Shunji Kusaka, MD,[5] recently developed a new sutureless ring system for MIVS. The silicone ring, strung between two cannulas, holds the metal ring of the contact lens in place (Figures 20.1A to C). The silicone band is easy to take on and off.

Challam[6] devised a self-stabilizing wide field contact lens for vitreous surgery. A standard wide-angle contact lens with the radius of curvature of 7.7 mm is modified with addition of four footplates to facilitate stability and centration. A drop of viscoelastic material is placed between the lens and the cornea. This induces negative suction, which helps to retain the lens in position and allows dynamic viewing of the retina.

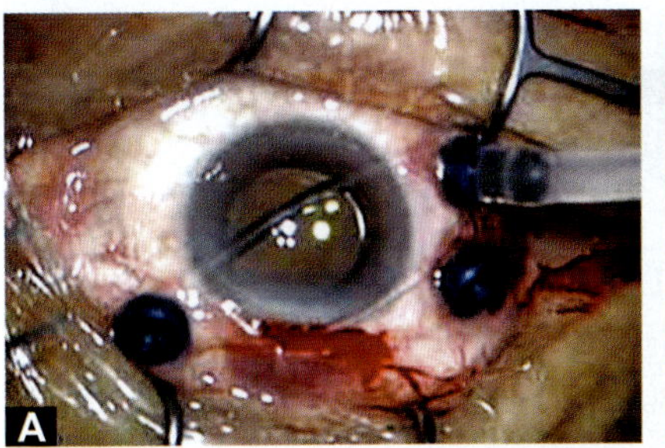

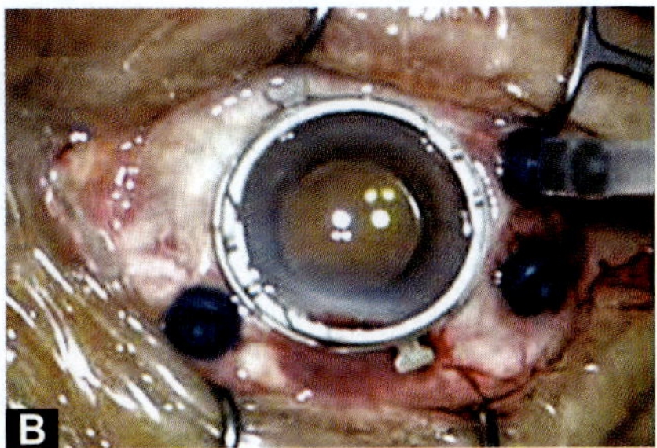

Figs 20.1A and B: (A) Silicone band between two cannulas; (B) The lens ring is held with the silicone band. (*Courtesy:* Retinal Imaging Fall 2006 I Retina Today I 23)

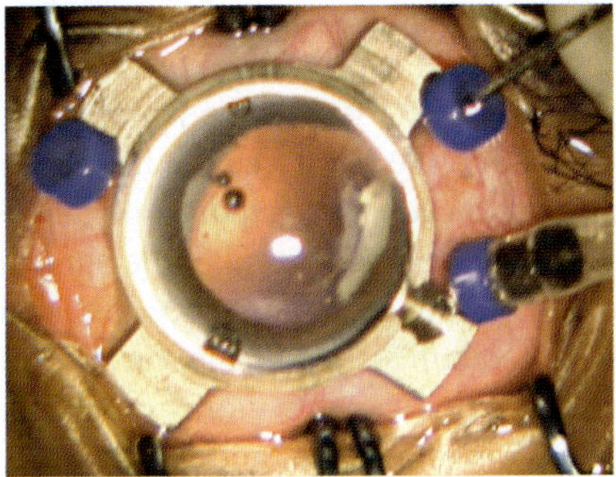

Fig. 20.1C: Sutureless ring for contact lens (*Courtesy*: Madhu Instruments, Delhi)

This specially designed lens reduces the need for a skilled assistant to stabilize the contact lens. It provides a stable, well-centered view of the peripheral fundus during vitreous surgery.

Noncontact Viewing

Noncontact viewing decreases axial (depth) and lateral resolution and, unlike contact-based viewing, does not compensate for pre-existing corneal asphericity (previous RK, LRI, cataract surgery, LASIK and PRK, as well as keratoconus and forme fruste keratoconus). Noncontact wide-angle viewing provides 10° less field of view than contact-based wide-angle viewing. In addition, noncontact wide-angle viewing of the periphery requires much greater ocular rotation; this increases instrument flex, which is especially a concern while using 25 gauge instruments.

Noncontact systems do not require a skilled assistant, and they cause fewer traumas to the corneal epithelium. Scleral depression is typically easier and manipulation of the microscope foot pedal remains consistent whether or not the image is inverted. The insight instruments binocular indirect ophthalmo microsope (Stuart, Fla) employs a stereoinverter above the microscope objective, while the Moeller erect indirect binocular ophthalmic system, or (Hamburg, Germany), uses an inverter below the objective.

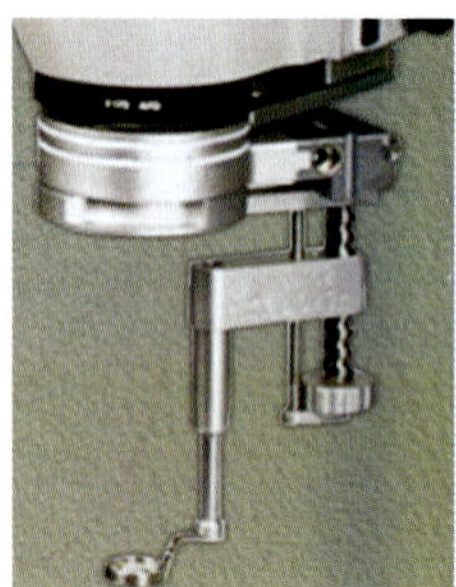

Fig. 20.2: BIOM 4 (Binocular Indirect Ophthalmo Microscope)

The BIOM (Binocular Indirect Ophthalmo Microscope)[7] holds a lens away from the eye allowing fine focus and a panoramic view, even through small pupils. When necessary, the BIOM can either be swung away from the operating field if another procedure is required or the lens can be changed to allow different procedures such as macula hole surgery. Wide field lenses invert the image, which is not acceptable, hence the use of the SDI (Stereo-diagonal Inverter) which rectifies the image for the surgeon. Wide-angle viewing systems have revolutionized vitrectomy procedures because surgeons now have access to the peripheral retina and vitreous base, the site of a vast amount of vitreoretinal pathology.

The noncontact system is simple with a large viewing angle of up to 130°. A long-lasting topical lubricant neutralizes corneal aberrations. There is no other lens or instrumentation to interfere with the globe during surgery. The smaller objective lens is ideal for manipulating the wide-angle view in a pediatric eyes.

Use of the BIOM is little influenced by: (1) Pupil size, (2) Corneal scars, (3) Lens opacities, (4) Vitreous substitutes including gas, (5) Surgery without contact to cornea, reducing corneal stress, (6) Improved mobility of the eye when required.

Second, the resolution is excellent. The view is more than adequate to peel complex peripheral membranes, create extensive retinotomies in PVR surgery or even peel obvious membranes in the macular region. When one views a wide-angle contact system, there is improved clarity from complete neutralization of the corneal aberrations. However, this small differential in image clarity does not make-up for the added manipulation and interference of the contact.

When used with the operating microscope, the SDI erects the inverted image of a wide-angle observation system while maintaining correct stereopsis, thus enabling bimanual vitreous surgery under panoramic viewing conditions.

The SDI is available in three different versions: Manually switched type, electrically switched, and electrically switched for hands-free focusing. The SDI fits below the oculars of most operating microscopes. In its neutral position, it does not interfere with the normal beam path of the microscope. Therefore, it can remain in place when the microscope is used for purposes other than vitreoretinal surgery.

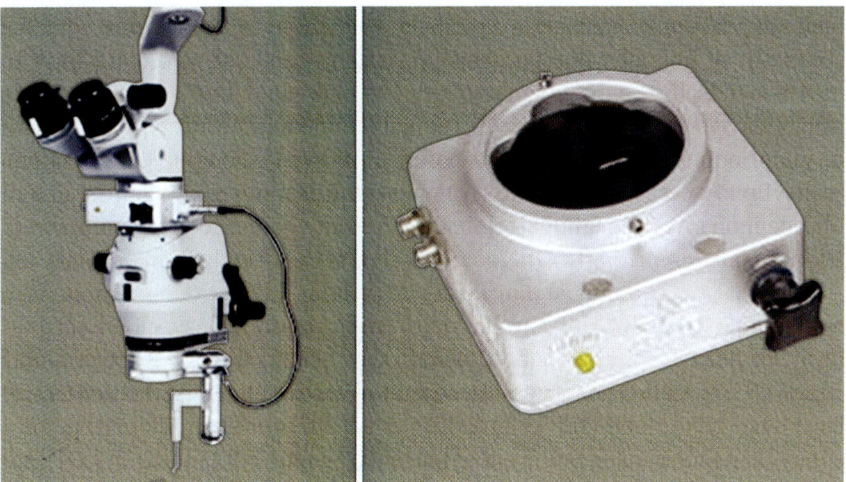

Fig. 20.3: SDI (Stereoscopic Diagonal Inverter)

The virtual image produced by a wide field BIOM lens lies a short distance above the lower lens, necessitating a reduction lens to shorten the normal focal length of the microscope. The focusing mechanism of the BIOM can then be used to adjust the virtual image to lie in the same plane as the new shorter focal point of the microscope.

Subsequent lowering or rising of the microscope will only increase or diminish the field of view without affecting the focus which is controlled by the BIOM.

New Disposable Lens Sets for VR Surgeons are now presented as a sterile, single use set of a reduction lens, and a wide field lens. These are available in a box of 6 individually wrapped sets. These new disposable wide field lenses give a superb image even under high magnification combined with a 130° field of view. After use, the arm of the lens is snapped off before it can be removed from the BIOM.

(To conform to American FDA requirements, the locating arm of the disposable noncontact wide field lens has been redesigned to ensure that the lens can only be used once.)

AUTOCLAVABLE LENSES

Autoclavable lenses are coated with amorphous carbon which protects against damage due to aggressive cleaning and mechanical wear giving longer life.

Lens description	Field
90 D Lens, autoclavable	89°
Wide Field (E) Lens, autoclavable	120°
Hi Resolution Macula Lens, autoclavable	60°

OFFISS (Optical Fiber-Free Intravitreal Surgery System)

OFFISS (Optical Fiber-Free Intravitreal Surgery System) was developed by Horiguchi, et al.[8] and presented in 2002. They used a wide-angle microscope combined with a newly designed aspheric 40 diopter lens and a prismatic inverting optical system. When the surgeon needs to perform bimanual surgery, the 40 diopter lens can be swung into place between the microscope and the patient's eye. The illumination of the microscope gives an inverted image of the fundus which may be returned to an upright position with the use of an inverting optical system. A commercial version of OFFISS became available in 2003; produced by Topcon Company, Tokyo, Japan.

The system consists of a high quality surgical microscope (OMS 800) additionally equipped with its own illumination. This allows the surgeon to use either usual coaxial illumination or the special OFFISS illumination (Figures 20.4A to C).

OFFISS illumination is especially designed to provide illumination of the fundus of the eye during vitrectomy without the use of any endoprobe or chandelier light.[9,10]

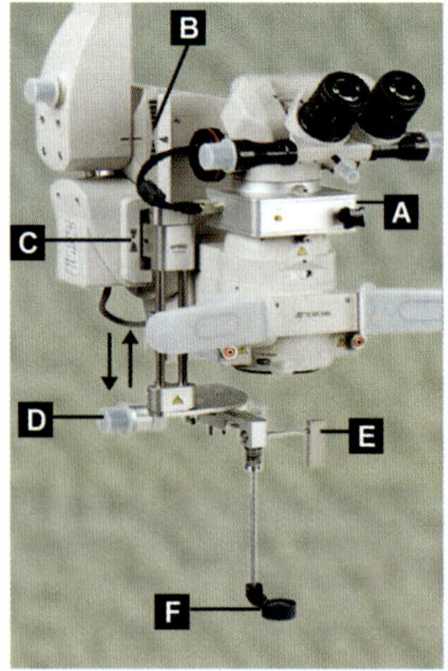

Fig. 20.4A: OFFISS attachment. (A) Inverter; (B) Focusing to move whole eye piece with OFFISS system allows anterior segment visualization without the need to move the lens system; (C) Fine focusing of OFFISS attachment; (D) Knob to unlock the OFFISS attachment; (E) Knob to move the attachment out; (F) 40 D posterior pole viewing lens

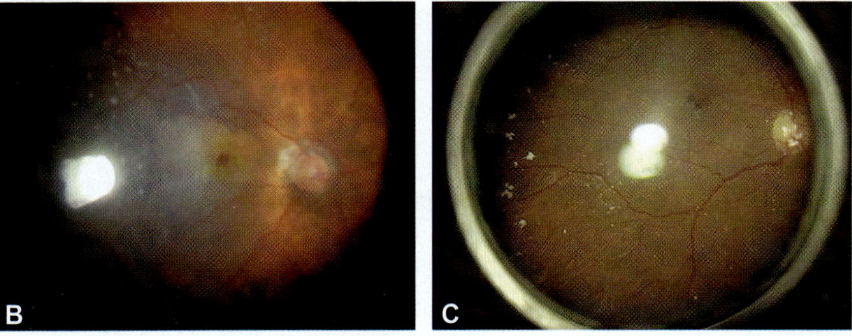

Figs 20.4B and C: (B) OFFISS system view through 40 diopter lens with endoilluminator; (C) OFFISS system view through 40 diopter lens without endoilluminator. (*Courtesy*: Dr Raju S)

The direction of the light is similar to binocular indirect ophthalmoscope in the upper central part of the field of view. The light may be in the form of full field or slit. Slit illumination is horizontal and may be moved through the operative field up and down without disturbing the surgeon.

The idea behind the system is similar to the idea of a binocular indirect ophthalmoscope. This means that we have two channels of viewing (one for each of the surgeon's eyes) and one channel for illumination. All three channels have to pass inside the wide pupil during surgery. Because the idea of the system is similar to a binocular indirect ophthalmoscope the achieved image is inverted. However, the microscope is also equipped with a stereoinverter which reinverts the image to achieve 'real' picture (Figure 20.5).

OFFISS itself is an attachment which hangs under the microscope as BIOM does. This attachment contains a 40 diopter lens which gives a visual field of approximately 50° inside the eye which is smaller than a wide-angle viewing system but wider than that obtained with a planoconcave contact lens The system is additionally equipped with a prismatic lens which may be put on the OFFISS lens with the aim of increasing the visual field up to 70°. Additional lenses may be used in a similar way to achieve visualization of anterior segment (for visualization of sclerotomies). An additional attachment —the OFFISS 120 diopter lens may be used to increase the field of view (Figures 20.6 to 20.9).

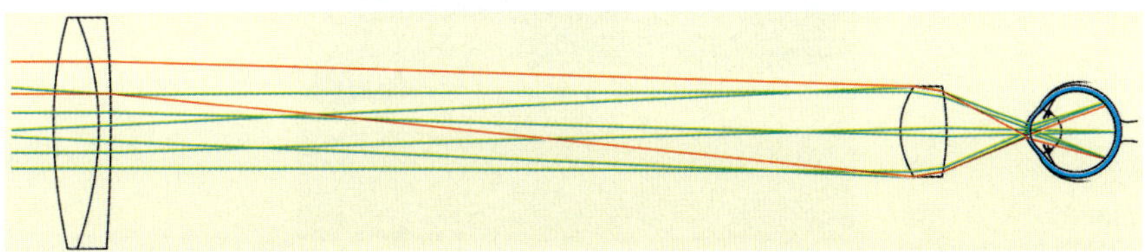

Fig. 20.5: Schematic drawing of illumination and observation light rays. Red line: Illumination path; Green line: Observation path

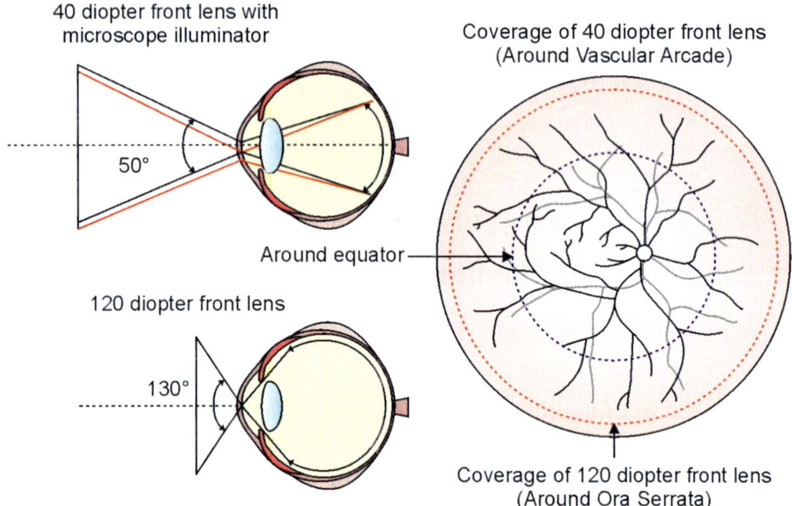

Fig. 20.6: Fundus coverage with various lenses
(*Courtesy:* M Horiguchi, Arch Ophthalmol 2002;120:491–4)

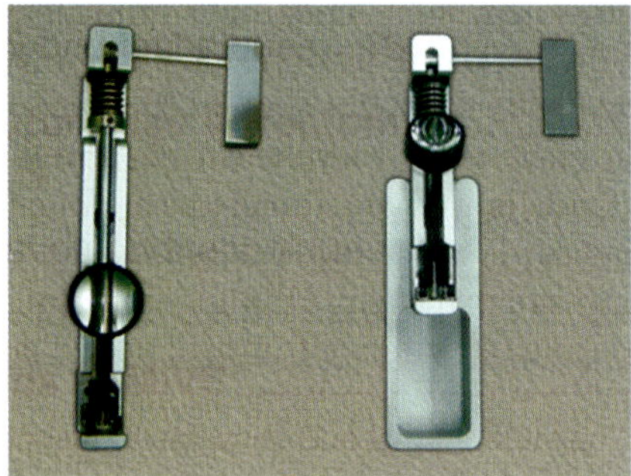

Fig. 20.7: OFFISS attachment

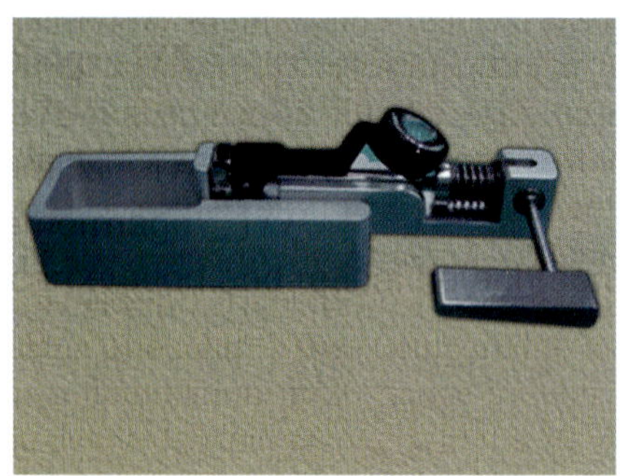

Fig. 20.8: OFFISS 120 diopter lens
(*Courtesy:* M Horiguchi, Arch Ophthalmol 2002;120:491–4)

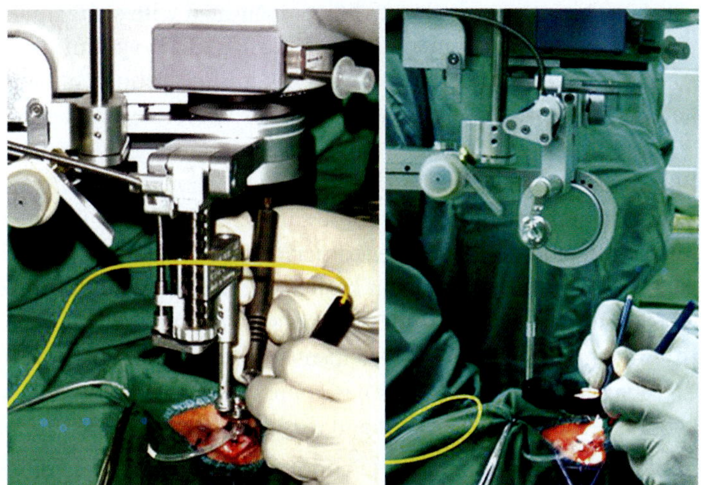

Fig. 20.9: Comparison of the distance from the microscope to the patients eye with OFFISS on the right side (please note that surgery is performed without endoillumination) and BIOM on the left side (*Courtesy:* M Horiguchi, Y Kojima, Y Shimada: New System for Fiberoptic-Free Bimanual Vitreous Surgery. Arch Ophthalmol. 2002;120:491–4)

An additional element of the system is the OFFISS 120 diopter lens which is a similar attachment mounted under the microscope. This allows wide field viewing inside the eye but with the use of endoillumination.[11]

The original construction did not allow for the use of BIOM (Oculus, Wetzlar, Germany) combined with OFFISS during the same surgery. The BIOM originally designed for Topcon's OMS 610 microscope may be mounted simultaneously with the OFFISS to the OFFISS OMS 800. To achieve this, the original OFFISS platform must be placed a few millimeters lower which is easily achieved with an adaptor a few millimeters longer than the original

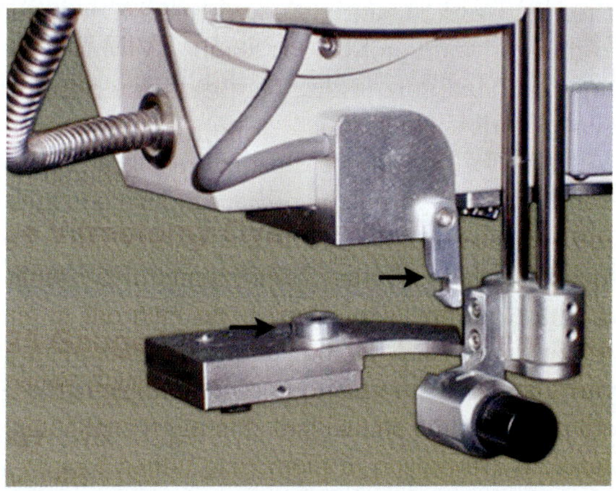

Fig. 20.10: Modifications to allow simultaneous use of BIOM and OFFISS. (*Courtesy:* M Horiguchi, Arch Ophthalmol 2002; 120:491–4)

(Figure 20.10) This movement has to be compensated with same thick button placed on the OFFISS platform to allow switch off of the system.

Another modification made is the use of slit illumination combined with flat contact lens. The use of slit illumination for vitrectomy was popularized by Bonnet and Ducournau and is widely used in France. This concept, along with OFFISS, allows you to perform vitrectomy without endoillumination.

This means that in some situations you can use one hand for other purposes than endoillumination, for example, to perform scleral depression. The use of flat contact lens as an observation system combined with slit illumination from OFFISS is specially useful for peripheral vitrectomy.

Slit illumination from OMS 800 is located horizontally not vertically as it is in case of surgical slit lamp. This has some disadvantages. With a vertical slit the picture seen by surgeons' left and right eyes are differently illuminated and therefore the effect of stereopsis is more noticeable when compared with horizontal slit. However, with horizontal slit from OMS 800 we can move the slit through the full field of view without disturbing the view. This allows surgery to be performed in both well-illuminated areas and in half-shadow. Observing the vitreous in half-shadow allows the surgeon to see additional details which are not visible in full field illumination. This may be of some value during peripheral vitrectomy with surgeon's own scleral depression. Another indication for use of OFFISS presented by Horio and Horiguchi may be the performance of intraoperative fluorescein videoangiography.

The use of the system has important advantages in everyday surgical practice. You can use it for complete or partial surgery. With the above modifications, we can use all known systems simultaneously during the same surgery. This means that for macula surgery we can use a flat contact lens which gives us the highest magnification but lowest field of view. However, for wide field viewing with lowest magnification we can use BIOM or OFFISS 120 diopter lens. This gives us good orientation in topography of the disease. For bimanual surgery we can use OFFISS. For peripheral vitrectomy both OFFISS and flat contact lens combined with OFFISS illumination give you the ability to see miniscule details.

As it is an illumination/observation system, it does not influence the gauge one chooses for the vitrectomy probe. It allows surgeons to change the system according to their judgment and to give the patient the best possible quality of surgery exactly appropriate to different surgical situations.

A disadvantage of the system is, the need to move the microscope up when you want to use OFFISS. Even if it is compensated for by moving the ocular the surgeon still has the feeling that the distance to the eye is different from what they are used to. It also takes sometime to carry out. Another disadvantage is the horizontal orientation of the slit, something many of us are not used to. Furthermore, we must consider the price. You cannot buy OFFISS alone you must buy a complete microscope because the special illumination is built into the microscope. However, you should remember that the system has no single-use parts and may be used for many years.

EIBOS

The noncontact wide-angle fundus observation system EIBOS can be adapted not only to MÖLLER microscopes but is also available for most microscopes of other manufacturers. The EIBOS is very easy to handle as it contains the inverter and an internal focus. Use of the EIBOS is associated with the following advantages:

1. Simultaneous observation of fundus and incision area
2. Spring-loaded suspension for safety
3. Internal focus ranging from retina to upper vitreous body operated via sterile lever
4. Swing-away device, rotatable around objective lens
5. Autoclavable front lens
6. Autoclavable silicon cover included.

For the EIBOS two lenses are available: Type 90 D: for approx. 90° viewing angle and Type SPXL (132 D): For approx. 124° viewing angle

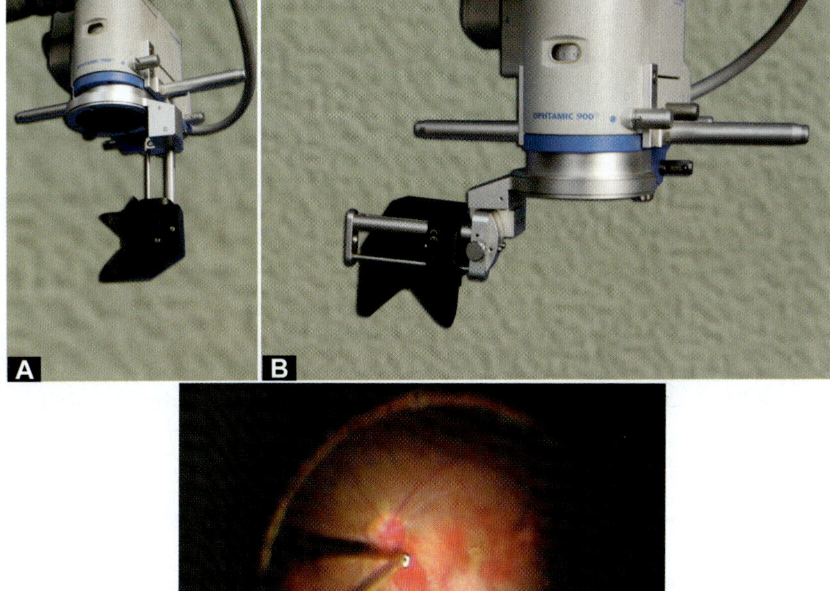

Figs 20.11A to C: (A) EIBOS; (B) EIBOS; (C) View through EIBOS (*Courtesy:* Dr Sharad Bhomaj)

PWL

The Peyman-Wessels-Landers 132 D Upright Vitrectomy Lens (PWL; Ocular Instruments, Bellevue, WA) provides wide field, upright images without an inverter because of an internal prismatic system.[12] It is less expensive than other noncontact systems. The focus can be adjusted with the footswitch.

One possible disadvantage of this system is that it may be difficult to maintain an appropriate x-y-z position with tilting when the device is attached to the wrist rest or to the microscope with the standard clamp, straight rods, and linkage system. Recently, Landers et al developed a holding system for the PWL lens to overcome this potential disadvantage.[13] The lens holder consists of three parts: The holding device, the rotating bar, and the lens holder. The holding device is fixed to the microscope and holds the rotating bar. The lens holder is fixed with a screw to the window at the lower part of the rotating bar.

When the surgeon sets up the new holding system, the lens holder can be easily and precisely held at the center of the light axis (Figures 20.12A and B). Surgeons obtain a wide field image of the fundus through the PWL lens held with the lens holder. It is easy to remove the lens temporarily when performing a procedure in the anterior segment without the fundus viewing system and to move it back to the center of the optical axis to see the fundus. Another advantage of the system is that surgeons can see the sclerotomy or 23 or 25 gauge cannula directly under the microscope by rotating the lens holder a little off the center of the optical axis.

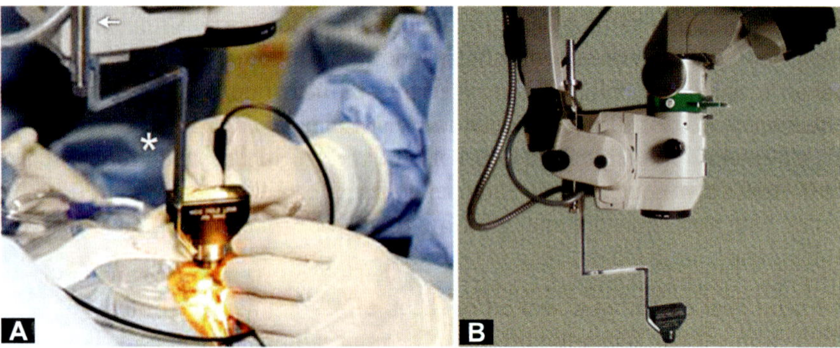

Figs 20.12A and B: (A) Rotating bar (arrow) and lens holder (asterisk). (*Courtesy*: Retinal Imaging Fall 2006 I Retina Today I 23); (B) Panoramic view of lens holder (*Courtesy*: Dr Bhushan Khare)

RESIGHT 700

The Resight 700 (Carl Zeiss Meditec AG, Jena, Germany) is the wide-angle viewing system incorporated into the Lumera 700 microscope (Carl Zeiss Meditec). This technology can hold two lenses, a 127.00 diopter lens for wide-angle viewing and a 60.00 diopter lens for magnifying images of the posterior pole. These lenses provide clear fundus images with minimal distortion. The fundus image is automatically inverted by Resight's Invertertube E. Users can also adjust the focus with the footswitch of the microscope through an internal focusing system (Figures 20.13A to C).

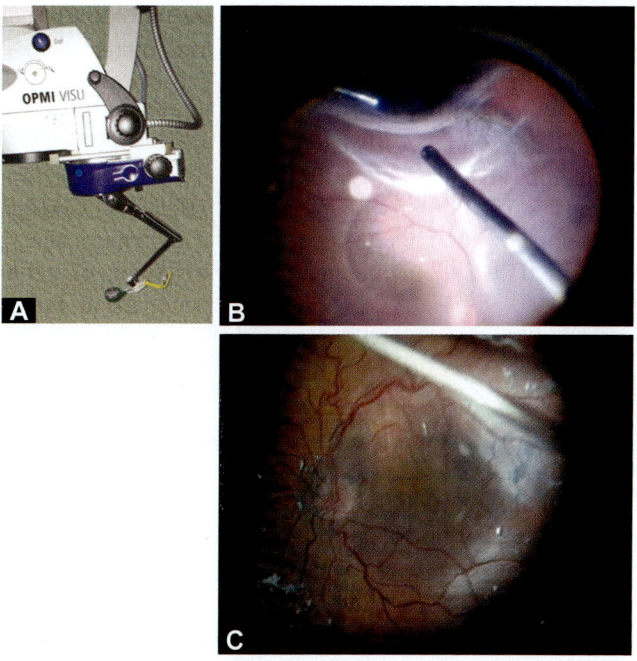

Figs 20.13A to C: (A) Resight system attached to microscope; (B) View through resight; (C) View of posterior pole. (*Courtesy:* Dr Suraj Pandya)

The wide-angle viewing systems are useful and, in my opinion, essential for MIVS. However, lower magnification makes it difficult to perform precise procedures in the macular area, such as internal limiting membrane removal. The Resight 700 has a magnifying lens as one of its two lens options, which is useful for this maneuver.

CONCLUSION

Improved visualization during vitrectomy surgery is one of the major factors that has improved surgical outcomes and allowed retinal physicians to approach more and more difficult cases. Wide-angle viewing has afforded surgeons a three-dimensional intraoperative view of the peripheral retina, vitreous base, ora serrata, pars plana and pars plicata, and ciliary body. Illumination systems have evolved along with smaller gauge surgery, and newer light sources allow for bimanual surgery, wider-angle viewing to visualize anterior ocular structures, and improved contrast for detecting subtle membranes and the ILM. Bullet light-pipe providing wide-angle illumination is used in conjunction with the wide-angle viewing system. Sometimes a xenon arc light source is preferred because of its bright, white illumination that gives a better contrast.

- Xenon illumination can and has been used safely in the real-world clinical setting.
- Any illumination system can be phototoxic, therefore usual precautions apply.
- Xenon illumination sources can significantly improve 25 gauge endoillumination (even beyond levels achieved with 20 gauge halogen endoillumination).
- New 25 gauge endoilluminators are more rigid and provide wider cone angles of illumination despite smaller light fibers.
- Chandelier endoilluminators work well in complex cases requiring bimanual maneuvers or peripheral scleral depression. Try first on an aphake or pseudophake and tape down the fiber for the best angle.

REFERENCES

1. Landers MB 3rd, Stefansson E, Wolbarsht ML. The optics of vitreous surgery. Am J Ophthalmol. 1981;91:611–4.
2. Bovey EH, Gonvers M. A new device for noncontact wide-angle viewing of the fundus during vitrectomy. Arch Ophthalmol. 1995;113:1572–3.
3. Chalam KV, Shah VA. Optics of wide-angle panoramic viewing system-assisted vitreous surgery. Surv Ophthalmol. 2004;49:437–45.
4. Ikuno Y, Ohji M, Kusaka S, et al. Sutureless contact lens ring system during vitrectomy. Am J Ophthalmol. 2002;133(6):847–8.
5. Kusaka S, Futamura H. New sutureless contact lens ring system for vitrectomy using cannula system. Retina. 2010;30(8):1318–9.
6. Shah VA, Chalam KV. Self-stabilizing wide-angle contact lens for vitreous surgery. Retina. 2003;23(5):667–9.
7. Spitznas M. A binocular indirect ophthalmo microscope (BIOM) for noncontact wide angle vitreous surgery. Graefes Arch Clin Exp Ophthalmol. 1987;225(1):13–5.
8. Horiguchi M, Kojima Y, Shima Y. Removal of lens matter dropped into the vitreous cavity during cataract surgery using an optical fiber-free intravitreal surgery system J. Cataract Refract Surg. 2003;29(7):1256–9.
9. Horiguchi M, Kojima Y, Shimada Y. New system for fiberoptic-free bimanual vitreous surgery. Arch Ophthalmol. 2002;120:491–4.
10. Horio N, Horiguchi M. Retinal blood flow analysis using intraoperative video fluorescein angiography combined with optical fiber-free intravitreal surgery system. Am J Ophthalmol. 2004;138(6):1082–3.
11. OFFISS (Optical fibre-free intravitreal surgery) in Retinology.
12. Landers MB, Peyman GA, Wessels IF, et al. A new, noncontact wide field viewing system for vitreous surgery. Am J Ophthalmol. 2003;136(1):199–201.
13. Kakinoki M, Hirakata A, Landers, MB, et al. The new ring holder for Peyman-Wessels-Landers 132D Upright Vitrectomy Lens. Retina. In press.

Index

Page numbers followed by *f* refer to figure

O